Neurological Assessment Scales: Clinical and Research Perspectives

Editors by

Nidhi Sharma
Department of Physiotherapy
Amity Institute of Health Allied Sciences
Amity University, Noida
Uttar Pradesh, India

Simranjeet Kaur
Pal Physiotherapy and Rehabilitation Centre
Pal Healthcare, Jandli, Ambala City
Haryana, India

&

Parveen Kumar
Pal Physiotherapy and Rehabilitation Centre
Pal Healthcare, Jandli, Ambala City
Haryana, India

Neurological Assessment Scales: Clinical and Research Perspectives

Editors: Nidhi Sharma, Simranjeet Kaur & Parveen Kumar

ISBN (Online): 979-8-89881-588-2

ISBN (Print): 979-8-89881-589-9

ISBN (Paperback): 979-8-89881-590-5

Published by Bentham Science Publishers Pte. Ltd. Singapore, in collaboration with Eureka Conferences, USA.

First published in 2026.

Bentham Science Publishers Pte. Ltd.
No. 9 Raffles Place
Office No. 26-01
Singapore 048619
Singapore
Email: subscriptions@benthamscience.net

BENTHAM SCIENCE

CONTENTS

PREFACE

The realm of neurology thrives at the intersection of science and humanity, where precise measurements of neurological function meet the unpredictable narratives of individual patients. Neurological assessment scales stand as the bridge between these two worlds, offering quantifiable, evidence-based insights while honoring the complexities of human experience. This book, ***Neurological Assessment Scales: Clinical and Research Perspectives,*** was born from the need to consolidate the vast landscape of these tools into a single, accessible resource for clinicians, researchers, and students alike.

Standardized assessment scales have revolutionized neurological practice by enabling clinicians to diagnose more effectively, monitor disease progression accurately, and evaluate treatment outcomes consistently. In research, these scales provide the rigor necessary for reproducibility and the comparability essential for global collaboration. Whether it is measuring spasticity with the Modified Ashworth Scale, evaluating coma recovery using the Glasgow Coma Scale, or assessing the quality of life with the SF-36, these tools form the backbone of both bedside care and benchside innovation.

This book brings together a diverse array of assessment scales spanning 15 chapters, each written by field experts. It offers an in-depth look at tools for evaluating conditions ranging from spasticity, coma, and vertigo to Parkinson's disease, multiple sclerosis, stroke, spinal cord injury, traumatic brain injury, and many more. The authors go beyond mere descriptions, presenting the clinical rationale, scoring, administration, interpretation, and psychometric properties of each scale. Also, the available modified version of the scales has been discussed. Readers will gain not only a reference guide but also a deeper understanding of how these tools shape decision-making in neurology.

Our aim is to make this book a cornerstone for those navigating the intricate pathways of neurological care and research. The content reflects a collaborative spirit, combining decades of clinical expertise and academic rigor. We hope this work will inspire confidence in its users, whether they are applying the tools in a bustling clinic, a quiet research lab, or a classroom filled with eager learners.

We extend our heartfelt gratitude to the contributors for their dedication to this endeavor and to Bentham Science Publishers for recognizing the significance of this compilation. We also thank the countless patients whose experiences have informed the creation and refinement of these scales; they remain the true focus of our collective efforts.

As neurology continues to evolve, so too will the tools we use to understand it. This book is not just a snapshot of the current state of neurological assessment but an invitation to future discoveries. We hope it serves as a trusted companion in your journey through the intricate world of neurological science.

Nidhi Sharma
Department of Physiotherapy
Amity Institute of Health Allied Sciences
Amity University, Noida
Uttar Pradesh, India

Simranjeet Kaur
Pal Physiotherapy and Rehabilitation Centre
Pal Healthcare, Jandli, Ambala City
Haryana, India

&

Parveen Kumar
Pal Physiotherapy and Rehabilitation Centre
Pal Healthcare, Jandli, Ambala City
Haryana, India

List of Contributors

Akanksha Saxena	Maharishi Markandeshwar Institute of Physiotherapy and Rehabilitation, Maharishi Markandeshwar (Deemed to be University), Mullana, Ambala, Haryana, India
Anshu Sharma	Maharishi Markandeshwar Institute of Physiotherapy and Rehabilitation, Maharishi Markandeshwar (Deemed to be University), Mullana, Ambala, Haryana, India Department of Physiotherapy, School of Health Care and Allied Science, G.D. Goenka University, Sohna, Haryana, India
Bhumika Kashyap	Maharishi Markandeshwar Institute of Physiotherapy and Rehabilitation, Maharishi Markandeshwar (Deemed to be University), Mullana, Ambala, Haryana, India
Gargi Sahu	Maharishi Markandeshwar Institute of Physiotherapy and Rehabilitation, Maharishi Markandeshwar (Deemed to be University), Mullana, Ambala, Haryana, India
Gurjant Singh	Maharishi Markandeshwar Institute of Physiotherapy and Rehabilitation, Maharishi Markandeshwar (Deemed to be University), Mullana, Ambala, Haryana, India Department of Physiotherapy, University Institute of Allied Health Sciences, Chandigarh University, Mohali, Punjab, India
Jayshankar Choudhary	Maharishi Markandeshwar Institute of Physiotherapy and Rehabilitation, Maharishi Markandeshwar (Deemed to be University), Mullana, Ambala, Haryana, India
Mandeep Jangra	Maharishi Markandeshwar Institute of Physiotherapy and Rehabilitation, Maharishi Markandeshwar (Deemed to be University), Mullana, Ambala, Haryana, India
Manpreet Kaur	Department of Physiotherapy, University Institute of Allied Health Sciences College, Chandigarh University, Mohali, Punjab, India Department of Physiotherapy, Mody University of Science and Technology, Lakshmangarh (Sikar), Rajasthan, India
Mayuri Thakur	Dolphin PG College of Life Science, Chunni Kalan, Punjab, India Maharishi Markandeshwar Institute of Physiotherapy and Rehabilitation, Maharishi Markandeshwar (Deemed to be University), Mullana, Ambala, Haryana, India
Naveeta Thakur	Maharishi Markandeshwar Institute of Physiotherapy and Rehabilitation, Maharishi Markandeshwar (Deemed to be University), Mullana, Ambala, Haryana, India
Nidhi Sharma	Maharishi Markandeshwar Institute of Physiotherapy and Rehabilitation, Maharishi Markandeshwar (Deemed to be University), Mullana, Ambala, Haryana, India Department of Physiotherapy, Amity Institute of Health Allied Sciences, Amity University, Noida, Uttar Pradesh, India
Parveen Kumar	Pal Physiotherapy and Rehabilitation Centre, Pal Healthcare, Ambala City, Haryana, India
Poornima Maurya	Maharishi Markandeshwar Institute of Physiotherapy and Rehabilitation, Maharishi Markandeshwar (Deemed to be University), Mullana, Ambala, Haryana, India Department of Physiotherapy, School of Allied and Healthcare Sciences, Lovely Professional University, Phagwara, Punjab, India
Preeti Kapri	Department of Physiotherapy, School of Allied Medical Sciences, Lovely Professional University, Phagwara, Punjab, India Maharishi Markandeshwar Institute of Physiotherapy and Rehabilitation, Maharishi Markandeshwar (Deemed to be University), Mullana, Ambala, Haryana, India

Priyanka Negi	Maharishi Markandeshwar Institute of Physiotherapy and Rehabilitation, Maharishi Markandeshwar (Deemed to be University), Mullana, Ambala, Haryana, India
Saumya Kothiyal	Department of Physiotherapy, University Institute of Allied Health Sciences, Chandigarh University, Mohali, Punjab, India
Sidharth Bansal	Department of Physiotherapy, School of Allied Medical Sciences, Lovely Professional University, Phagwara, Punjab, India
Simranjeet Kaur	Maharishi Markandeshwar Institute of Physiotherapy and Rehabilitation, Maharishi Markandeshwar (Deemed to be University), Mullana, Ambala, Haryana, India Pal Physiotherapy and Rehabilitation Centre, Pal Healthcare, Ambala City, Haryana, India
Sudhamoy Maity	Maharishi Markandeshwar Institute of Physiotherapy and Rehabilitation, Maharishi Markandeshwar (Deemed to be University), Mullana, Ambala, Haryana, India
Sukhpal Singh	Maharishi Markandeshwar Institute of Physiotherapy and Rehabilitation, Maharishi Markandeshwar (Deemed to be University), Mullana, Ambala, Haryana, India
Sukhpreet Kaur	Sri Guru Granth Sahib World University, Fatehgarh Sahib, Punjab, India Maharishi Markandeshwar Institute of Physiotherapy and Rehabilitation, Maharishi Markandeshwar (Deemed to be University), Mullana, Ambala, Haryana, India
Yashleen Kaur Sandhu	University School of Physiotherapy and Radiology, Rayat Bahra University, Mohali-140301, Punjab, India Maharishi Markandeshwar Institute of Physiotherapy and Rehabilitation, Maharishi Markandeshwar (Deemed to be University), Mullana, Ambala, Haryana, India
Yukta Sharma	Department of Physiotherapy, University Institute of Allied Health Sciences, Chandigarh University, Mohali, Punjab, India Maharishi Markandeshwar Institute of Physiotherapy and Rehabilitation, Maharishi Markandeshwar (Deemed to be University), Mullana, Ambala, Haryana, India

CHAPTER 1

Scales for Spasticity

Gargi Sahu[1], **Parveen Kumar**[2] and **Nidhi Sharma**[1,3,*]

[1] *Maharishi Markandeshwar Institute of Physiotherapy and Rehabilitation, Maharishi Markandeshwar (Deemed to be University), Mullana, Ambala, Haryana, India*

[2] *Pal Physiotherapy and Rehabilitation Centre, Pal Healthcare, Ambala City, Haryana, India*

[3] *Department of Physiotherapy, Amity Institute of Health Allied Sciences, Amity University, Noida, Uttar Pradesh, India*

Abstract: Spasticity, a neurological condition characterized by increased muscle tone, is a common sequel of various neurological disorders. Accurate assessment of spasticity is crucial for effective management. This chapter provides an overview of three commonly used scales for spasticity assessment: the Modified Ashworth Scale (MAS), the Penn Spasm Frequency Scale (PSFS), and the Tardieu Scale. The MAS is a simple, clinician-administered scale that assesses passive range of motion resistance due to spasticity. It is widely used but has limitations in quantifying the velocity-dependent nature of spasticity. The Tardieu Scale addresses this limitation by evaluating spasticity at different speeds. It consists of three components: a reflex component, a tonic component, and a clonus component. The PSFS is a self-report measure that assesses the frequency and severity of muscle spasms. This chapter also discusses the psychometric properties of each scale, which are essential for ensuring their accuracy and usefulness in clinical practice.

Keywords: Catch, Cerebral palsy, Extension, Flexion, Grade, Movement, Multiple sclerosis, Muscle, Range of motion, Release, Reliability, Resistance, Scale, Spasm, Spasticity, Spinal cord injury, Stroke, Tone, Traumatic brain injury, Velocity.

INTRODUCTION

Spasticity is a complex motor disorder characterized by an abnormal increase in muscle tone and exaggerated reflexes, often resulting from upper motor neuron lesions. As the understanding of spasticity evolves, so too does the need for effective assessment tools that can accurately measure its severity and impact on

* **Corresponding author Nidhi Sharma:** Department of Physiotherapy, Amity Institute of Health Allied Sciences, Amity University, Noida, Uttar Pradesh, India; E-mail: sharmanidhiphysio@gmail.com

patient function. This chapter explores the various scales used to assess spasticity, highlighting their development, application, and relevance in clinical practice. By understanding the characteristics and applications of these scales, healthcare professionals can make informed decisions regarding the diagnosis, prognosis, and treatment of spasticity.

MODIFIED ASHWORTH SCALE

The Modified Ashworth scale is among the most widely used clinical instruments for determining muscle spasticity, or more precisely, measures tonus abnormalities. The original Ashworth Scale was developed by Bryan Ashworth in 1964 to assess the effectiveness of anti-spasticity medications in patients with Multiple Sclerosis.

There are five possible grades on the scale between zero (no resistance) and four (a stiff limb in flexion or extension) [1]. In 1987, to improve the sensitivity of the measure and simplify scoring, Bohannon and Smith added the grade "1+" and suggested minor changes [2]. The Modified Ashworth Scale, as it was called after modification, has been considered the gold standard for measuring spasticity. In 2006, to improve reliability, grade "1+" was omitted and grade "2" was slightly redefined, resulting in the Modified Modified Ashworth Scale [3].

The comparison of the scores of available modifications of the Ashworth Scale has been depicted in Table **1**.

Table 1. Comparison of grades of ashworth, modified ashworth and modified modified ashworth scale.

Score	Ashworth Scale (Ashworth, 1964)	Modified Ashworth Scale (Bohannon & Smith, 1987)	Modified Modified Ashworth Scale (Ansari *et al*, 2006)
0	No increase in tone	No increase in muscle tone	No increase in muscle tone
1	Slight increase in tone, giving a catch when the limb was moved in flexion or extension.	Slight increase in muscle tone, with a catch and release or minimal resistance at the end of the range of motion when an affected part(s) is moved in flexion or extension.	Slight increase in muscle tone, manifested by a catch and release or by minimal resistance at the end of the range of motion when the affected part(s) is moved in flexion or extension.
1+	N/A	Slight increase in muscle tone, manifested as a catch, followed by minimal resistance through the remainder (less than half) of the range of motion.	N/A

(Table 1) cont.....

Score	Ashworth Scale (Ashworth, 1964)	Modified Ashworth Scale (Bohannon & Smith, 1987)	Modified Modified Ashworth Scale (Ansari *et al*, 2006)
2	More marked increase in tone, but the limb easily flexed.	A marked increase in muscle tone throughout most of the range of motion, but the affected part(s) are still easily moved.	Marked increase in muscle tone, manifested by a catch in the middle range and resistance throughout the remainder of the range of motion, but the affected part (s) easily moved.
3	Considerable increase in tone, passive movement difficult.	Considerable increase in muscle tone, and passive movement difficult.	Considerable increase in muscle tone, passive movement difficult.
4	The limb is rigid in flexion or extension.	Affected part(s) are rigid in flexion or extension.	Affected part(s) are rigid in flexion or extension.

Population:

- Stroke
- Spinal cord injury (SCI)
- Traumatic brain injury (TBI)
- Multiple sclerosis (MS)
- Cerebral palsy
- Pediatric hypertonia
- Central nervous system lesions

Administration

It is performed by first stretching the patient's limb from maximum flexion to maximum extension (the point at which the first gentle resistance is encountered). It is then evaluated while transitioning from extension to flexion [2].

It was reported that the upper-limb evaluation should occur when the client is in the supine position. The upper limbs should be aligned with the trunk, with extended elbows and neutral wrist positions, while the lower limbs are parallel to each other. There are specific adjustments for the shoulder extensors, where the arm should transition from extension to 90 degrees of flexion, and for the shoulder internal rotators, where the arm should move from a neutral position to the maximum external rotation [4].

For assessment of the lower limbs, it is recommended that the client assume a side-lying position. Specifically, for testing the soleus muscle, the hips and knees should be flexed to 45 degrees, and the ankle should be taken through the range of motion from maximum plantar flexion to maximum dorsiflexion. In case of the gastrocnemius muscle, the hips should be flexed at 45 degrees, the knees in maximum extension, and the ankle moved from maximum plantar flexion to maximum dorsiflexion. To assess the quadriceps femoris muscle, both knees and hips should be in full extension, and the knee should be moved from maximum extension to maximum flexion [5].

Time to Administer

It has not been reported, but it will change depending on how many muscles are examined.

Scoring and Interpretation

The six-point Modified Ashworth Scale ranges from 0 to 4, with lower values indicating normal muscle tone and higher values indicating spasticity or increased resistance to passive movement.

Psychometric properties: The psychometric properties of the Ashworth scale and its modifications are presented in Tables **2-4**.

Table 2. Psychometric properties of the ashworth scale.

Author	Population	Age Group	Muscles Used	Psychometric Property
Mutlu *et al* [6]	children with spastic diplegic CP	38 children 52.9 months (SD: 19.6)	Hip flexors, adductors, internal rotators, hamstrings, gastrocnemius	Inter-rater reliability ICC = 0.54 and 0.78 Test-retest reliability ICC = 0.31 and 0.82

Table 3. Psychometric properties of modified ashworth scale.

Author	Population	Age Group	Muscles Used	Psychometric Property
Bohannon *et al*, 1987 [2]	One patient had multiple sclerosis, 5 had closed head injuries, and 24 had cerebrovascular accidents. [The paretic or weaker side of each patient]	30 patients (17 men and 13 women) (59.3 ± 17.6 years)	NA	Inter-rater reliability: Kendall's tau = 0.847
Allison *et al*, 1995 [7]	Traumatic brain injuries (Mean = 3.8 years)	34 Patients (30.32±10.81) years		Concurrent validity Timed toe tapping (r = -0.042) Reflex Threshold Angle (r = 0.49) H-reflex during dorsiflexion (r = 0.47) H-wave during vibration (r = 0.39)
Allison *et al*, 1996 [8]	Chronic TBI time since injury = 56 ± 48.4 months	30 Patients, (28.3±10.8) years	Plantar flexor	Interrater reliability (r = 0.727) for plantar flexor spasticity

(Table 3) cont.....

Author	Population	Age Group	Muscles Used	Psychometric Property
Gregson *et al*, 1999 [9]	Acute stroke	32 Patients (18 men and 14 women)	NA	Inter-Rater (kappa= 0.84), Intra-rater (kappa= 0.83)
Blackburn *et al*, 2002 [5]	20 patients were tested 2 weeks after their stroke, and 12 patients were tested 12 weeks after their stroke.	32 Patients (76.1 ±7.89) years	Gastrocnemius, soleus, and quadriceps femoris muscles on the hemiplegic side	Intra-rater reliability (Kendall tau-b= 0.567, percentage of agreement73.3%) Inter-rater reliability (Kendall tau-b= 0.062, percentage of agreement= 45%)
Fosang *et al*, 2003 [10]	Cerebral palsy	11 females and 7 males (6 years 4 months ± 2 years 4 months)	Hamstring, Calf, Hip adductors	Inter-rater reliability Hamstrings (ICC = 0.37-0.48) Calf (ICC= 0.27-0.45) Adductors (ICC= 0.54-0.56) Test-retest reliability Hamstrings (ICC = 0.66-0.80) Calf (ICC= 0.21-0.70) Adductors (ICC=0.59-0.72)
Mehrholz *et al*, 2005 [4]	Impaired consciousness due to severe cerebral damage	30 Patients	Shoulder, elbow, wrist, hip, knee and ankle	Test-retest reliability (kappa = 0.47-0.62) Inter-rater reliability (kappa = 0.16-0.42)
Yam *et al*, 2005 [11]	Children with spastic diplegic cerebral palsy	17(mean age=7.9 years)	Hip adductors, ankle plantar flexors	Inter-rater reliability hip adductors, [knee flexed (ICC = 0.41), knee extended (ICC = 0.73)] ankle plantar flexors, [knee extended (ICC = 0.56), knee flexed (ICC = 0.46)]
Clopton *et al*, 2005 [12]	Children with hypertonia	17 children	Elbow flexor, hip adductor, quadriceps, hamstring, gastrocnemius, and soleus muscles were tested bilaterally.	Inter-rater reliability [ICC >0.75) for elbow flexors and hamstrings (ICC <0.50) for other muscles Intra-rater reliability (ICC >0.75) for hamstrings (ICC = 0.50 to 0.75) for other muscles
Ansari N *et al*, 2008 [13]	Patients with spastic hemiplegia	30 subjects with upper and lower limb muscle spasticity	Shoulder adductor, elbow flexor, wrist flexor, hip adductor, knee extensor, and ankle plantar flexor	Inter-rater reliability (kappa=0.514) Intra-rater reliability (kappa=0.590)

(Table 3) cont.....

Author	Population	Age Group	Muscles Used	Psychometric Property
Mutlu *et al*, 2008 [6]	Children with spastic diplegic CP	38 children (52.9±9.6) months	Hip flexors, adductors, internal rotators, hamstrings, gastrocnemius	Inter-rater reliability [ICC= 0.61-0.87] hamstrings (ICC = 0.76, 0.73) hip adductors (ICC = 0.83, 0.87) hip internal rotators (ICC = 0.61, 0.84) hip flexors (ICC = 0.71, 0.74) gastrocnemius (ICC = 0.64, 0.68) Intra-rater reliability [ICC= 0.36 and 0.83] , hip internal rotators (ICC = 0.36), hip flexors (ICC = 0.83)
Nakhostin *et al*, 2009 [14]	Brain injury on average 33.3 ± 26.2 months earlier	15 patients with a mean age of (57.3 ± 14.4) years.	Elbow flexor and wrist flexor	Inter-rater reliability κw =0.61 for elbow flexor and κw =0.78 for wrist flexor.
Ghotbi *et al*, 2009 [15]	Different neurological conditions	22 adults with (17 women, 5 men (44 ± 18) years	Hip adductor, knee extensor and ankle plantar flexor	For the hip adductor and the knee extensor (weighted kappa = 0.82, $p < 0.0001$) and for the ankle plantarflexor (weighted kappa = 0.74, $p < 0.0001$).
Craven BC *et al*, 2010 [16]	Chronic SCI (C5–T10 AIS A–D>12 months)	20 subjects	NA	Intra-rater reliability ($0.2<\kappa<1.0$) Inter-rater reliability ($\kappa<0.6$) for all muscle groups except the hip adductors. Test-retest reliability (0.4<ICC<0.75) for all muscle groups.
Waninge *et al*, 2011 [17]	Profound intellectual and multiple disabilities	35 participants	NA	Test-retest reliability Arm ICC= 0.853 (kw= 0.82) Leg ICC= 0.813 (kw= 0.78) Inter-rater reliability Arm ICC= 0.894 (kw= 0.88) Leg ICC= 0.895 (kw= 0.88)
Li F *et al*, 2014 [18]	hemiplegic stroke.	51 inpatients	Elbow flexors, Dorsi flexors	Inter- rater reliability: Elbow flexors (kappa= 0.66), Plantar flexors (kappa= 0.48) Intra-rater reliability Elbow flexors (kappa= 0.69), Planter flexors (kappa= 0.48)
Akpinar *et al*, 2017 [19]	SCI with spasticity	65 participants age between 18 and 88 years)	Hip adductor, hip extensor muscles and knee extensor muscles, knee extensors, and ankle plantar flexor muscles	Test-retest reliability (κ=0.580 for hip adductor) (κ= 0.636 to 0.716) Inter-rater reliability (κ= 0.531 to 0.774)

Table 4. Psychometric properties of modified ashworth scale.

Author	Population	Age Group	Muscles Used	Psychometric Property
Ansari NK *et al*, 2009 [14]	First-ever stroke	More than 18	Quadriceps femoris	Inter-rater (k= 0.72), Intra-rater (k= 0.82)
Naghdi *et al* 2008 [20]	Upper motor neuron lesions resulted in hemiplegia	30 hemiplegic patients (55.6±7.8) years	Wrist flexor muscle	Inter-rater reliability weighted kappa=0.92
Ghotbi *et al*, 2011 [15]	Eighteen patients had MS and five patients had hemiplegia due to a single stroke	23 patients with an average age of 37.3 ± 14.1 years	Hip adductors, Knee Extensors, and ankle plantar flexors	Inter-rater reliability Hip adductors (kw= 0.45) Knee Extensors(kw= 0.62), Ankle Plantar flexors (kw= 0.85), Overall (kw= 0.87)
Kaya *et al*, 2011 [21]	Poststroke hemiplegia 15.7±10.2 weeks	64 patients (60.5±11.9) years	Elbow flexor	Inter-rater reliability (kw= 0.892)
Mishra *et al*, 2014 [22]	Spinal cord injury	38 subjects (32 males and 6 females, (31.9±12.6) years	Calf muscle	Inter-rater reliability soleus (κ=0.75) gastrocnemius (κ= 0.70)

PENN SPASM FREQUENCY SCALE

The Penn Spasm Frequency Scale (PSFS) is a self-report tool consisting of two components, designed to assess the frequency of reported muscle spasms. It is widely used for quantifying spasticity [23].

The PSFS is frequently influenced by concurrent subclinical factors, such as bladder fullness, the onset of symptomatic urinary tract infections, anxiety levels, room temperature, and subject comfort, among other conditions [24].

The frequency of spasms tends to be reported more frequently than the severity of spasms [24].

Population:

Spinal Injury

Administration:

- Self-reported outcome measure
- Consists of two components-
- A self-report assessment utilizing 5-point scales was created to enhance clinical evaluations of spasticity, offering a more thorough evaluation of spasticity.

- A severity assessment for spasms, utilizing a 3-point scale.

Time to administer:

1 minute

Scoring and interpretation [24]:

A. Spasm Frequency:

- 0 = No spasm
- 1 = Mild spasms induced by stimulation
- 2 = Infrequent full spasms occurring less than once per hour
- 3 = Spasms occurring more than once per hour
- 4 = Spasms occurring more than 10 times per hour

B. Spasm Severity:

- 1 = Mild
- 2 = Moderate
- 3 = Severe

If the patient reports no spasms in the first component, then they do not proceed to the second component.

Psychometric properties: Table **5** showed the available psychometric properties of the Penn Spasm Frequency Scale.

Table 5. Psychometric properties of penn spasm frequency scale.

Author	Population	Age Group	Muscles Used	Psychometric Property
Adams *et al*, 2007 [25]	Chronic spinal cord injury	NA	NA	Internal Consistency ICC = 0.90 PSFS and SCI-SET correlations (r = -0.66) PSFS and Spasticity Severity correlations (r = 0.58*) PSFS and Spasticity Impact correlations (r = 0.67*) PSFS and FIM Motor Score correlations (r = -0.05) PSFS and QLI Health and Functioning Subscale correlations (r = -0.46*)
Mills *et al*, 2018 [26]	Chronic traumatic spinal cord injury	NA	NA	PSFS Part 1: Intra-rater reliability = 0.822 (5-10 days) and 0.734 (4-6 weeks after baseline) PSFS Part 1 and 2: 0.812 (5-10 days) and 0.729 (4-6 weeks after baseline)

TARDIEU SCALE

The Tardieu Scale was first created by Tardieu and colleagues in 1954. In 1969, Held and Pierrot-Deseilligny modified it, and in 1999 Boyd and Graham further revised the scale [27]. These scales aim to measure spasticity by evaluating how muscles respond to different stretch speeds and identifying the spasticity angle [28].

Population:

- Stroke
- Cerebral Palsy
- Brain Injury

Administration:

A standard goniometer is used to measure R2 and R1. The patient is positioned for testing based on the muscle being examined. The stretching velocities of V1 and V3 are applied to measure R2 and R1, respectively. Additionally, the quality of the muscle reaction is graded at the stretching velocity of V3. The difference between R2 and R1 serves as the measure of the dynamic component of spasticity [29].

Time to administer:

Depends on the number of joints being tested.

Scoring and interpretation [29]:

A. Quality of Muscle Reaction

- Grade 0: No resistance throughout the course of the passive movement
- Grade 1: Slight resistance throughout the course of the passive movement, followed by release
- Grade 2: Clear catch at a precise angle, interrupting the passive movement, followed by release
- Grade 3: Fatigable clonus (< 10 seconds when maintaining pressure) occurring at a precise angle
- Grade 4: Infatigable clonus (> 10 seconds when maintaining pressure occurring at a precise angle

B. Speed Definitions

- V1 involves moving as slowly as possible.
- V2 entails the speed at which the limb falls under gravity.
- V3 requires moving as quickly as possible.

C. Joint Angle

The Modified Tardieu scale defines R1 as the muscle reaction angle and R2 as the full passive range of motion (PROM). The full ROM angle (R2) is measured at a very slow speed (V1). The muscle reaction angle (R1) is identified as the angle where a catch or clonus occurs during a rapid stretch (V3). Subtracting R1 from R2 gives the dynamic tone component of the muscle.

Psychometric Properties: Table 6 exhibited the available psychometric properties of the Modified Tardieu Scale.

Table 6. Psychometric properties of modified tardieu scale.

Author	Population	Age Group	Muscles Used	Psychometric Property
Akpinar *et al*, 2017 [19]	SCI with spasticity	65 participants aged between 18 and 88 years.	Hip adductor, hip extensor muscles and knee extensor muscles, knee extensors, and ankle plantar flexor muscles.	Inter-rater and test–retest reliability (κ=0.692–0.917)
Yam *et al*, 2005 [11]	Children with spastic diplegic cerebral palsy	17(mean age=7.9 years)	Hip adductors, ankle plantar flexors	Inter-rater reliability hip adductors, [knee flexed (ICC = 0.66), knee extended (ICC = 0.71)] ankle plantar flexors, [knee extended (ICC = 0.22), knee flexed (ICC = 0.44)]
Mehrholz *et al*, 2005 [4]	Patients with impaired consciousness due to severe cerebral damage	30 patients	Shoulder, elbow, wrist, hip, knee, and ankle.	Test-retest reliability (kappa = 0.52-0.87) Inter-rater reliability (kappa = 0.29- 0.53)
Li F *et al*, 2014 [18]	Hemiplegic stroke.	51 inpatients	Elbow flexors, Plantar flexors	Inter- rater Elbow flexors (kappa= 0.73), Plantar flexors (kappa= 0.82) Intra-rater Elbow flexors (kappa= 0.73), Planter flexors (kappa= 0.79)

(Table 6) cont.....

Author	Population	Age Group	Muscles Used	Psychometric Property
Fosang *et al*, 2003 [10]	Cerebral palsy (CP)	11 females and seven males (mean age 6 years 4 months, SD 2 years 4 months	Hamstring, Calf, Hip adductors	Inter-rater reliability Hamstrings (ICC = 0.72- 0.74) Calf (ICC= 0.55- 0.71) Adductors (ICC= 0.58- 0.64) Test-retest reliability Hamstrings (ICC = 0.68- 0.90) Calf (ICC= 0.38- 0.90) Adductors (ICC= 0.61- 0.93)
Waninge *et al*, 2011 [17]	Profound intellectual and multiple disabilities	35 participants	NA	Test-retest reliability Arm (ICC= 0.627- 0.815) Leg (ICC= 0.741- 0.850) Inter-rater reliability Arm (ICC= 0.806- 0.851) Leg (ICC= 0.766- 0.877)

CLINICAL CONSIDERATIONS, STRENGTHS, LIMITATIONS, AND EMERGING TRENDS

Spasticity is a common and often disabling consequence of upper motor neuron lesions, encountered across a wide range of neurological conditions such as stroke, spinal cord injury, traumatic brain injury, multiple sclerosis, and cerebral palsy. Although it is traditionally defined as a velocity-dependent increase in muscle tone, clinical experience suggests that spasticity is rarely an isolated phenomenon. Instead, it frequently coexists with muscle weakness, altered motor control, soft tissue stiffness, and functional limitations. This complexity makes its assessment particularly challenging and explains why multiple clinical scales have been developed to capture different aspects of the condition [30].

The Modified Ashworth Scale (MAS) remains the most widely used tool for the clinical assessment of spasticity, largely because of its simplicity and ease of administration. In routine practice, the MAS allows rapid bedside evaluation without the need for specialized equipment, making it particularly useful in busy outpatient and inpatient rehabilitation settings. Its widespread use has also enabled comparison across studies and clinical populations. However, it is important to acknowledge that the MAS primarily reflects resistance to passive movement and does not reliably differentiate between neural components of spasticity and non-neural factors such as muscle stiffness or contracture. As a result, changes in MAS scores may not always correspond to meaningful functional improvement, especially following interventions aimed at improving activity or participation rather than tone reduction alone. Inter-rater variability, particularly among less experienced examiners, further limits its precision and highlights the need for cautious interpretation.

The Tardieu Scale addresses some of these limitations by incorporating the velocity-dependent nature of spasticity into its assessment framework. By examining muscle response at different stretch velocities and identifying the angle at which a catch or clonus occurs, the Tardieu Scale provides valuable insight into whether increased resistance is primarily neural or mechanical in origin [31]. This distinction is clinically relevant when planning interventions such as botulinum toxin injections, casting, or surgical procedures. Despite its conceptual advantages, the Tardieu Scale is more time-consuming and requires careful standardization of testing speed and joint positioning. Consequently, its use is often limited to specialized neurorehabilitation settings, and it may be less practical for routine screening or large-scale clinical studies.

The Penn Spasm Frequency Scale (PSFS) complements clinician-rated measures by capturing the patient's subjective experience of involuntary spasms. In conditions such as spinal cord injury and multiple sclerosis, spasm frequency and severity can significantly affect sleep, comfort, mobility, and overall quality of life. By focusing on these patient-reported outcomes, the PSFS adds an important dimension to spasticity assessment that is not adequately reflected by tone-based measures alone. However, as with all self-reported tools, responses may be influenced by cognitive status, mood, and individual perception, which can affect reliability. Therefore, the PSFS is most informative when used alongside objective or clinician-administered assessments.

A common limitation across traditional spasticity scales is their limited ability to reflect functional impact. While increased tone and spasms are defining features of spasticity, their clinical relevance ultimately depends on how they interfere with movement, daily activities, and participation. In many cases, patients may demonstrate functional improvement without substantial changes in tone scores, or conversely, show reduced tone without meaningful gains in function. This mismatch underscores the importance of interpreting spasticity measures within the broader context of functional assessment and patient-centered goals.

Recent years have seen growing interest in instrumented and technology-assisted approaches to spasticity assessment. Wearable sensors, inertial measurement units, and surface electromyography have shown promise in objectively quantifying muscle activation patterns, stretch reflex thresholds, and movement velocity. These tools may enhance the sensitivity and reliability of spasticity assessment, particularly in detecting subtle changes over time or in response to treatment. Additionally, the expansion of tele-rehabilitation has increased the relevance of digital assessment platforms, allowing standardized clinical scales to be administered remotely and facilitating long-term monitoring in chronic neurological conditions [32]. While these approaches are not yet routine in everyday clinical practice, they represent important complementary strategies rather than replacements for established clinical scales.

In clinical and research settings, selecting an appropriate spasticity assessment tool should be guided by the purpose of the evaluation, patient characteristics, and the care context. For rapid screening or documentation, the MAS remains practical and widely accepted. For detailed treatment planning and differentiation between neural and mechanical contributors, the Tardieu Scale offers greater specificity. Patient-reported measures such as the PSFS are particularly valuable when symptom burden and quality of life are primary concerns. Rather than relying on a single scale, a combined approach often provides a more comprehensive understanding of spasticity and its functional implications.

To support informed decision-making, a comparative summary Table 7 outlining the domains assessed, strengths, limitations, and ideal clinical applications of commonly used spasticity scales can serve as a practical reference for clinicians and researchers. Such an integrative use of assessment tools aligns with contemporary rehabilitation practice, which emphasizes individualized, goal-oriented evaluation over reliance on isolated impairment measures.

Table 7. Comparative summary of commonly used spasticity scales.

Scale	Primary Domain Assessed	Key Strengths	Major Limitations	Ideal Clinical Use
Modified Ashworth Scale (MAS)	Resistance to passive movement.	Quick, simple, widely accepted; minimal equipment.	Poor differentiation between neural and mechanical stiffness; inter-rater variability; limited sensitivity to change	Rapid screening in outpatient and inpatient settings.
Tardieu Scale	Velocity-dependent muscle response.	Differentiates spasticity from contracture; physiologically sound.	Requires training and precise velocity control; time-consuming.	Detailed assessment and treatment planning in neurorehabilitation.
Penn Spasm Frequency Scale (PSFS)	Frequency and severity of involuntary spasms.	Captures patient perspective; relevant to quality of life	Subjective; influenced by cognition and mood.	Monitoring spasm burden in SCI and MS.
Instrumented Measures (Emerging)	Objective muscle activity and reflex response.	High sensitivity; objective quantification.	Limited availability; higher cost.	Research settings and advanced clinical assessment.

CONCLUSION

Accurate evaluation of spasticity is essential for assessing the extent of neuromuscular dysfunction and guiding targeted therapeutic interventions. The Modified Ashworth Scale (MAS) remains the most widely used clinical measure owing to its simplicity and ease of administration, despite its limitations in sensitivity to velocity-dependent changes. The Tardieu Scale complements this by incorporating assessments at varying stretch velocities, providing a more comprehensive understanding of the reflex and non-reflex components of spasticity. The Penn Spasm Frequency Scale (PSFS), as a patient-reported measure, offers valuable insights into the subjective experience of spasticity and its impact on daily function. Collectively, these tools enable clinicians to evaluate motor impairment more effectively, monitor treatment outcomes, and tailor management strategies to individual patient needs. Ongoing efforts to improve their reliability, validity, and responsiveness will continue to enhance their clinical utility in neurorehabilitation.

AI DISCLOSURE STATEMENT

During the preparation of this chapter, the authors used ChatGPT (OpenAI) as a support tool for language refinement, structural organisation, and clarification of ideas. All content generated with AI assistance was carefully reviewed, verified, and revised by the authors to ensure factual accuracy, originality, and consistency with the scientific literature. The authors take full responsibility for the integrity, interpretation, and final content of the published chapter.

ACKNOWLEDGEMENTS

The authors gratefully acknowledge the contributions of neurologists, physiatrists, and rehabilitation specialists whose work in spasticity assessment and management has advanced clinical practice and research. Their continued efforts have improved diagnostic accuracy and therapeutic outcomes for individuals with spasticity resulting from neurological disorders.

REFERENCES

[1] Ashworth B. Preliminary trial of carisoprodol in multiple sclerosis. Practitioner 1964; 192: 540-2. [PMID: 14143329]

[2] Bohannon R W, Smith M B. Interrater reliability of a modified Ashworth scale of muscle spasticity. Phys Ther 1987; 67(2): 206-7. [PMID: 14143329]

[3] Ansari N N, Naghdi S, Moammeri H, Jalaie S. Ashworth Scales are unreliable for the assessment of muscle spasticity. Physiother Theory Pract 2006; 22(3): 119-25. [http://dx.doi.org/10.1093/ptj/67.2.206] [PMID: 3809245]

[4] Mehrholz J, Wagner K, Meissner D, *et al.* Reliability of the Modified Tardieu Scale and the Modified Ashworth Scale in adult patients with severe brain injury: a comparison study. Clin Rehabil 2005; 19(7): 751-9.
[http://dx.doi.org/10.1080/09593980600724188] [PMID: 16848350]

[5] Blackburn M, van Vliet P, Mockett S. Reliability of measurements obtained with the Modified Ashworth Scale in the lower extremities of people with stroke. Phys Ther 2002; 82: 25-34.
[http://dx.doi.org/10.1191/0269215505cr889oa] [PMID: 16250194]

[6] Mutlu A, Livanelioglu A, Gunel M K. Reliability of Ashworth and Modified Ashworth scales in children with spastic cerebral palsy. BMC Musculoskelet Disord 2008; 9: 44.
[http://dx.doi.org/10.1093/ptj/82.1.25] [PMID: 11784275]

[7] Allison S C, Abraham L D. Correlation of quantitative measures with the modified Ashworth scale in the assessment of plantar flexor spasticity in patients with traumatic brain injury. J Neurol 1995; 242(10): 699-706.
[http://dx.doi.org/10.1186/1471-2474-9-44] [PMID: 18402701] [PMCID: PMC2330046]

[8] Allison S C, Abraham L D, Petersen C L. Reliability of the Modified Ashworth Scale in the assessment of plantarflexor muscle spasticity in patients with traumatic brain injury. Int J Rehabil Res Int Zeitschrift fur Rehabil Rev Int Rech Readapt 1996; 19(1): 67-78.
[http://dx.doi.org/10.1007/BF00866923] [PMID: 8568534]

[9] Gregson J M, Leathley M, Moore A P, Sharma A K, Smith T L, Watkins C L. Reliability of the Tone Assessment Scale and the modified Ashworth scale as clinical tools for assessing poststroke spasticity. Arch Phys Med Rehabil 1999; 80(9): 1013-6.
[http://dx.doi.org/10.1097/00004356-199603000-00007] [PMID: 8730545]

[10] Fosang A L, Galea M P, McCoy A T, Reddihough D S, Story I. Measures of muscle and joint performance in the lower limb of children with cerebral palsy. Dev Med Child Neurol 2003; 45(10): 664-70.
[http://dx.doi.org/10.1016/s0003-9993(99)90053-9] [PMID: 10489001]

[11] Yam W, Leung M. Interrater reliability of Modified Ashworth Scale and Modified Tardieu Scale in children with spastic cerebral palsy. J Child Neurol 2007; 21: 1031-5.
[http://dx.doi.org/10.1017/s0012162203001245] [PMID: 14515937]

[12] Clopton N, Dutton J, Featherston T, Grigsby A, Mobley J, Melvin J. Interrater and intrarater reliability of the Modified Ashworth Scale in children with hypertonia. Pediatr Phys Ther Off Publ Sect Pediatr Am Phys Ther Assoc 2005; 17(4): 268-74.
[http://dx.doi.org/10.1177/7010.2006.00222] [PMID: 17156693]

[13] Ansari N N, Naghdi S, Arab T K, Jalaie S. The interrater and intrarater reliability of the Modified Ashworth Scale in the assessment of muscle spasticity: limb and muscle group effect. NeuroRehabilitation 2008; 23(3): 231-7.
[http://dx.doi.org/10.1097/01.pep.0000186509.41238.1a] [PMID: 16357682]

[14] Ansari N N, Naghdi S, Hasson S, Fakhari Z, Mashayekhi M, Herasi M. Assessing the reliability of the Modified Modified Ashworth Scale between two physiotherapists in adult patients with hemiplegia. NeuroRehabilitation 2009; 25(4): 235-40.
[http://dx.doi.org/10.3233/NRE-2008-23304]

[15] Ghotbi N, Nakhostin Ansari N, Naghdi S, Hasson S. Measurement of lower-limb muscle spasticity: intrarater reliability of Modified Modified Ashworth Scale. J Rehabil Res Dev 2011; 48(1): 83-8.
[http://dx.doi.org/10.3233/NRE-2009-0520] [PMID: 20037215]

[16] Craven B C, Morris A R. Modified Ashworth scale reliability for measurement of lower extremity spasticity among patients with SCI. Spinal Cord 2010; 48(3): 207-13.
[http://dx.doi.org/10.1682/jrrd.2010.02.0020] [PMID: 21328165]

[17] Waninge A, Rook R A, Dijkhuizen A, Gielen E, van der Schans C P. Feasibility, test-retest reliability,

and interrater reliability of the Modified Ashworth Scale and Modified Tardieu Scale in persons with profound intellectual and multiple disabilities. Res Dev Disabil 2011; 32(2): 613-20. [http://dx.doi.org/10.1038/sc.2009.107. Epub 2009 Sep 29] [PMID: 19786977]

[18] Li F, Wu Y, Li X. Test-retest reliability and inter-rater reliability of the Modified Tardieu Scale and the Modified Ashworth Scale in hemiplegic patients with stroke. Eur J Phys Rehabil Med 2014; 50(1): 9-15. [http://dx.doi.org/10.1016/j.ridd.2010.12.013. Epub 2011 Jan 12] [PMID: 21232915]

[19] Akpinar P, Atici A, Ozkan F U, *et al.* Reliability of the Modified Ashworth Scale and Modified Tardieu Scale in patients with spinal cord injuries. Spinal Cord 2017; 55(10): 944-9. [PMID: 24309501]

[20] Naghdi S, Ansari N N, Azarnia S, Kazemnejad A. Interrater reliability of the Modified Modified Ashworth Scale (MMAS) for patients with wrist flexor muscle spasticity. Physiother Theory Pract 2008; 24(5): 372-9. [http://dx.doi.org/10.1038/sc.2017.48. Epub 2017 May 9] [PMID: 28485384]

[21] Kaya T, Karatepe A G, Gunaydin R, Koc A, Altundal Ercan U. Inter-rater reliability of the Modified Ashworth Scale and modified Modified Ashworth Scale in assessing poststroke elbow flexor spasticity. Int J Rehabil Res Int Zeitschrift fur Rehabil Rev Int Rech Readapt 2011; 34(1): 59-64. [http://dx.doi.org/10.1080/09593980802278959] [PMID: 18821443]

[22] Mishra C, Ganesh G S. Inter-rater reliability of modified modified Ashworth scale in the assessment of plantar flexor muscle spasticity in patients with spinal cord injury. Physiother Res Int J Res Clin Phys Ther 2014; 19(4): 231-7. [http://dx.doi.org/10.1097/MRR.0b013e32833d6cdf] [PMID: 20671560]

[23] Penn R D, Savoy S M, Corcos D, *et al.* Intrathecal baclofen for severe spinal spasticity. N Engl J Med 1989; 320(23): 1517-21. [http://dx.doi.org/10.1002/pri.1588. Epub 2014 Mar 12] [PMID: 24619735]

[24] Hugos C L, Cameron M H. Assessment and measurement of spasticity in MS: state of the evidence. Curr Neurol Neurosci Rep 2019; 19(10): 79. [http://dx.doi.org/10.1056/NEJM198906083202303] [PMID: 2657424]

[25] Adams M M, Ginis K A M, Hicks A L. The spinal cord injury spasticity evaluation tool: development and evaluation. Arch Phys Med Rehabil 2007; 88(9): 1185-92. [http://dx.doi.org/10.1007/s11910-019-0991-2] [PMID: 31471769] [PMCID: PMC6948104]

[26] Mills P B, Vakil A P, Phillips C, Kei L, Kwon B K. Intra-rater and inter-rater reliability of the Penn Spasm Frequency Scale in people with chronic traumatic spinal cord injury. Spinal Cord 2018; 56(6): 569-74. [http://dx.doi.org/10.1016/j.apmr.2007.06.012] [PMID: 17826466]

[27] Abolhasani H, Ansari N N, Naghdi S, Mansouri K, Ghotbi N, Hasson S. Comparing the validity of the Modified Modified Ashworth Scale (MMAS) and the Modified Tardieu Scale (MTS) in the assessment of wrist flexor spasticity in patients with stroke: protocol for a neurophysiological study. BMJ Open 2012; 2(6): e001394. [http://dx.doi.org/10.1038/s41393-018-0063-5. Epub 2018 Jan 25] [PMID: 29371700]

[28] Balci B P. Spasticity measurement. Noro Psikiyatr Ars 2018; 55(Suppl 1): S49-53. [http://dx.doi.org/10.1136/bmjopen-2012-001394] [PMID: 23166123] [PMCID: PMC3532966]

[29] Boyd R N, Graham H K. Objective measurement of clinical findings in the use of botulinum toxin type A for the management of children with cerebral palsy. Eur J Neurol 1999; 6(S4): s23-35. [http://dx.doi.org/10.29399/npa.23339] [PMID: 30692856] [PMCID: PMC6278623]

[30] Gal O, Baude M, Deltombe T, *et al.* Clinical outcome assessments for spasticity: review, critique, and recommendations. Mov Disord 2025; 40(1): 22-43. [http://dx.doi.org/10.1111/J.1468-1331.1999.TB00031.X]

[31] Shu X, Lin D, Lin Y, Wu T, Wu Y, Li S. Validity and reliability of the Modified Tardieu Scale in adults with upper limb spasticity. BMJ Open 2021; 11(12): e050711.
[http://dx.doi.org/10.1002/mds.30062. Epub 2024 Dec 4] [PMID: 39629752] [PMCID: PMC11752990]

[32] He J, Porland C Z, He X, *et al.* Quantitative assessment of spasticity: a narrative review of novel approaches and technologies. Front Neurol 2023; 14: 1121323.
[http://dx.doi.org/10.3389/fneur.2023.1121323] [PMID: 37475737] [PMCID: PMC10354649]

CHAPTER 2

Scales for Dizziness and Vertigo

Sukhpreet Kaur[1,2], **Sukhpal Singh**[2] and **Simranjeet Kaur**[2,3,*]

[1] *Sri Guru Granth Sahib World University, Fatehgarh Sahib, Punjab, India*

[2] *Maharishi Markandeshwar Institute of Physiotherapy and Rehabilitation, Maharishi Markandeshwar (Deemed to be University), Mullana, Ambala, Haryana, India*

[3] *Pal Physiotherapy and Rehabilitation Centre, Pal Healthcare, Ambala City, Haryana, India*

Abstract: Dizziness and vertigo are complex symptoms that can have a substantial influence on a person's quality of life. An accurate assessment of these symptoms is essential for appropriate diagnosis and therapy. This chapter provides a detailed review of the scales and questionnaires used to assess dizziness and vertigo, including the Dizziness Handicap Inventory (DHI), the Amer Dizziness Diagnostic Scale, the Vertigo Symptom Scale, the Visual Vertigo Analogue Scale, and the and Numeric Dizziness Scale. The chapter covers each scale's introduction, its method of use, and its psychometric features, and provides advice on choosing the best instrument for your clinical requirements and patient population. This chapter seeks to synthesize current research and therapeutic practices.

Keywords: Assessment tools, Dizziness, Dizziness handicap inventory, Vertigo, Vertigo symptom scale, Vestibular disorders.

INTRODUCTION

Dizziness is a broad term that encompasses sensations such as light-headedness, imbalance, or unsteadiness, whereas vertigo is a specific type of dizziness characterized by a false sense of movement or spinning. Both symptoms have a substantial impact on a patient's quality of life and can be caused by a variety of variables such as vestibular dysfunction, neurological problems, cardiovascular concerns, and psychological factors [1].

Because dizziness and vertigo are multidimensional, it is critical to have reliable and valid evaluation measures to determine the severity, frequency, and impact of these many scales and questionnaires have been designed to help clinicians evalu-

* **Corresponding author Simranjeet Kaur:** Pal Physiotherapy and Rehabilitation Centre, Pal Healthcare, Ambala City, Haryana, India; E-mail: Simranjeetkaursaini825@gmail.com

Nidhi Sharma, Simranjeet Kaur & Parveen Kumar (Eds.)

ate patients with dizziness and vertigo, provide insights into their condition, and aid in diagnosis and therapy planning. These measures enable a consistent approach to evaluate dizziness-related impairments, disability, and health-related quality of life (HRQoL) [2].

DIZZINESS HANDICAP INVENTORY (DHI)

Introduction

The Dizziness Handicap Inventory (DHI) was developed by Jacobson and Newman in 1990 to measure the self-perceived level of handicap associated with dizziness. In addition to being used to assess subjective dizziness impairment, it has primarily been employed in patients with peripheral and central vestibular pathology in individuals who have severe brain injuries, chronic whiplash-related problems, severe anxiety disorders in the elderly, as well [1].

Number of Items

The DHI consists of 25 items with three response options, divided into three domains: functional, emotional, and physical.

- Functional (9 items): Assesses the impact of dizziness on everyday activities (*e.g.*, walking, reading).
- Emotional (9 items): Examines emotional responses to dizziness (*e.g.*, frustration, fear).
- Physical (7 items): Evaluates dizziness triggered by movement or physical actions (*e.g.*, looking up, bending over) [2].

Administration

Administering the questionnaires requires no additional training and takes only 5 to 10 minutes to complete. Scores for the Physical (28 points), Emotional (36 points), and Functional (36 points) subdomains are calculated (Table **1**).

Table 1. Dizziness handicap inventory (DHI) [1].

P1. Does looking up increase your problem?	Yes	Sometimes	No
E2. Because of your problem, do you feel frustrated?	Yes	Sometimes	No
F3. Because of your problem, do you restrict your travel for business or recreation?	Yes	Sometimes	No
P4. Does walking down the supermarket aisle increase your problems?	Yes	Sometimes	No
F5. Because of your problem, do you have difficulty getting into or out of bed?	Yes	Sometimes	No
F6. Does your problem significantly restrict your participation in social activities, such as going out to dinner, going to the movies, dancing, or going to parties?	Yes	Sometimes	No

(Table 1) cont.....

F7. Because of your problem, do you have difficulty reading?	Yes	Sometimes	No
P8. Does performing more ambitious activities, such as sports, dancing, or household chores (sweeping or putting dishes away), increase your problems?	Yes	Sometimes	No
E9. Because of your problem, are you afraid to leave your home without someone accompanying you?	Yes	Sometimes	No
E10. Because of your problem, have you been embarrassed in front of others?	Yes	Sometimes	No
P11. Do quick head movements make your problem worse?	Yes	Sometimes	No
F12. Because of your problem, do you avoid heights?	Yes	Sometimes	No
P13. Does turning over in bed make your problem worse?	Yes	Sometimes	No
F14. Because of your problem, is it difficult for you to do strenuous homework or yard work?	Yes	Sometimes	No
E15. Because of your problem, are you afraid people may think you are intoxicated?	Yes	Sometimes	No
F16. Because of your problem, is it difficult for you to go for a walk by yourself?	Yes	Sometimes	No
P17. Does walking down a sidewalk increase your problem?	Yes	Sometimes	No
E18. Because of your problem, is it difficult for you to concentrate?	Yes	Sometimes	No
F19. Because of your problem, is it difficult for you to walk around your house in the dark?	Yes	Sometimes	No
E20. Because of your problem, are you afraid to stay home alone?	Yes	Sometimes	No
E21. Because of your problem, do you feel handicapped?	Yes	Sometimes	No
E22. Has the problem placed stress on your relationships with members of your family or friends	Yes	Sometimes	No
E23. Because of your problem, are you depressed?	Yes	Sometimes	No
F24. Does your problem interfere with your job or household responsibilities?	Yes	Sometimes	No
P25. Does bending over increase your problem?	Yes	Sometimes	No

Scoring and Interpretation Total Score = 100

The following scores may be given to each item:

Score 0 = No; Score 2 = Sometimes; Score 4 = Yes. Hence, a score of 16-34 = mild handicap, 36-52 = moderate handicap, 54+ = severe handicap. The total possible score ranges from 0 (no handicap) to 100 (maximum handicap), with higher scores indicating greater perceived disability due to dizziness.

Indications

Vestibular Disorder, Multiple Sclerosis, Brain Injury, Older adults and Geriatric care, Movement and Gait Disorders [2].

Languages

This scale is available in many languages such as English [1], Dutch [3], Norwegian [4], Swedish [5], Chinese [6], German [7], Arabic [8], Italian [9], Japanese [10], Persian [11], Turkish [12] (Table **2**).

Table 2. Internal consistency (Cronbach's alpha) of different versions/ languages of DHI.

Version	Overall DHI Score (Cronbach's Alpha)	Functional Score (Cronbach's Alpha)	Physical Score (Cronbach's Alpha)	Emotional Score (Cronbach's Alpha)
Persian [11]	0.79	0.90	0.83	0.82
Turkish [12]	0.92	0.88	0.67	0.83
Italian [9]	0.92	0.82	0.75	0.84
German [7]	0.90	0.80	0.71	0.82
Swedish [5]	0.63	-	-	-
Arabian [8]	0.92	0.87	0.81	0.79
Chinese [6]	>0.7	-	-	-
Norwegian [4]	0.95	-	-	-

Psychometric Properties

Reliability: Test-retest reliability for the total score was excellent ($r = 0.97$, $p<0.001$). Correlation coefficients associated with the functional ($r = 0.94$), emotional ($r = 0.97$), and physical ($r = 0.92$) subscales were high [13].

AMER DIZZINESS DIAGNOSTIC SCALE

Introduction

The Amer Dizziness Diagnostic Scale is used to assess and make a differentiating diagnosis for patients with vestibular problems. Thus, the ADDS offers doctors a measure that is objective to aid in clinical decision-making, and it can be utilized as in general clinics as a primary assessment technique so that even individuals who are an adequately examine individuals who are not specialists in these fields can direct them to the right expertise if they complain of dizziness seeking a second opinion and additional treatment [14].

Number of Items

There are a total of 5 sections, which include a total of 17 questions under the Amer Dizziness Diagnostic Scale.

- Section 1 (no score) includes 1-7 questions
- Section 2 (where, Yes = 1, no = 0) includes 8-10 questions
- Section 3 (where, Yes = 5, no = 0) includes 11-12 questions
- Section 4 (where, Yes = 20, no = 0) includes 13-16 questions
- Section 5 (where, No = 0, S = 1, M = 5 and H = 20) includes 17 questions

Description

The ADDS includes seventeen questions, which are divided into five categories:

General Information: The first seven questions collect demographic information and medical history on hypertension, diabetes, balance difficulties, and partial hearing loss for research purposes (Table **3**).

- Unilateral Vestibular Hypofunction (UVH): Three questions are asked about recent infections, hazy vision with or without vomiting, and whether the patient leans to one side while walking.
- Benign Paroxysmal Positional Vertigo (BPPV): Two questions address dizziness caused by head movements and body positions, such as bending forward or sleeping on one side.
- Central Mediated Problems (CM): Four questions assess neurological problems, prior concussions, lightheadedness or fainting while shifting positions, and ear tinnitus.
- General Vestibular Disorders: The last question concerns the frequency and character of dizzy episodes, which encompasses all preceding vestibular diseases, including Cervicogenic dizzy (CGD).

Table 3. AMER dizziness diagnostic scale (ADDS).

Name: **Date:**

	Question	Yes	No
	Section 1 (no score)		
1	Gender?	[M]	[F]
2	Age?	Above 50	Below 50
3	Are you Hypertensive?		
4	Are you Diabetic?		
5	Do you have a balance problem?		
6	Do you experience double vision or blurred vision that cause vomiting?		
7	Have you ever experienced partial hearing loss associated with dizziness?		
	Section 2 (yes = 1, no = 0)		

(Table 3) cont.....

	Question	Yes		No	
8	Have you been diagnosed with the viral or bacterial infection in the last 2 weeks (cold, flu)?				
9	Do you experience double vision or blurred vision?				
10	Do you drift to one side when walking?				
	Section 3 (yes = 5, no = 0)				
11	Do you experience dizziness while moving your head?				
12	Do you experience dizziness with different body movements, like bending forward or sleeping on your side?				
	Section 4 (yes = 20, no = 0)				
13	Have you been diagnosed with any neurological disorder (Stroke, MS)?				
14	Have you had a head Concussion before experiencing dizziness?				
15	Do you experience lightheadedness or fainting when moving from sitting to standing position?				
16	Do you have ear Tinnitus?				
	Section 5 (No = 0, S = 1, M = 5 and H = 20)				
17	How long does your dizziness last?	No	S	M	H
	Total (max 113) =				

- Therapist:
- Diagnosis:
- CGD ☐ UVH ☐
- BPPV ☐ CM ☐

Scoring and Interpretation

Score 0 = Cervicogenic Dizziness
Score 1- 4 = Unilateral Vestibular Hypofunction (UVH)
Score 5-19 = Benign Paroxysmal Positional Vertigo (BPPV)
Score 20 or higher = Centrally Mediated Problem

Psychometric Properties

Sensitivity = 96%
Specificity = 96%
ADDS strongly correlated with the "true-positive" and "true-negative" results ($r=0.95$, $p<0.05$) [14].

VERTIGO SYMPTOM SCALE

The Vertigo Symptom Scale is a tool used to assess the severity of vertigo symptoms. It typically involves a questionnaire where individuals rate the frequency and intensity of their vertigo episodes, helping healthcare professionals better understand and manage the condition [15].

Number of Items

There are two subscales in the short form of the Vertigo Symptom scale.

- 8 items relating to vertigo-balance (VSS-V score ranging from 0-32)
- 7 items relating to autonomic anxiety symptoms (VSS-A, score ranging 0-28)

Measurement Domain

Emotion, General health, Motor

Intended Population

Brain Injury Recovery, Vestibular Disorders

Description

Frequency of symptoms is rated on a Likert scale: (Fig. **1**)

- 0 point: "never"
- 1 point: "a few times (1-3 times a year)."
- 2 points: "several times (4-12 times a year)."
- 3 points: "quite often (on average, more than once a month)."
- 4 points: "very often (on average more than once a week)"

Scoring

- Vertigo/balance sub scale score range: 0-76
- Autonomic/Anxiety subscale score range: 0-60
- Maximum score: 136 (severe vertigo)
- Minimum score: 0 (no symptoms)

Psychometric Properties

Test/Retest Reliability for Vestibular Dysfunction [16]:

Excellent test-retest reliability for vertigo symptom scale score (r=0.94)

Excellent test-retest reliability for Autonomic/Anxiety symptom scale (r=0.95).

Vertigo Symptom Scale (short form)

We would like to know what dizziness-related symptoms you have had just recently. Please circle the appropriate number to indicate about how many times you have experienced each of the symptoms listed below *during the past month*. The range of responses is:

0	1	2	3	4
Never	A few times	Several times	Quite often (every week)	Very often (most days)

How often in the past month have you had the following symptoms:

1. A feeling that either you, or things around you, are spinning or moning, lasting less than 20 minutes	0	1	2	3	4
2. Hot or cold spells	0	1	2	3	4
3. Nausea (feeling sick), vomiting	0	1	2	3	4
4. A feeling that either you, or things around you, are spinning or moning, lasting more than 20 minutes	0	1	2	3	4
5. Heart pounding or fluttering	0	1	2	3	4
6. A feeling of being dizzy, disoriented or "swimmy," lasting *all day*	0	1	2	3	4
7. Headache, or feeling of pressure in the head	0	1	2	3	4
8. Unable to stand or walk properly without support, vearing or staggering to one side	0	1	2	3	4
9. Difficulty breathing, short of breath	0	1	2	3	4
10. Feeling unsteady, about to lose balance, lasting more than 20 minutes	0	1	2	3	4
11. Excessive sweating	0	1	2	3	4
12. Feeling faint, about to black out	0	1	2	3	4
13. Feeling unsteady, about to lose balance, lasting less than 20 minutes	0	1	2	3	4
14. Pains in the heart or chest region	0	1	2	3	4
15. A feeling of being dizzy, disoriented or "swimmy." lasting *less* than 20 minutes	0	1	2	3	4

Fig. (1). Vertigo symptom scale [17].

VISUAL VERTIGO ANALOGUE SCALE

The Visual Vertigo Analogue Scale (VVAS) assesses the degree of visual vertigo in nine demanding conditions that might cause dizziness. Participants rated their dizziness in various situations (*e.g.*, walking in a supermarket, being a passenger in a car, *etc.*) by drawing a vertical line on a ten-centimeter line anchored at 0 [18].

Instructions for Administration and Scoring

Administration:

- The VVAS is made up of nine visual analogue scales that participants rated. Each scale is based on a distinct visual vertigo-causing condition (Fig. **2**).
- The individual marks a vertical line on a 10 cm line to indicate the amount of dizziness provoked by each of 9 situations.
- Zero anchor representing no dizziness and 10 anchor representing extreme dizziness or activity avoided due to dizziness.

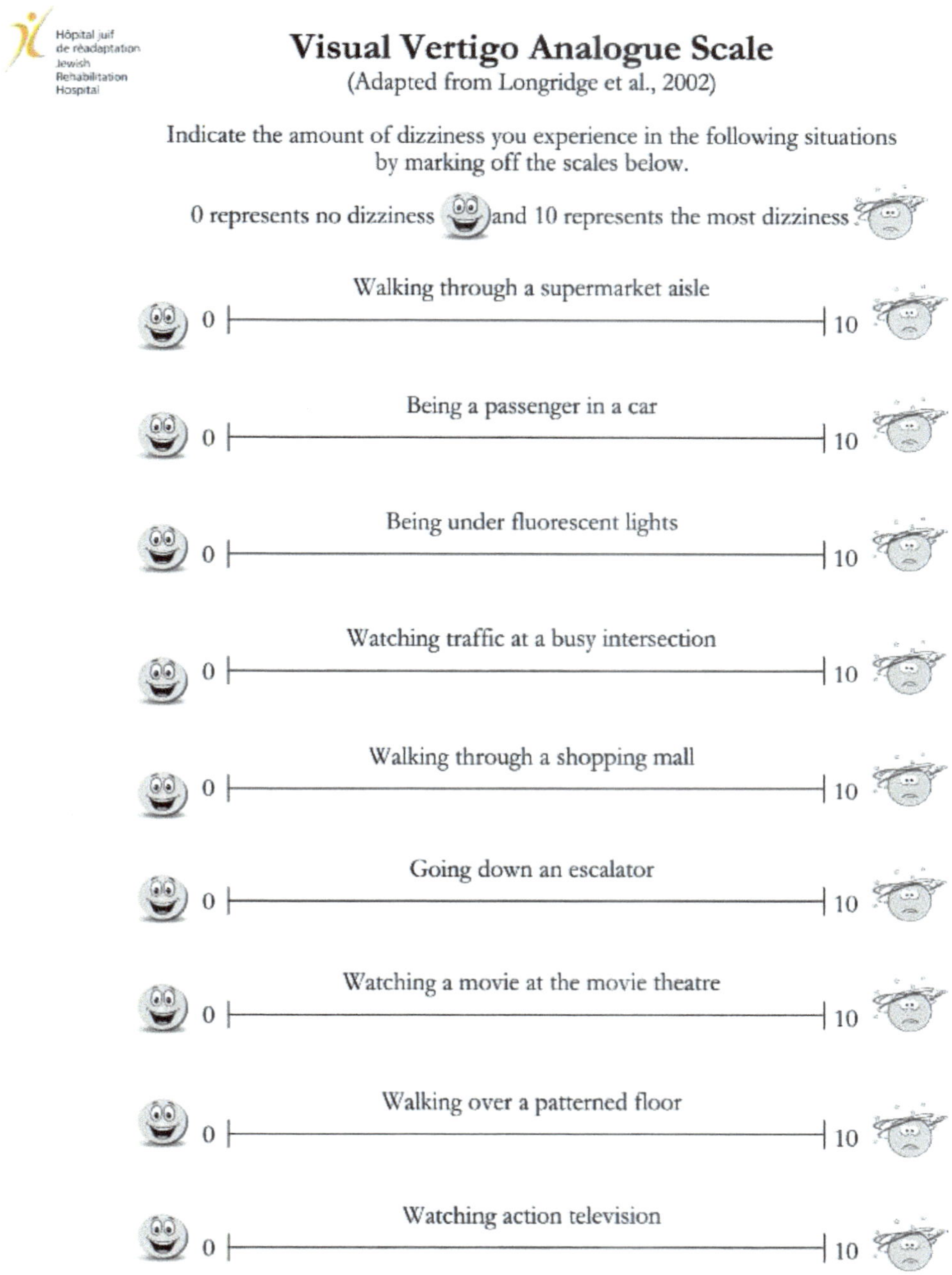

Hôpital juif de réadaptation Jewish Rehabilitation Hospital

Visual Vertigo Analogue Scale

(Adapted from Longridge et al., 2002)

Indicate the amount of dizziness you experience in the following situations by marking off the scales below.

0 represents no dizziness and 10 represents the most dizziness

Walking through a supermarket aisle — 0 to 10

Being a passenger in a car — 0 to 10

Being under fluorescent lights — 0 to 10

Watching traffic at a busy intersection — 0 to 10

Walking through a shopping mall — 0 to 10

Going down an escalator — 0 to 10

Watching a movie at the movie theatre — 0 to 10

Walking over a patterned floor — 0 to 10

Watching action television — 0 to 10

Fig. (2). Visual vertigo analogue scale.

Intended Population

Vestibular Disorders

Time to Administer

5 to 10 minutes

Psychometric Properties

Excellent Internal Consistency (Cronbach alpha = 0.94)

Excellent predictive validity between VVAS and total DHI ($r = 0.67$, $p < 0.0001$) as well as VAS and functional ($r = 0.71$, $p < 0.0001$), emotional ($r = 0.65$, $p < 0.0001$) and Adequate predictive validity with physical DHI subscale score ($r= 0.45$, $p < 0.0001$) [19].

NUMERIC DIZZINESS SCALE (NDS)

The Numeric Dizziness Scale is where individuals rate their dizziness on a scale from 0 to 10, with 0 being no dizziness and 10 being the worst possible dizziness [20].

Instructions for Administration and Scoring

The NPRS is an 11-point scale scored from 0 to 10 (Fig. **3**):

1) "0" = no pain

2) "10" = the most intense pain imaginable

Patients verbally select a value that best reflects the intensity of pain they have experienced in the last 24 hours.

Required Training: No training required

Time to Administer: Less than 3 minutes

Psychometric Properties

All components of the NDS (current, best, worst) demonstrated good to excellent test-retest reliability (ICC $r = 0.68$-0.93) [22].
The NDS was found to have good reliability with ICC=0.73.
The NDS worst was found to have excellent reliability with ICC=0.93.
The NDS current was found to have the lowest ICC value, but good reliability with ICC=0.68.

Dizziness
Participant Number________________ Date________________ Time________________
On a scale from 0 to 10, with 0 being no dizziness at all and 10 being your worst imaginable dizziness, how would you rate your current level of dizziness? *Please circle one:* 0 1 2 3 4 5 6 7 8 9 10 (no dizziness) (worst imaginable dizziness)
On a scale from 0 to 10, with 0 being no dizziness at all and 10 being your worst imaginable dizziness, how would you rate your worst level of dizziness in the past 24-hours? *Please circle one:* 0 1 2 3 4 5 6 7 8 9 10 (no dizziness) (worst imaginable dizziness)
On a scale from 0 to 10, with 0 being no dizziness at all and 10 being your worst imaginable dizziness, how would you rate your best level of dizziness in the past 24-hours? *Please circle one:* 0 1 2 3 4 5 6 7 8 9 10 (no dizziness) (worst imaginable dizziness)

Fig. (3). Numeric dizziness scale (NDS) [21].

CLINICAL CONSIDERATIONS, STRENGTHS, LIMITATIONS, AND EMERGING TRENDS

Dizziness and vertigo are among the most common yet challenging symptoms encountered in neurological and rehabilitation practice. Their subjective nature, multifactorial etiology, and frequent overlap with psychological and sensory disturbances make accurate assessment particularly complex. The scales included in this chapter, such as the Dizziness Handicap Inventory (DHI), Amer Dizziness Diagnostic Scale, Vertigo Symptom Scale, Visual Vertigo Analogue Scale, and Numeric Dizziness Scale, reflect different conceptual approaches to evaluation, ranging from symptom severity to functional impact and diagnostic differentiation [23].

The Dizziness Handicap Inventory (DHI) is one of the most widely used tools for assessing the perceived impact of dizziness on daily life. Its strength lies in its ability to capture physical, functional, and emotional consequences, thereby offering a holistic view of symptom burden from the patient's perspective. This makes the DHI especially useful in chronic vestibular disorders and during rehabilitation, where changes in participation and quality of life are key outcome measures [24]. However, because the DHI is entirely self-reported, scores may be influenced by anxiety, depression, or fear of movement, which are commonly associated with dizziness. As a result, elevated scores do not always reflect vestibular dysfunction alone and should be interpreted in conjunction with clinical examination and objective testing [25].

The Amer Dizziness Diagnostic Scale attempts to address one of the major limitations of purely symptom-based tools by aiding in the clinical differentiation of dizziness subtypes. By guiding clinicians toward possible peripheral, central, or non-vestibular causes, this scale has a practical value in initial assessment and referral decision-making. Its structured format can be particularly helpful for less experienced clinicians or in primary care settings. Nevertheless, diagnostic scales rely heavily on accurate symptom reporting and clinician interpretation, and they cannot replace detailed vestibular examination or neuroimaging when central pathology is suspected.

The Vertigo Symptom Scale offers a more nuanced assessment by distinguishing vestibular-balance symptoms from autonomic and anxiety-related complaints. This distinction is clinically relevant, as persistent dizziness is frequently maintained by psychological factors even after the resolution of the primary vestibular insult. By capturing this overlap, the scale supports a more comprehensive management approach that may include vestibular rehabilitation, behavioral strategies, and psychological intervention. However, its length and emphasis on symptom frequency may limit feasibility in acute care settings or in patients with cognitive fatigue.

The Visual Vertigo Analogue Scale addresses a specific but increasingly recognized domain of dizziness—visual dependence and visually induced vertigo. This tool is particularly useful for patients who report symptom exacerbation in visually complex environments such as shopping malls or crowded streets. While it provides valuable insight into visual–vestibular interaction, its application is relatively narrow and may be less informative in patients with purely peripheral vestibular disorders. Therefore, it is best used as an adjunct rather than a primary assessment measure [26].

The Numeric Dizziness Scale (NDS) offers a quick and simple method for quantifying perceived dizziness intensity. Its ease of administration makes it suitable for repeated measurements, monitoring symptom fluctuation, and assessing short-term response to interventions. However, like other single-item scales, it lacks specificity and does not capture the multidimensional impact of dizziness on function or participation. Consequently, the NDS is most effective when combined with more comprehensive tools such as the DHI.

A common limitation across dizziness and vertigo scales is their dependence on subjective reporting, which can be influenced by psychological state, coping strategies, and individual symptom interpretation. Additionally, many scales demonstrate limited sensitivity in acute vestibular conditions, where symptoms may fluctuate rapidly, or in distinguishing central from peripheral etiologies. These challenges highlight the importance of using symptom scales as part of a broader assessment framework that includes clinical examination, vestibular function testing, and functional evaluation.

Recent advancements in dizziness assessment have increasingly focused on technology-assisted and objective measures. Virtual reality–based environments are being explored to systematically provoke and quantify visually induced dizziness, while mobile applications allow real-time symptom tracking in natural environments. Wearable sensors and balance platforms are also being integrated to correlate subjective symptom severity with objective postural control measures. These emerging approaches hold promise for improving diagnostic precision and treatment monitoring, particularly in patients with persistent or complex dizziness syndromes [27, 28].

In clinical practice, the selection of dizziness assessment tools should be guided by the clinical objective. For evaluating overall symptom impact and monitoring rehabilitation outcomes, the DHI remains highly valuable. Diagnostic-oriented scales may be more appropriate during initial assessment, whereas symptom intensity scales such as the NDS are useful for tracking short-term changes. Using a combination of scales allows clinicians to capture both the subjective experience and functional consequences of dizziness, leading to more targeted and effective management strategies.

A comparative summary in Table 4 outlining the focus, strengths, and ideal clinical applications of commonly used dizziness and vertigo scales can further assist clinicians in selecting the most appropriate tool for a given patient and setting. Such integrative assessment aligns with contemporary vestibular rehabilitation practice, which emphasizes individualized, patient-centered evaluation over reliance on a single outcome measure.

Table 4. Comparative overview of dizziness and vertigo assessment scales.

Scale	Focus of Assessment	Strengths	Limitations	Best Clinical Application
Dizziness Handicap Inventory (DHI)	Functional, physical, and emotional impact.	Comprehensive; sensitive to rehabilitation outcomes	Influenced by anxiety and depression, subjective	Chronic dizziness and vestibular rehabilitation
Amer Dizziness Diagnostic Scale	Diagnostic differentiation	Guides clinical reasoning; useful in initial assessment.	Cannot replace detailed vestibular testing.	Early screening and referral decisions

(Table 4) cont.....

Scale	Focus of Assessment	Strengths	Limitations	Best Clinical Application
Vertigo Symptom Scale	Vestibular and autonomic symptoms	Differentiates physical and anxiety-related symptoms	Lengthy; limited use in acute care	Persistent or recurrent dizziness
Visual Vertigo Analogue Scale	Visually induced dizziness	Targets the visual–vestibular interaction	Narrow application scope	Visual dependence and complex environments
Numeric Dizziness Scale (NDS)	Symptom intensity	Simple; suitable for repeated measures	Lacks a multidimensional assessment	Short-term monitoring and symptom tracking
Technology-Based Tools (Emerging)	Objective balance and symptom provocation	Enhanced sensitivity; real-world data	Limited clinical availability	Research and advanced clinical settings

CONCLUSION

A precise evaluation of vertigo and dizziness is essential to a successful diagnosis and course of treatment. The DHI, ADDS, VVAS, NDS, and Vertigo Symptom Scale are the scales that were examined and offer important information about the intensity and effects of these symptoms. Strong psychometric qualities are demonstrated by each instrument, which makes them dependable options for medical professionals. Choosing the right scale can improve patient care and guide focused treatment plans.

AI DISCLOSURE STATEMENT

During the preparation of this chapter, the authors used ChatGPT (OpenAI) as a support tool for language refinement, structural organisation, and clarification of ideas. All content generated with AI assistance was carefully reviewed, verified, and revised by the authors to ensure factual accuracy, originality, and consistency with the scientific literature. The authors take full responsibility for the integrity, interpretation, and final content of the published chapter.

ACKNOWLEDGEMENT

The authors would like to acknowledge the contributions of all researchers and clinicians whose work on vestibular assessment scales has enriched this field of study. Their collective efforts have significantly advanced the understanding and management of dizziness and vertigo.

REFERENCES

[1] Jacobson G P, Newman C W. The development of the dizzinesshandicap inventory. Archivesof Otolaryngology–Head & Neck Surgery 1990; 116(4): 424-7. [http://dx.doi.org/10.1001/archotol.1990.01870040046011] [PMID: 2317323]

[2] Enloe L J, Shields R K. Evaluation of health-related quality of life in individuals with vestibular disease using disease-specific and general outcome measures. Phys Ther 1997; 77(9): 890-903. [http://dx.doi.org/10.1093/ptj/77.9.890] [PMID: 9291947]

[3] Vereeck L, Truijen S, Wuyts F L, Van De Heyning P H. Internal consistency and factor analysis of the Dutch version of the Dizziness Handicap Inventory. Acta Otolaryngol 2007; 127(8): 788-95. [http://dx.doi.org/10.1080/00016480601075464] [PMID: 17729178]

[4] Tamber A L, Wilhelmsen K T, Strand L I. Measurement properties of the DizzinessHandicap Inventory by cross-sectional and longitudinal designs. Health Qual Life Outcomes 2009; 7: 101. [http://dx.doi.org/10.1186/1477-7525-7-101] [PMID: 20025754]

[5] Jarlsäter, S., & Mattsson, E. Test of reliability of the Dizziness Handicap Inventory and The Activities-specific Balance Confidence Scale for Use in Sweden. Advances in Physiotherapy 2003, 5(3), 137–144. [http://dx.doi.org/10.1080/14038190310004385]

[6] Poon D M, Chow L C, Hui Y, Au D K, Leung M C. Translation of the dizziness handicap inventory into Chinese, validation of it, and evaluation of the quality of life of patients with chronic dizziness. Annals of Otology,Rhinology & Laryngology 2004; 113(12): 1006-1. [http://dx.doi.org/10.1177/000348940411301212] [PMID: 15633905]

[7] Kurre A, van Gool C J, Bastiaenen C H, Gloor-Juzi T, Straumann D, de Bruin E D. Translation, cross-cultural adaptation and reliability of the german version of the dizziness handicap inventory. Otol Neurotol 2009; 30(3): 359-67. [http://dx.doi.org/10.1097/MAO.0b013e3181977e09] [PMID: 19225437]

[8] Alsanosi AA. Adaptation of the dizziness handicap inventory for use in the Arab population. Neurosciences (Riyadh). 2012; 17(2):139–144. PMID: 22465888.

[9] Nola G, Mostardini C, Salvi C, Ercolani AP, Ralli G. Validity of Italian adaptation of the Dizziness Handicap Inventory (DHI) and evaluation of the quality of life in patients with acute dizziness. Acta Otorhinolaryngol Ital. 2010; 30(4): 190. PMID: 21253284; PMCID: PMC3008147.

[10] Goto F, Tsutsumi T, Ogawa K. The Japanese version of the Dizziness Handicap Inventory as an index of treatment success: exploratory factor analysis. Acta oto-laryngologica 2011; 131(8): 817-25. [http://dx.doi.org/10.3109/00016489.2011.565423] [PMID: 21762004]

[11] Jafarzadeh S, Bahrami E, Pourbakht A, Jalaie S, Daneshi A. Validity and reliability of the Persian version of the dizziness handicap inventory. Journal of research in medical sciences: the official journal of Isfahan University of Medical Sciences. 2014 19(8): 769. PMID: 25422664; PMCID: PMC4235099.

[12] Karapolat H, Eyigor S, Kirazlı Y, Celebisoy N, Bilgen C, Kirazlı T. Reliability, validity and sensitivity to change of Turkish Dizziness Handicap Inventory (DHI) in patients with unilateral peripheral vestibular disease. The Journal of International Advanced Otology. 2009; 5(2):237-45.

[13] Mutlu B, Serbetcioglu B. Discussion of the dizziness handicap inventory. Journal of vestibular research 2013; 23(6): 271-7. [http://dx.doi.org/10.3233/VES-130488] [PMID: 24447966]

[14] Al Saif A, Alsenany S. Sensitivity and specificity of the amer dizziness diagnostic scale (adds) for patients with vestibular disorders. J Phys Ther Sci 2015; 27(1): 91-6. [http://dx.doi.org/10.1589/jpts.27.91] [PMID: 25642046]

[15] Alsaif AA, Alsenany SA. Balance and prevention of fall among elderly. MOJ Gerontol Ger. 2018; 3(1): 65-69.

[http://dx.doi.org/10.15406/mojgg.2018.03.00087]

[16] Cohen H S, Kimball K T, Adams A S. Application of the vestibular disorders activities of daily living scale. The Laryngoscope 2000; 110(7): 1204-9.
[http://dx.doi.org/10.1097/00005537-200007000-00026] [PMID: 10892697]

[17] Yardley L, Masson E, Verschuur C, Haacke N, Luxon L. Symptoms, anxiety and handicap in dizzy patients: development of the vertigo symptom scale. Journal of psychosomatic research 1992; 36(8): 731-41.
[http://dx.doi.org/10.1016/0022-3999(92)90131-K] [PMID: 1432863]

[18] Wilhelmsen K, Strand L I, Nordahl S H, Eide G E, Ljunggren A E. Psychometric properties of the Vertigo symptom scale–Short form. BMC Ear, Nose and Throat Disorders 2008; 8: 1-9.
[http://dx.doi.org/10.1186/1472-6815-8-2] [PMID: 18371190]

[19] Yardley L, Donovan-Hall M, Smith H E, Walsh B M, Mullee M, Bronstein A M. Effectiveness of primary care–based vestibular rehabilitation for chronic dizziness. Annals of internalmedicine 2004; 141(8): 598-605.
[http://dx.doi.org/10.7326/0003-4819-141-8-200410190-00007] [PMID: 15492339]

[20] Dannenbaum E, Chilingaryan G, Fung J. Visual vertigo analogue scale: an assessmentquestionnaire for visual vertigo. J Vestib Res 2011; 21(3): 153-9.
[http://dx.doi.org/10.3233/VES-2011-0412] [PMID: 21558640]

[21] Verdecchia D H, Hernandez D, Andreu M F, Salzberg S. Translation and cross-cultural adaptation of the Visual Vertigo AnalogueScale for use in Argentina. Acta Otorrinolaringologica (English Edition) 2020; 71(5): 289-95.
[http://dx.doi.org/10.1016/j.otoeng.2019.10.003] [PMID: 32204877]

[22] Rice T, Mancinelli C, Utzman R, Cassis A, Wetmore S. Reliability of the numeric dizziness scale for the quantification of dizziness. West Virginia Medical Journal. 2018; 114(3): 30-5.

[23] Staab J P. Chronic subjective dizziness. Continuum (Minneapolis, Minn) 2012; 18(5): 1118-41.
[http://dx.doi.org/10.1212/01.CON.0000421622.56525.58] [PMID: 23042063]

[24] Jacobson G P, Newman C W. The development of the Dizziness Handicap Inventory. Archives of Otolaryngology–Head & Neck Surgery 1990; 116(4): 424-7.
[http://dx.doi.org/10.1001/archotol.1990.01870040046011] [PMID: 2317323]

[25] Yardley L, Redfern M S. Psychological factors influencing recovery from balance disorders. Journal of Anxiety Disorders 2001; 15(1–2): 107-19.
[http://dx.doi.org/10.1016/S0887-6185(00)00045-1] [PMID: 11388354]

[26] Pavlou M, Davies RA, Bronstein AM. The assessment of increased sensitivity to visual stimuli in patients with chronic dizziness. J Vestib Res. 2006; 16(4-5): 223-31. PMID: 17538212.

[27] Whitney SL, Sparto PJ. Principles of vestibular physical therapy rehabilitation. NeuroRehabilitation. 2011; 29(2): 157-66. doi: 10.3233/NRE-2011-0690. PMID: 22027077; PMCID: PMC4894843.

[28] Pérez-Fernández N, Ramos-Macías A. Recent advances in the diagnosis and treatment of vestibular disorders. Journal of clinical medicine 2023; 12(16): 52.
[http://dx.doi.org/10.3390/jcm12165281] [PMID: 37629323]

CHAPTER 3

Scales for Coma

Mayuri Thakur[1,2] and **Akanksha Saxena**[2,*]

[1] *Dolphin PG College of Life Science, Chunni Kalan, Punjab, India*

[2] *Maharishi Markandeshwar Institute of Physiotherapy and Rehabilitation, Maharishi Markandeshwar (Deemed to be University), Mullana, Ambala, Haryana, India*

Abstract: Coma is a state of profound unresponsiveness characterized by the inability to awaken or respond to stimuli, often resulting from severe brain injury, metabolic disturbances, or other critical medical conditions. Assessing the level of consciousness and potential recovery in comatose patients is essential for guiding treatment and rehabilitation strategies. Various scales are employed for this purpose, each providing unique insights into the patient's condition. The Glasgow Coma Scale (GCS) evaluates eye, verbal, and motor responses to determine the depth of coma and potential recovery. The Full Outline of Unresponsiveness (FOUR) scale combines neurological assessments and vital signs to provide a comprehensive overview of the patient's status. The Rappaport Disability Rating Scale (DRS) assesses overall functioning and disability in individuals recovering from coma, helping track rehabilitation progress. Lastly, the Western Neuro Sensory Stimulation Profile (WNSSP) evaluates sensory and motor responses, which can guide therapeutic interventions for those with significant cognitive impairments. Together, these scales form a robust framework for understanding and managing coma, aiding in both clinical decision-making and patient care.

Keywords: Assessment, Brain injury, Brainstem, Cognitive, Coma, Consciousness, Healthcare, Illness, Neuro, Reflexes, Rehabilitation, Respiration, Sensory, Treatment, Unconsciousness.

INTRODUCTION

A coma is a profound state of unconsciousness characterized by a lack of awareness of self and the environment, along with an inability to respond to stimuli [1]. This condition represents a critical medical emergency and can arise from various causes, including traumatic brain injuries, strokes, infections, metabolic imbalances, and drug overdoses. Understanding coma is essential not

* **Corresponding author Akanksha Saxena:** Maharishi Markandeshwar Institute of Physiotherapy and Rehabilitation, Maharishi Markandeshwar (Deemed to be University), Mullana-Ambala (Haryana), India; E-mail: akankshasaxena623@gmail.com

Nidhi Sharma, Simranjeet Kaur & Parveen Kumar (Eds.)

only for medical professionals but also for families and caregivers grappling with the implications of such a severe condition [2].

When a person enters a coma, they exhibit no signs of wakefulness or awareness, which can be distressing for loved ones. Unlike sleep, a comatose state is prolonged and involves a significant disruption in normal brain function [3]. Comas are typically assessed using the Glasgow Coma Scale (GCS), a tool that evaluates a patient’s responsiveness through eye, verbal, and motor responses. The depth and duration of a coma can vary widely, with some individuals emerging with full recovery, while others may transition into a vegetative state or suffer permanent neurological damage [4].

The underlying causes of coma are diverse, and prompt medical intervention is critical for improving outcomes. For instance, traumatic brain injuries from accidents can lead to swelling and pressure in the brain, while strokes may disrupt blood flow, affecting cognitive function [5]. Metabolic disorders, such as severe hypoglycaemia or liver failure, can also result in coma by altering brain chemistry. Identifying the cause is crucial, as targeted treatments can often prevent further damage [6].

The journey of recovery from a coma is highly individualized. Some patients may regain consciousness within days, while others may take weeks or even months. Rehabilitation plays a significant role in this process, as physical, occupational, and speech therapies help patients regain lost functions [7]. Families are often left to navigate an emotional landscape of uncertainty, hope, and despair, making support systems and resources essential [8].

In recent years, advances in neuroimaging and monitoring techniques have enhanced our understanding of coma, revealing the brain's potential for recovery and rehabilitation. As research continues to evolve, it is imperative to foster awareness and compassion around this complex condition, empowering families to advocate for the best possible care while promoting a deeper understanding of the human brain's resilience [9].

GLASGOW COMA SCALE (GCS)

Introduction

Glasgow Coma Scale (GCS) is a clinical scale that can be used to accurately gauge a person's level of consciousness following a head injury. It was first published in 1974 at the University of Glasgow by neurosurgery professors Graham Teasdale and Bryan Jennett [1]. It examines a person's capacity to speak, move their body, and perform eye movements.

Population

This score is used to provide emergency medical care following a brain injury (such as one sustained in a vehicle accident), as well as to monitor and track patients' level of awareness in hospitals [4, 11].

Description

The scale's three components—eye, verbal, and motor are made up of these three behaviours. The GCS scale runs from 3 (totally nonresponsive) to 15 for an individual. (Responsive) [10]. The Glasgow Coma Scale is reported as a combined score (ranging from 3 to 15) and the scores for each test (E for eye, V for Verbal, and M for Motor) (Table **1**). The best response should determine the value for each test that the subject can give.

Table 1. Glasgow Coma Scale (GCS).

Eye open	Spontaneously To speech To pain None	4 3 2 1
Verbal response	Oriented Confused Inappropriate words Incomprehensible sounds None	5 4 3 2 1
Motor response	Obey commands Localises to pain Withdraws from pain Flexion to pain Extension to pain None	6 5 4 3 2 1
Maximum score		/15

Time to Administration

Less than 5 minutes

Psychometric Properties

Sensitivity: 79 to 97% [10]; **Specificity:** 84-97% [11]

Advantage:

- Most commonly accepted conscious level scoring system in the world has face validity (seems to work).

- Repeatable (this is debatable because in one study, 38% of the time the GCS scores were the same, and in 33% of the time the results varied by more than two points).
- Biased towards the motor score, which is advantageous because it is the most accurate indicator of the short-term prognosis in TBI.
- The differential between motor scores of 2, 3, and 4 is a highly helpful clinical predictor of TBI severity, and the area of brain function that has been damaged corresponds with negative neurological outcomes, such as brain injury, neurosurgical intervention, and mortality.

Disadvantage:

- Does not take into account brain-stem reflexes.
- The M score does not take into account unilateral pathophysiology.
- Unreliable in patients between the ages of 9 and 12.
- Depending on the components, the same GCS score will forecast various TBI mortality rates.
- Generally predictive but unable to correctly predict results in specific patients.

Interpretation: It is crucial to consider all the individual components and the overall score.

- Severe, GCS ≤ 8
- Moderate, GCS 9–12
- Minor, GCS ≥ 13

FULL OUTLINE OF UNRESPONSIVENESS

Introduction

A recently developed and clinically tested technique called the "Full Outline of Unresponsiveness" is used to evaluate patients with diminished degrees of consciousness. It was created at the Mayo Clinic in Rochester, Minnesota, in the Neurocritical Care unit [12]. It allows for a straightforward assessment of the neurological condition of critically sick patients, in particular, in terms of identifying signs of oncoming neurological decline (such as brainstem herniation) and making finer distinctions between comatose states. (*e.g.*, minimal conscious state, locked-in syndrome) [13].

Population

Brain injury recovery, cardiac dysfunction, stroke recovery.

Description

The FOUR Score measures vital brainstem reflexes and offers data on the severity of brainstem injury that is not available with the GCS. It consists of 4 types of responses that help assess the patient's severity. It includes the eye, motor (upper extremity), brainstem reflex, and respiratory pattern [12]. It consists of a total of 16 points, *i.e.*, 4 points for each domain. The lower the score, the higher the level of severity (Table **2**).

Table 2. Full outline of unresponsiveness.

Eye response	Eyelids open or opened, tracking, or blinking to command. Eyelids open but not tracking. Eyelids closed, but open to a loud voice. Eyelids closed but open to pain. Eyelids remain closed with pain.	+4 +3 +2 +1 0
Motor response (upper extremities)	Thumbs-up, fist, or peace sign. Localizing to pain. Flexion response to pain. Extension response to pain. No response to pain.	+4 +3 +2 +1 0
Brainstem Reflexes	Pupil and corneal reflexes present. One pupil wide and fixed. Pupil or corneal reflex absent Pupil and corneal reflexes absent. Absent pupil, corneal, and cough reflexes.	+4 +3 +2 +1 0
Respiration Pattern	Not intubated, regular breathing pattern. Not intubated, Cheyne-Stokes breathing pattern. Not intubated, irregular breathing. Breathes above the ventilatory rate. Breathes at ventilator rate or apnea.	+4 +3 +2 +1 0
Total score		/16

Time to Administration

Less than 5 minutes

Psychometric properties

Validity and reliability for this scale have not been established yet.

Interpretation

The lower the score, the higher the level of severity.

GLASGOW-LIEGE SCALE (GLS)

The Glasgow-Liege Scale (GLS), a coma scale created in 1982, which combines the Glasgow Coma Scale (GCS) with the quantitative examination of five brain stem reflexes [14] (Table **3**).

Table 3. Glasgow-Liege Scale (GLS).

E	
Best Eye Response	
Eye open spontaneously	4
Eye opening to verbal command	3
Eye opening to pain	2
No eye opening	1
V	
Best Verbal Response	
Orientated	5
Confused	4
Inappropriate words	3
Incomprehensible sounds	2
No verbal response	1
M	
Best Motor Response	
Obeys commands	6
Localizing pain	5
Withdrawal from pain	4
Stereotyped flexion to pain	3
Stereotyped extension to pain	2
No motor response	1
R	
Brainstem Reflexes	
Fronto-orbicular reflex	5
Vertical oculocephalic or oculovestibular reflex	4
Pupillary light reflex	3
Horizontal oculocephalic or oculovestibular reflex	2
Oculocardiac reflex	1

(Table 3) cont.....

E	
Best Eye Response	
No brainstem reflex	0

Population

This score is used to provide emergency medical care following a brain injury (such as one sustained in a vehicle accident), as well as to monitor and track patients' level of awareness in hospitals.

Interpretation

- Under 8: coma
- Between 12 and 8: critical, case-by-case evaluation

Time to Administration

Less than 10 minutes

Psychometric properties

Validity and reliability for this scale have not been established yet.

RAPPAPORT DISABILITY RATING SCALE (DRS)

Introduction

The Disability Rating Scale (DRS) was created to follow traumatic brain injury (TBI) patients from "Coma to Community." The scale was used to evaluate the impact of the injury and estimate how long recovery may take. The ranking sheds light on the TBI victim's cognitive impairment [15].

Population

It was initially created to evaluate TBI victims throughout their rehabilitation phase of recovery. The scale was designed to track the patient's overall functional changes as they occurred during the course of their recuperation.

Description

The DRS shares similarities with the Glasgow Outcome Scale (GOS). However, its primary objective is to monitor a patient's progression over time, unlike the GOS, which primarily assesses the severity of a brain injury. In several respects, the DRS effectively addresses many of the limitations of the GOS [16] (Table **4a** and Table **4b**).

Table 4a. Rappaport Disability Rating Scale (DRS).

Category	Item	Instructions	Score
Arousability, Awareness, and Responsivity	Eye Opening	0 = spontaneous 1 = to speech 2 = to pain 3 = none	
	Communication Ability	0 = oriented 1 = confused 2= inappropriate 3= incomprehensible 4 = none	
	Motor Response	0 = obeying 1 = localizing 2 = withdrawing 3 = flexing 4 = extending 5 = none	
Cognitive Ability for Self-care Activities	Feeding	0 = complete 1 = partial 2 = minimal 3 = none	
	Toileting	0 = complete 1 = partial 2 = minimal 3 = none	
	Grooming	0 = complete 1 = partial 2 = minimal 3 = none	
Dependence on Others	Level of Functioning	0 = completely independent 1= independent in a special environment 2 = mildly dependent 3 = moderately dependent 4 = markedly dependent 5 = totally dependent	
Psychosocial Adaptability	Employability	0 = not restricted 1 = selected jobs 2= sheltered workshop (non-competitive) 3 = not employable	
Total DR Score			

Table 4b. Interpretation of rappaport Disability Rating Scale (DRS).

0	None
1	Mild
2-3	Partial
4-6	Moderate
7-11	Moderately Severe
12-16	Severe
17-21	Extremely Severe
22-24	Vegetative State
25-29	Extreme Vegetative State

It is a 30-point continuous scale that provides quantitative information to document the progress of patients with severe head injury from coma to community reintegration.

Time to Administration

30 minutes

Advantages

1. The DRS aids in monitoring a patient's recovery journey efficiently. Its adaptability and simplicity in evaluating a patient make progress tracking highly accessible. Little training is needed for accurate completion, taking approximately fifteen minutes to score. The assessment can be conducted retrospectively or based on medical records.
2. The scale effectively measures progress. It is particularly robust and sensitive in assessing overall behavioral disability. When used alongside the Functional Independence Measure (FIM), which provides more detailed functionality insights, the DRS enhances accuracy.

Disadvantages

1. The reliability of different raters' agreement on the DRS varies according to sources. Some indicate it is firmly established, while others highlight significant variability.
2. Using the DRS requires raters to undergo more specialized training. Its primary strength lies in broad assessments rather than specific functional evaluations, which pose challenges in assessing mild to severe functional impairments.
3. This limitation can be effectively addressed by supplementing the DRS assessment with the FIM, which provides a more detailed measurement of functionality.

Psychometric Properties

In the confirmatory factor analysis, DRS had good factor loadings of 0.32–0.80 [17]. A reliability coefficient above 0.92 indicates strong internal consistency. External validity was shown by good sensitivity (0.95) and specificity (0.94) [18].

WESTERN NEURO SENSORY STIMULATION PROFILE (WNSSP)

Introduction

The Western Neuro Sensory Stimulation Profile (WNSSP) is a comprehensive assessment tool designed to evaluate sensory and motor responses in individuals with severe cognitive impairments [19]. Developed to support caregivers and healthcare professionals, the WNSSP aims to facilitate tailored interventions that enhance sensory processing and improve the overall quality of life for affected individuals. By systematically assessing responses to various stimuli, the WNSSP provides valuable insights into an individual's cognitive state and potential for rehabilitation [20].

Population

The WNSSP is primarily intended for use with individuals who have significant cognitive impairments, including: patients in a coma, severe developmental disabilities, patients in a persistent vegetative state, and neurological disorders.

- **Arousal/Attention**

1. **Arousability:** (eye opening/facial or body movement to voice/touch or shaking/raising bed/wet cloth on face)
   0 = require REPEATED presentation of two or more stimuli
   1 = TWO OR MORE stimuli
   2 = ONE stimulus
   3 = SPONTANEOUSLY AWAKE
2. **Wakefulness:** Longest period without being re-aroused
   0 = < 10 min
   1 = 11-20 min
   2 = > 21 min (or all throughout testing session)
3. **Eye Contact:**
   0 = Eyes CLOSED
   1 = Eyes OPEN but not focused on the examiner

2 = Eyes FOCUSED on examiner (50% or more) N = Physically unable to open eyes (CN III paralysis)

4. **Attention to Task:** Visual attention or the ability to attend to tasks
   0 = Attends <50% of time
   1 = Attends >50% of time

- **Auditory Response**

Localization

1. **Voice**: Response to introductory remarks: "Hello my name is …"
   0 = NO response < 20 s
   1 = UNDIFFERENTIATED (does not awaken and then = to all stimuli: posturing, hyperventilation, chewing)
   2= DIFFERENTIATED (awakens or ≠ to various stimuli: eye movement/head turn)
2. **Sound:** Best response to non-verbal sound (music/bell/clicker/tape recorder/sneeze/door slam out of visual field)
   0 = NO response < 20 s
   1 = UNDIFFERENTIATED (= to all stimuli: posturing, hyperventilation, blinking, chewing,)
   2 = DIFFERENTIATED (≠ to various stimuli: eye movement/head turn, movement of part touched or named)

Comprehension (of single-stage auditory commands, repeat once without penalty, then use ≠ cues, score only coinciding responses, penalty for perseveration)

0 = NO response < 20 s
1 = Incorrect response
2 = Cued (prior visual modelling /touching /moving intended body part) delayed (>5 s) response 3 = Cued, prompt response
4 = Spontaneous, delayed response (response after more than 5 s) 5 = Spontaneous, prompt response

1. **Shake my Hand**

2. **Open/close mouth** (if mouth is usually closed, use "open" for command)
3. Stick out tongue
4. **Close/open eyes** (if eyes are usually opened, use "closed" for command)
5. Raise eyebrows
6. **Move body part** (that the patient can move spontaneously)

Vocalization:

0 = NO response
1 = Best spontaneous, non-meaningful VOCALIZATION (moaning, sighing, crying, other vocal noises)
2= Best spontaneous, INAPPROPRIATE VERBALIZATION or mouthing of words irrelevant to the stimulus or unintelligible)
3 = Vocalizes on COMMAND (repetition of sound or word) or mouths words or verbalizes APPROPRIATELY either spontaneously or on command (intelligible, relevant speech)

Facial/Gestural expression for communication: (except for yes/no head nods)

0 = No response during the entire session (only RANDOM grimaces/reflex or involuntary behaviours)
1=ONE(smiling/frowning/eyebrow/eyewidening/pointing/reaching/shoulders/waving/pushing away)
2 = Uses > ONE gesture/facial expression with communicative intent

Yes/No Response: Verbal or nonverbal (finger signals, eye gaze, buzzer system) to 3 verbal or written questions, spontaneous responses may be given credit (Are you married?/Do you live in/ Were you born in the year…)

0= NEITHER response observed
1= Either "Yes" OR "No" response observed (does not need to be accurate, only present)
2= BOTH responses observed (does not need to be accurate, only present)

- **Visual Response Tracking** (repeat several times)

Horizontal Tracking

0= NO response < 20 s
1= Follows (from midline) to the left OR right side
2= Follows (from midline) to the left AND right side
3 = Follows across midline from one side to the other

Horizontal Mirror – Visual Fixation

1. **Horizontal individual** (slowly walk from one side of the bed/chair around to the opposite side, examiner or other person)
2. **Horizontal picture** (large, brightly colored familiar personality/greeting card/family picture)

3. **Horizontal object** (no-sound producing, brightly colored puppet/snow globe with moving parts)

Horizontal Mirror – Visual Tracking

0 = NO response < 20 s
1 = Follows (from midline) up OR down
2 = Follows (from midline) up AND down

VERTICAL PICTURE

Vertical object

COMPREHENSION: Best response to single-stage written commands, "Read card & do what it says"; direction may be repeated once & attention directed to the card by pointing without penalty; then use ≠ cues. Do not read the card

0= NO response < 20 s
1= Incorrect response
2= Cued (prior visual modeling /touching or moving intended body part) delayed (>5 s) response
3 = Cued, prompt response
4 = Spontaneous, delayed response (response after more than 5 s)
5 = Spontaneous, prompt response

1. **Open mouth** (if mouth is usually closed, use "open" for command)
2. **Stick out tongue**
3. **Close eyes** (if eyes are usually opened, use "closed" for command)
4. **Raise eyebrows**
5. **Move body part** (that patient can move spontaneously)

Tactile Response

Localization

1. Touch: (non-painful tap on shoulder outside vision/ stimulation of ≠ body parts with brush, rough towel, comb)

0 = NO response 20 s
1 = UNDIFFERENTIATED (= to all stimuli: reflexive posturing, hyperventilation, blinking, chewing,)
2 = DIFFERENTIATED (≠ to various stimuli: eye movement/head turn, movement of part touched or named)

2. Oral Stimulation: (stimulate the external surface of the upper and lower lips with a Q-tip)

0 = WITHDRAWAL/ABNORMAL reflexes (tonic bite, tongue or jaw thrust, lip retraction or pursing)
1= PRIMITIVE REFLEXES (chewing, sucking, phasic bite, rooting)
2= TOLERATES stimulation

Object Manipulation ("This is a -. Show me how you use it")

0= No response 20 s
1= Holds/releases object
2= Moves object/uses it inappropriately
3 = Reaches for/pushes away object
4 = Uses appropriately cued (demonstrate correct use, help initiate by touching/raising arm)
5 = Uses appropriately spontaneously
N = Both arms cast or splinted
3. **Manipulation spoon** (present in the field of vision or in hand if unable to take it)
4. **Manipulation comb** (if score 3 thought related to motor rather than cognitive limitations, circle the score)
5. **Manipulation pencil** (try to elicit understanding of object's use by alternate means such as yes/no questions)

Olfactory Response (pleasant and unpleasant: cologne/foods: vinegar, cinnamon, coffee, garlic

0 = No response 20 s
1 = UNDIFFERENTIATED (= to all stimuli: reflexive posturing, hyperventilation, blinking, chewing,)
2 = DIFFERENTIATED (≠ to various stimuli: eye movement/head turn, movement of part touched or named) N = Not applicable (tracheostomy)

Interpretation

The WNSSP has a total score range of 0 to 113, with higher scores indicating better cognitive function.

Time of Administration

The administration of the WNSSP typically takes 30-60 minutes, depending on the individual's responsiveness and the specific sensory modalities being assessed. The evaluation can be conducted in a single session or spread over multiple sessions to ensure a thorough assessment without overwhelming the individual.

Advantages

1. **Comprehensive Assessment**: The WNSSP evaluates multiple sensory modalities, providing a holistic view of an individual's sensory processing capabilities.
2. **Guides Interventions**: Results from the assessment can inform personalized therapeutic strategies tailored to the individual's specific needs.
3. **Standardized Tool**: The structured nature of the WNSSP allows for consistent application and comparison across different populations and settings.
4. **Supports Communication**: Provides caregivers and healthcare professionals with insights that help them better communicate with and understand the individual's needs.
5. **Documentation of Progress**: Regular assessments can track changes over time, aiding in evaluating the effectiveness of interventions.

Disadvantages

1. **Limited Responsiveness**: Some individuals may show minimal or no response to sensory stimuli, which can limit the effectiveness of the assessment.
2. **Time-Consuming**: The assessment process may require significant time and resources, especially if multiple sessions are needed.
3. **Subjectivity in Interpretation**: Responses can vary widely among individuals, making it challenging to interpret results uniformly.
4. **Requires Training**: Proper administration and interpretation of the WNSSP necessitate trained personnel, which may not always be available in all settings.
5. **Cultural Sensitivity**: The assessment may not fully account for cultural differences in sensory perception and response, potentially affecting its applicability across diverse populations.

Psychometric properties

Internal consistency reliability, α = 0.933 [21]

Concurrent validity is found to be less significant when compared to other scales (-0.146) [22].

RAPPAPORT COMA/NEAR COMA SCALE

Introduction

The Rappaport Coma/Near Coma Scale is a clinical assessment tool designed to evaluate and categorize the levels of consciousness in patients experiencing coma or near-coma states. This scale is instrumental in assessing the severity of a patient's condition and tracking changes over time, aiding clinical decision-making and patient management [22].

Population

The Rappaport scale is primarily utilized in populations affected by severe brain injuries, strokes, traumatic brain injuries, and other neurological disorders that impair consciousness. It is commonly used in emergency and intensive care settings, where rapid, accurate assessments are crucial for effective patient care.

Description

The Rappaport Coma/Near Coma Scale consists of a series of criteria that assess a patient's responsiveness to stimuli, including eye opening, verbal responses, and motor reactions [23]. The scale categorizes patients based on their ability to respond to external stimuli, ranging from full coma (no response) to varying degrees of near-coma states where some responsiveness is observed. This structured approach provides clinicians with a systematic way to evaluate and document consciousness levels [24].

Time Administration

Administering the Rappaport scale typically takes about 5 to 10 minutes, allowing healthcare providers to assess the patient's state quickly. This rapid assessment is particularly valuable in critical care settings, where timely information can influence treatment strategies and patient outcomes. Regular assessments can also be conducted to monitor changes and recovery.

Advantages

- **Standardized Assessment**: Provides a consistent framework for evaluating consciousness and improving communication among healthcare professionals.
- **Facilitates Decision-Making**: Helps guide clinical interventions based on the severity of the patient's condition, aiding in treatment planning and prognosis.

- **Tracking Progress**: Allows for ongoing monitoring of a patient's responsiveness, making it easier to detect improvements or declines in condition.

Disadvantages

- **Subjective Interpretation**: The assessment can be influenced by the clinician's judgment, leading to variability in results among different evaluators.
- **Narrow Focus**: Primarily concentrates on consciousness levels and may not adequately address other important aspects of neurological function, such as cognitive or emotional states.
- **Potential for Misclassification**: Patients with fluctuating consciousness may be inaccurately assessed, which can result in inappropriate treatment or care decisions.

Psychometric Properties

Inter-rater reliability = 0.95 [25]

CLINICAL CONSIDERATIONS, STRENGTHS, LIMITATIONS, AND EMERGING PERSPECTIVES

Glasgow Coma Scale (GCS) is the most widely used tool for rapid assessment of consciousness in acute settings such as emergency departments and ICUs. Its strengths lie in its simplicity, speed, and universal acceptance, making it valuable for initial triage and communication. However, it has limited sensitivity to subtle neurological changes, relies on verbal responses (which are problematic in intubated or aphasic patients), and does not assess brainstem reflexes or respiration. Emerging perspectives emphasize supplementing GCS with more comprehensive tools, particularly in neurocritical care.

Full Outline of UnResponsiveness (FOUR) Score was developed to address key limitations of the GCS by including brainstem reflexes and respiratory patterns while eliminating the verbal component. It is especially useful for intubated patients and in detecting conditions such as locked-in syndrome. Although slightly more complex and less universally familiar than GCS, the FOUR score is increasingly favored in neuro-ICUs and is gaining recognition for its improved prognostic value.

Glasgow–Liège Scale (GLS) extends the GCS by incorporating brainstem reflex assessment, improving sensitivity in severe coma and enhancing prognostic accuracy in deep unconsciousness. Its clinical use is largely limited to specialized neurocritical settings due to its complexity, limited standardization, and reduced global adoption. In recent practice, the GLS has been largely overshadowed by the FOUR score, which offers similar advantages with greater practicality.

Disability Rating Scale (DRS) is primarily used to measure functional recovery and disability across the continuum from coma to community reintegration. It captures physical, cognitive, and psychosocial aspects of recovery and is useful for rehabilitation planning and outcome monitoring. However, it is not sensitive to early coma states or subtle cognitive deficits and may show ceiling effects in mildly impaired individuals. Current perspectives support its continued use alongside broader participation- and quality-of-life measures.

Western Neuro Sensory Stimulation Profile (WNSSP) is a detailed behavioral assessment designed to evaluate responsiveness to structured sensory stimuli in patients with disorders of consciousness, particularly in rehabilitation settings. Its major strength is sensitivity to subtle and inconsistent responses, making it valuable for treatment planning and monitoring gradual recovery. Limitations include time demands, need for specialized training, and susceptibility to patient fatigue. Emerging approaches integrate WNSSP findings with advanced rehabilitation technologies and neurophysiological data.

Rappaport Coma/Near Coma Scale (CNCS) is specifically designed to differentiate coma, vegetative state, and minimally conscious states during recovery. It is highly sensitive to small behavioral changes and is well-suited for tracking recovery in subacute and chronic disorders of consciousness. Its limitations include limited applicability in acute care and the need for repeated observations. Emerging perspectives emphasize its role within multimodal assessment frameworks that combine behavioral evaluation with neuroimaging and electrophysiological techniques.

A comparative summary of commonly used coma assessment scales, including their core components, clinical utility, and preferred applications, is presented in Table **5**.

Table 5. Summary of various scales used in Coma assessment.

Scale	Primary Purpose	Domains Assessed	Score Range	Typical Setting	Acute/ Chronic Use	Reliability and Validity
Glasgow Coma Scale (GCS)	Assess the level of consciousness	Eye-opening, Verbal response, Motor response	3–15	Emergency, ICU, trauma	**Acute**	good to excellent reliability and validity (r =.75-.95)

(Table 5) cont.....

Scale	Primary Purpose	Domains Assessed	Score Range	Typical Setting	Acute/ Chronic Use	Reliability and Validity
Full Outline of UnResponsiveness (FOUR) Score	Assess consciousness incl. brainstem function	Eye response, Motor response, Brainstem reflexes, Respiration	0–16	ICU, neurocritical care	**Acute**	excellent reliability and strong validity (r = .93)
Glasgow–Liège Scale (GLS)	Modify GCS by adding brainstem reflexes	GCS components: brainstem reflexes	3–20 (varies by version)	ICU, severe brain injury	**Acute**	Good reliability and validity (r = .77)
Disability Rating Scale (DRS)	Measure overall disability & functional change	Arousal, awareness, cognitive ability, self-care, and employability	0–29	Rehab, long-term care	**Subacute–Chronic**	excellent inter-rater reliability and good predictive validity (r = .90)
Western Neuro Sensory Stimulation Profile (WNSSP)	Assess responsiveness to sensory stimuli	Auditory, visual, tactile, olfactory, motor responses	0–113	Rehabilitation settings	**Subacute–Chronic**	High reliability and strong concurrent validity (r = .93)
Rappaport Coma/Near Coma Scale (CNCS)	Differentiate coma vs near-coma states	Auditory, visual, motor, communication responses	0–4.9 (lower = better)	Rehabilitation	**Subacute–Chronic**	High reliabilityand validity(r = .95)

CONCLUSION

A comprehensive evaluation of coma requires tools that integrate the neurological, physiological, and functional dimensions of consciousness. Scales such as the GCS and FOUR Scale are indispensable for acute neurological assessment, while the DRS and WNSSP extend this evaluation into the recovery and rehabilitation phases. Together, they enable clinicians to track changes in consciousness, anticipate outcomes, and plan interventions tailored to patient needs. Future research should continue refining these instruments for enhanced sensitivity, cross-cultural applicability, and predictive validity across diverse clinical settings.

AI DISCLOSURE STATEMENT

During the preparation of this chapter, the authors used ChatGPT (OpenAI) as a support tool for language refinement, structural organisation, and clarification of ideas. All content generated with AI assistance was carefully reviewed, verified, and revised by the authors to ensure factual accuracy, originality, and consistency with the scientific literature. The authors take full responsibility for the integrity, interpretation, and final content of the published chapter.

ACKNOWLEDGEMENT

The authors extend their sincere appreciation to clinicians and researchers contributing to the development and validation of coma assessment tools. Their continuous efforts in refining neurological and functional scales have significantly improved the understanding, prognosis, and rehabilitation of patients with disorders of consciousness.

REFERENCES

[1] Huff JS, Tadi P. Coma StatPearls. Treasure Island, FL: StatPearls Publishing 2025. Internet

[2] Weiglein T, Zimmermann M, Niesen WD, Hoffmann F, Klein M. Acute Onset of Impaired Consciousness. Dtsch Arztebl Int. 2024 Jul 26; 121(15): 508-518. doi: 10.3238/arztebl.m2024.0079. PMID: 38867660; PMCID: PMC11526356.

[3] Ichim TE, Ramos RA, Rath A, Castellano J, Azimi N, Veltmeyer JD, Koumjian M, Ma NE, Bajnath A, Lin E, Ichim GE, Woods EJ, Jothen J, Reznik BN. Reversing coma by senolytics and stem cells: the future is now. J Transl Med. 2025 Oct 7; 23(1): 1060. doi: 10.1186/s12967-025-07099-6. PMID: 41057934; PMCID: PMC12502250.

[4] Omar WM, Khader IRA, Hani SB, ALBashtawy M. The Glasgow Coma Scale and Full Outline of Unresponsiveness score evaluation to predict patient outcomes with neurological illnesses in intensive care units in West Bank: a prospective cross-sectional study. Acute Crit Care 2024; 39(3): 408-19. [http://dx.doi.org/10.4266/acc.2024.00570] [PMID: 39266276]

[5] Rakhit S, Nordness MF, Lombardo SR, Cook M, Smith L, Patel MB. Management and Challenges of Severe Traumatic Brain Injury. Semin Respir Crit Care Med 2021; 42(1): 127-44. [http://dx.doi.org/10.1055/s-0040-1716493] [PMID: 32916746]

[6] Mason E, Hindmarch CCT, Dunham-Snary KJ. Medium-chain Acyl-COA dehydrogenase deficiency: Pathogenesis, diagnosis, and treatment. Endocrinol Diabetes Metab. 2023 Jan; 6(1): e385. doi: 10.1002/edm2.385. Epub 2022 Oct 27. PMID: 36300606; PMCID: PMC9836253.

[7] Ponsford J, Carrier S, Hicks A, McKay A. Assessment and management of patients in the acute stages of recovery after traumatic brain injury in adults: a worldwide survey. J Neurotrauma 2021; 38(8): 1060-7. [http://dx.doi.org/10.1089/neu.2020.7299]

[8] Yoshikawa MH, Rabelo NN, Welling LC, Telles JPM, Figueiredo EG. Brain death and management of the potential donor. Neurol Sci 2021; 42(9): 3541-52. [http://dx.doi.org/10.1007/s10072-021-05360-6] [PMID: 34138388]

[9] Sanz LRD, Laureys S, Gosseries O. Towards modern post-coma care based on neuroscientific evidence. Int J Clin Health Psychol 2023; 23(3): 100370. [http://dx.doi.org/10.1016/j.ijchp.2023.100370] [PMID: 36817874]

[10] Heydari F, Azizkhani R, Ahmadi O, Majidinejad S, Nasr-Esfahani M, Ahmadi A. Physiologic Scoring Systems versus Glasgow Coma Scale in Predicting In-Hospital Mortality of Trauma Patients; a Diagnostic Accuracy Study. Arch Acad Emerg Med 2021; 9(1): e64. [http://dx.doi.org/10.22037/aaem.v9i1.1376] [PMID: 34870230]

[11] Bodien YG, Barra A, Temkin NR, Barber J, Foreman B, Vassar M, Robertson C, Taylor SR, Markowitz AJ, Manley GT, Giacino JT, Edlow BL; TRACK-TBI Investigators. Diagnosing Level of Consciousness: The Limits of the Glasgow Coma Scale Total Score. J Neurotrauma. 2021 Dec; 38(23): 3295-3305. doi: 10.1089/neu.2021.0199. PMID: 34605668; PMCID: PMC8917895.

[12] Adcock AK, Kosiorek H, Parikh P, Chauncey A, Wu Q, Demaerschalk BM. Reliability of Robotic Telemedicine for Assessing Critically Ill Patients with the Full Outline of UnResponsiveness Score and Glasgow Coma Scale. Telemed J E Health 2017; 23(7): 555-60. [http://dx.doi.org/10.1089/tmj.2016.0225] [PMID: 28085631]

[13] Helbok R, Rass V, Beghi E, *et al*; Curing Coma Campaign and its Contributing Members. The Curing Coma Campaign International Survey on Coma Epidemiology, Evaluation, and Therapy (COME TOGETHER). Neurocrit Care. 2022 Aug; 37(1): 47-59. doi: 10.1007/s12028-021-01425-8. Epub 2022 Feb 9. PMID: 35141860; PMCID: PMC9283177.

[14] Schey JE, Schoch M, Kerr D. The Predictive Validity of the Full Outline of UnResponsiveness Score Compared to the Glasgow Coma Scale in the Intensive Care Unit: A Systematic Review. Neurocrit Care. 2025 Oct; 43(2): 645-658. doi: 10.1007/s12028-024-02150-8. Epub 2024 Nov 5. PMID: 39496882; PMCID: PMC12436514.

[15] Chesnut R, Temkin N, Pridgeon J, *et al.* Development of a Randomized Trial Comparing ICP-Monitor-Based Management of Severe Pediatric Traumatic Brain Injury to Management Based on Imaging and Clinical Examination Without ICP Monitoring-Study Protocol. Neurosurgery. 2024 Jan 1; 94(1): 65-71. doi: 10.1227/neu.0000000000002582. Epub 2023 Jul 6. PMID: 37409817; PMCID: PMC12245298.

[16] Machamer J, Temkin NR, Manley GT, Dikmen S. Functional Status Examination in Patients with Moderate-to-Severe Traumatic Brain Injuries. J Neurotrauma 2018; 35(10): 1132-7. [http://dx.doi.org/10.1089/neu.2017.5460] [PMID: 29415608]

[17] Williams MW, Smith EL. Clinical utility and psychometric properties of the Disability Rating Scale with individuals with traumatic brain injury. Rehabil Psychol 2017; 62(3): 407-8. [http://dx.doi.org/10.1037/rep0000168] [PMID: 28836811]

[18] Kang Y, Jamison K, Jaywant A, *et al.* Longitudinal alterations in gamma-aminobutyric acid (GABAA) receptor availability over ~ 1 year following traumatic brain injury. Brain Commun. 2022 Jun 15; 4(4): 159. doi: 10.1093/braincomms/fcac159. PMID: 35794871; PMCID: PMC9253887.

[19] Cataford G, Monton LA, Karzon S, *et al.* Cognitive and Motor Function Effects of Antipsychotics in Traumatic Brain Injury: A Systematic Review of Pre-Clinical Studies. Neurotrauma Rep. 2024 Mar 5; 5(1): 181-193. doi: 10.1089/neur.2023.0108. PMID: 38463417; PMCID: PMC10924062.

[20] Bodien YG, LaRovere K, Kondziella D, Taran S, Estraneo A, Shutter L. Curing Coma Campaign, its Contributing Members. Common Data Elements for Disorders of Consciousness: Recommendations from the Working Group on Outcomes and Endpoints. Neurocrit Care. 2024 Oct;41(2):357-368. doi: 10.1007/s12028-024-02068-1. Epub 2024 Aug 14. Erratum in: Neurocrit Care. 2025 Feb; 42(1): 324. doi: 10.1007/s12028-024-02134-8. PMID: 39143375.

[21] Molteni E, Colombo K, Pastore V, *et al.* Joint Neuropsychological Assessment through Coma/Near Coma and Level of Cognitive Functioning Assessment Scales Reduces Negative Findings in Pediatric Disorders of Consciousness. Brain Sci 2020; 10(3): 162. [http://dx.doi.org/10.3390/brainsci10030162] [PMID: 32178348]

[22] Vitello MM, Rosenfelder MJ, Cardone P, *et al.* A protocol for a multicenter randomized and personalized controlled trial using rTMS in patients with disorders of consciousness. Front Neurol. 2023 Jul 21; 14: 1216468. doi: 10.3389/fneur.2023.1216468. PMID: 37545735; PMCID:

PMC10401598.

[23] Mulvaney SW, Lynch JH, Mahadevan S, Dineen KJ, Rae Olmsted KL. The Effect of Bilateral, Two-Level Cervical Sympathetic Chain Blocks on Specific Symptom Clusters for Traumatic Brain Injury, Independent of Concomitant PTSD Symptoms. Brain Sci. 2024 Nov 27; 14(12): 1193. doi: 10.3390/brainsci14121193. PMID: 39766392; PMCID: PMC11674670.

[24] Overbeek BUH, Lavrijsen JCM, van Gaal S, Kondziella D, Eilander HJ, Koopmans RTCM. Towards consensus on visual pursuit and visual fixation in patients with disorders of consciousness. A Delphi study. J Neurol. 2022 Jun; 269(6): 3204-3215. doi: 10.1007/s00415-021-10905-y. Epub 2022 Jan 10. PMID: 35001197.

[25] Duan X, Zhang T, Chen Y, *et al.* Natural course and predictors of consciousness recovery in children with prolonged disorder of consciousness. Sci Rep. 2024 Jul 29; 14(1): 17417. doi: 10.1038/s41598-024-68370-2. PMID: 39075188; PMCID: PMC11286944.

CHAPTER 4

Scales for the Elderly

Mayuri Thakur[1,2] and **Akanksha Saxena**[2,*]

[1] *Dolphin PG College of Life Science, Chunni Kalan, Punjab, India*

[2] *Maharishi Markandeshwar Institute of Physiotherapy and Rehabilitation, Maharishi Markandeshwar (Deemed to be University), Mullana, Ambala, Haryana, India*

Abstract: Ageing is a complex process characterised by progressive physiological changes that can affect mobility, mental health, and overall quality of life. As individuals age, they may experience a decline in physical function, cognitive abilities, and emotional well-being, necessitating effective assessment tools to monitor these changes. The Elderly Mobility Scale (EMS) evaluates functional mobility in older adults, helping identify those at risk for falls and mobility limitations. The Balance Outcome Measure for Elder Rehabilitation (BOOMER) assesses balance capabilities, guiding interventions to enhance stability and prevent injuries. The Karnofsky Performance Scale Index provides a standardised measure of functional status, enabling healthcare providers to evaluate a patient's ability to perform daily activities. The Geriatric Depression Scale screens for depressive symptoms, addressing mental health issues that are prevalent in the elderly population. Lastly, the Clinical Frailty Scale (CFS) offers a holistic view of frailty, helping to stratify risk and tailor care for older adults. Together, these scales facilitate a comprehensive assessment of age-related changes, guiding effective interventions and improving seniors' overall health and well-being.

Keywords: Ageing, Chronic illness, Cognitive, Elderly, Emergency, Health, Patients, Physical, Physiological, Population, Psychological, Quality of life, Treatment.

INTRODUCTION

Ageing is an intricate and universal process that every individual experiences, encompassing a myriad of biological, psychological, and social changes [1]. As populations around the globe continue to age due to advances in healthcare, nutrition, and overall living standards, understanding the implications of Ageing has become increasingly vital. The journey of Ageing is not merely a linear prog-

* **Corresponding Author Akanksha Saxena:** Maharishi Markandeshwar Institute of Physiotherapy and Rehabilitation, Maharishi Markandeshwar (Deemed to be University), Mullana, Ambala, Haryana, India;
E-mail: akankshasaxena623@gmail.com

Nidhi Sharma, Simranjeet Kaur & Parveen Kumar (Eds.)

ression of years but a complex interplay of experiences that shape individuals and societies [2].

Biologically, Ageing is marked by a gradual decline in physiological functions, with cells and tissues undergoing changes that affect everything from skin elasticity to organ efficiency [3]. These changes can lead to age-related conditions, such as arthritis, cardiovascular diseases, and cognitive decline. However, the biological aspects of Ageing are accompanied by a range of psychological dimensions [4]. Ageing can bring about reflections on identity, purpose, and the legacy one leaves behind. It is often a time of introspection, where individuals reassess their life goals and relationships, leading to both challenges and opportunities for personal growth [5].

Socially, the Ageing population significantly influences economic structures, healthcare systems, and cultural norms. As societies age, they must adapt to ensure adequate support systems are in place, from pensions to healthcare services [6]. This demographic shift challenges stereotypes about Ageing, highlighting the capabilities and contributions of older individuals. Many remain active participants in their communities, engaging in volunteer work, mentorship, and even second careers [7].

Moreover, Ageing is often culturally constructed; perceptions of Ageing vary widely across different societies. In some cultures, older adults are revered and respected for their wisdom, while in others, they may face marginalisation. This cultural lens shapes the Ageing experience, influencing how individuals perceive their own Ageing and how they are treated by others [8].

In essence, Ageing is a multifaceted phenomenon that goes beyond physical decline to encompass emotional resilience, societal roles, and cultural narratives. By exploring these dimensions, we can foster a more nuanced understanding of Ageing, promoting a positive perspective that embraces the richness of the later stages of life. As we navigate the challenges and opportunities of Ageing, it becomes essential to cultivate environments that celebrate the contributions of older adults and enhance their quality of life [9].

ELDERLY MOBILITY SCALE (EMS)

Introduction

Through seven functional tasks, including bed mobility, transfers, and body response to disturbance, EMS assesses a person's mobility issues. Analysis is done on the sit-to-stand and walking speeds [10]. According to studies, walking pace slows down with age; for healthy women over 75, the average walking speed is 1 metre per second [10, 11]. Walking speed will be further decreased when frailty increases.

Population

Older people in a hospital setting, either in a ward or in a day hospital.

Description

Table **1** shows that the Elderly Mobility Scale (EMS) is a 20-item, validated assessment tool for evaluating frail older adults. It is an ordinal scale [12].

Table 1. Elderly mobility scale score.

TASK		Score		
Lying to Sitting	2 Independent 1 Needs the help of 1 person. 0 Needs help of 2+ people			
Sitting to Lying	2 Independent 1 Needs the help of 1 person 0 Needs help of 2+ people			
Sitting to Standing	3 Independent in under 3 seconds 2 Independent in over 3 seconds 1 Needs the help of 1 person 0 Needs help of 2+ people			
Standing	3 Stands without support and able to reach 2 Stands without support, but needs support to reach 1 Stands but needs support 0 Stands only with the physical support of another person			
Gait	3 Independent (+ / - stick) 2 Independent with frame 1 Mobile with walking aid but erratic/unsafe 0Needs physical help to walk or constant supervision			
Timed Walk (6 metres)	3 Under 15 seconds 2 16 – 30 seconds 1 Over 30 seconds 0 Unable to cover 6 metres Recorded time in seconds.			
Functional Reach	4 Over 20 cm 2 10 - 20 cm. 0 Under 10 cm Actual reach			
		/20	**/20**	**/20**

Time to Administration

15 minutes

Psychometric Property

Inter-rater Reliability: By comparing the researcher's findings to those of clinical physiotherapists, reliability was proven. Clinical staff of various levels were employed. Results of the Mann-Whitney test were 196, and a p-value of 0.75 indicated that there was no significant difference between the testers [13].

Concurrent validity: Results from the EMS were compared with those from the Functional Independence Measure and the Barthel Index to evaluate concurrent validity. At 0.948 and 0.962, the EMS scores showed a strong correlation [14].

Sensitivity: not established.

Benefits

- Thought to be useful
- Has both personal and clinical relevance
- A small amount of training is required.

Limitation

- In communal settings, 6 metres are not frequently available
- Disturbances in functional reach distances from the initial functional reach test
- Not a particularly sensitive tool for those who struggle with a lack of confidence

Interpretation

Scores under 10 – generally, these patients are dependent on mobility manoeuvres and require help with basic ADLs, such as transfers, toileting, and dressing.

Scores between 10 –13 – generally these patients are borderline in terms of safe mobility and independence in ADL, *i.e.*, they require some help with some mobility manoeuvres.

Scores over 14 – Generally, these patients can perform mobility manoeuvres alone and safely, and are independent in basic ADL.

BALANCE OUTCOME MEASURE FOR ELDER REHABILITATION (BOOMER)

Introduction

The Balance Outcome Measure for Elder Rehabilitation (BOOMER) is designed to evaluate standing balance and functional mobility among elderly individuals. It serves as a comprehensive assessment tool that encompasses static, dynamic, and functional balance across various settings of elder rehabilitation [15] as exhibited in Table **2**. By integrating multiple commonly used outcome measures into a single tool, the BOOMER ensures practicality and applicability while optimising time and resources. This makes it particularly advantageous in clinical practice for efficiently assessing and monitoring balance improvements in elderly patients undergoing rehabilitation interventions. The BOOMER's holistic approach supports tailored rehabilitation strategies to enhance overall balance and mobility in this population [16, 17].

Table 2. Balance Outcome Measure for Elder Rehabilitation (BOOMER).

Test	Description
Step Test	One foot is repeatedly placed on top of a 7.5cm step and returned to the ground as many times as possible in 15 sec. The average between legs is then calculated for scoring.
Time Up and Go	From a seated position, the individual stands, walks 3m, turns 180°, walks back 3m to the chair, and sits down with the back resting against the backrest.
Functional Reach	The individual reaches as far forward as possible in a standing position without losing balance.
Timed Static Stance	Standing with feet together and eyes closed.

Population

Older adults with issues in standing balance.

Time to Administration

5-10 minutes

Psychometric Property

Concurrent Validity

The BOOMER correlates significantly with the Functional Independence Measure and Modified Elderly Mobility Scale. It demonstrates a strong correlation with the

Berg Balance Scale upon admission (ρ=.91; P<.01) and at discharge (ρ=.68; P<.01) in geriatric rehabilitation settings (n=134) [17].

Construct Validity

Research indicates high associations between BOOMER scores and Berg Balance Scale scores ($r = .93$, $p < 0.001$), as well as with raw scores from the de Morton Mobility Index ($r = .89$, $p < 0.001$) [18].

However, it shows only moderate correlations with perceived confidence on the Activities-specific Balance Confidence scale ($r > .52$, $p < 0.001$) [19].

Interpretation

- Scores range from 0 to 16
- Each item (4 items) can score between 0 and 4, as shown in Table **3**.
- The overall score is created by summing the scores for each item.
- The scale ranges from 0 (unable to perform the test) to 4 (excellent), with a maximum score of 16.

Table 3. Scoring criteria for balance outcome measure for elder rehabilitation.

Test	Scoring				
	0	**1**	**2**	**3**	**4**
Step Test	Unable	0-5	5-8	8-12	>12
Time Up and Go	Unable	≥30	29-20	19-10	<10
Functional Reach	0	1-15	16-20	21-30	>30
Timed Static Stance	Unable	0-30	30-60	60-<90	90

KARNOFSKY PERFORMANCE SCALE INDEX (KPS)

Introduction

The Karnofsky Performance Scale (KPS) is a widely used clinical tool for assessing a patient's functional status and overall well-being, as shown in Table **4**. Developed in the late 1940s, the KPS provides a standardised method for evaluating how a disease affects a patient's ability to perform daily activities. It is particularly valuable in oncology, geriatrics, and palliative care, offering healthcare providers insights into prognosis, treatment decisions, and the effectiveness of therapeutic interventions [20, 21].

Table 4. Karnofsky performance status scale definitions rating (%) Criteria.

Able to carry on normal activity and to work; no special care needed.	**100**	**Normal, no complaints; no evidence of disease.**
	90	Able to carry on normal activity; minor signs or symptoms of disease.
	80	Normal activity with effort; some signs or symptoms of disease.
Unable to work; able to live at home and care for most personal needs; varying amount of assistance needed.	70	Cares for self; unable to carry on normal activity or to do active work.
	60	Requires occasional assistance, but can care for most of his personal needs.
	50	Requires considerable assistance and frequent medical care.
Unable to care for self; requires equivalent of institutional or hospital care; disease may be progressing rapidly.	40	Disabled; requires special care and assistance.
	30	Severely disabled; hospital admission is indicated, although death is not imminent.
	20	Very sick; hospital admission necessary; active supportive treatment necessary.
	10	Moribund; fatal processes progressing rapidly.
	0	Dead

Population Description

The KPS is applicable to a broad range of patient populations, including: cancer patients, geriatric patients, patients with chronic illnesses, and palliative care patients.

Time of Administration

The KPS is quick to administer, typically requiring **5 to 10 minutes** to complete. It can be easily integrated into routine clinical assessments, making it convenient for healthcare providers.

Advantages

1. **Simplicity and Ease of Use**: The KPS is straightforward, allowing healthcare professionals to quickly assess functional status without extensive training.
2. **Standardisation**: Provides a consistent framework for evaluating patient performance, facilitating comparison across studies and clinical settings.
3. **Prognostic Value**: Correlates well with clinical outcomes, helping predict survival and treatment response.
4. **Holistic Assessment**: Addresses various aspects of patient functioning, including physical, psychological, and social factors.

5. **Widely Respected**: The KPS is a well-established tool used in clinical research and practice, enhancing its credibility.

Disadvantages

1. **Subjectivity**: The assessment can be somewhat subjective, as it relies on the evaluator's interpretation of the patient's abilities, potentially leading to variability.
2. **Ceiling Effect**: In patients with high performance status, the KPS may not capture subtle declines in function.
3. **Limited Detail**: While it provides a general overview, the KPS lacks specificity regarding the underlying causes of functional decline.
4. **Not Comprehensive**: It may not account for all factors affecting a patient's quality of life, such as psychological or emotional well-being.
5. **Cultural Sensitivity**: The scale may not fully capture performance differences across diverse cultural contexts, impacting its applicability.

Psychometric Property

Inter-rater reliability- 0.97 [22]

Construct validity- less than 0.97 [22]

Interpretation

The lower the Karnofsky score, the worse the survival for most serious illnesses.

GERIATRIC DEPRESSION SCALE(GDS)

Introduction

The Geriatric Depression Scale (GDS) Short Form is a widely utilised screening tool designed to identify depression in older adults. Developed specifically for the elderly population, the GDS helps clinicians assess depressive symptoms while minimising the risk of misdiagnosis due to the unique presentation of depression in this age group [23]. The Short Form consists of 15 items, making it a brief yet effective way to evaluate mood and emotional well-being among seniors, as shown in Table **5**.

Population Description

The GDS short form is primarily intended for older adults, patients with chronic illnesses, and geriatric psychiatry.

Table 5. Geriatric depression scale.

Circle the answer that best describes how you felt over the past week.		
1.	Are you basically satisfied with your life?	Yes/ No
2.	Have you dropped many of your activities and interests?	Yes/ No
3.	Do you feel that your life is empty?	Yes/ No
4.	Do you often get bored?	Yes/ No
5.	Are you in good spirits most of the time?	Yes/ No
6.	Are you afraid that something bad is going to happen to you?	Yes/ No
7.	Do you feel happy most of the time?	Yes/ No
8.	Do you often feel helpless?	Yes/ No
9.	Do you prefer to stay at home, rather than going out and doing things?	Yes/ No
10.	Do you feel that you have more problems with memory than most?	Yes/ No
11.	Do you think it is wonderful to be alive now?	Yes/ No
12.	Do you feel worthless the way you are now?	Yes/ No
13.	Do you feel full of energy?	Yes/ No
14.	Do you feel that your situation is hopeless?	Yes/ No
15.	Do you think that most people are better off than you are?	Yes/ No
Total Score		Yes/ No

Time of Administration

The GDS Short Form is quick to administer, typically taking about 5 to 10 minutes to complete. Its brevity makes it easy to incorporate into routine clinical assessments without disrupting patient care.

Advantages

1. **Simplicity and Ease of Use**: The GDS Short Form is straightforward and user-friendly, allowing healthcare providers to administer it with minimal training.
2. **Quick Assessment**: Its brevity ensures that it can be completed in a short time, making it practical for busy clinical settings.
3. **High Reliability and Validity**: The scale is reliable and valid for detecting depression in older adults, making it a trusted tool in geriatric care.
4. **Focus on Geriatric Population**: Tailored specifically for older adults, it considers the unique aspects of depression in this demographic, enhancing diagnostic accuracy.
5. **Supports Early Intervention**: By identifying depressive symptoms early, the GDS can facilitate timely interventions and improve patient outcomes.

Disadvantages

1. **Limited Scope**: The GDS primarily focuses on depressive symptoms and may not capture other mental health issues, such as anxiety or cognitive impairment.
2. **Self-Report Bias**: As a self-report measure, the results may be influenced by the patient's insight or willingness to disclose their feelings.
3. **Potential Cultural Sensitivity**: Responses may vary across different cultural backgrounds, which could affect the applicability of the scale.
4. **Not Diagnostic**: While the GDS is a useful screening tool, it is not intended for diagnosing depression; further assessment may be necessary for a comprehensive evaluation.
5. **Ceiling Effect**: In highly functional older adults, the scale may not detect subtle depressive symptoms, leading to under-identification.

Psychometric Property

Sensitivity = 92% [24]

Specificity = 89% [24]

Interpretation

0–4: Normal
5–8: Mild depression
9–11: Moderate depression
12–15: Severe depression

CLINICAL FRAILTY SCALE (CFS)

Introduction

The Clinical Frailty Scale (CFS) is a validated assessment tool used to evaluate frailty in older adults. Frailty is characterised by decreased physiological reserve and increased vulnerability to stressors, making it a critical factor in assessing the health and care needs of elderly individuals [25]. The CFS provides a simple, straightforward way to categorise patients based on their level of functioning and frailty, helping healthcare providers tailor interventions and optimise care [26].

Population Description

The CFS is primarily intended for older adults, patients with chronic conditions, and geriatric medicine.

Time of Administration

The CFS is quick to administer, typically taking about **5** minutes to complete. The assessment can be done through clinical observation and a brief interview, making it efficient for busy healthcare settings (Fig. **1**).

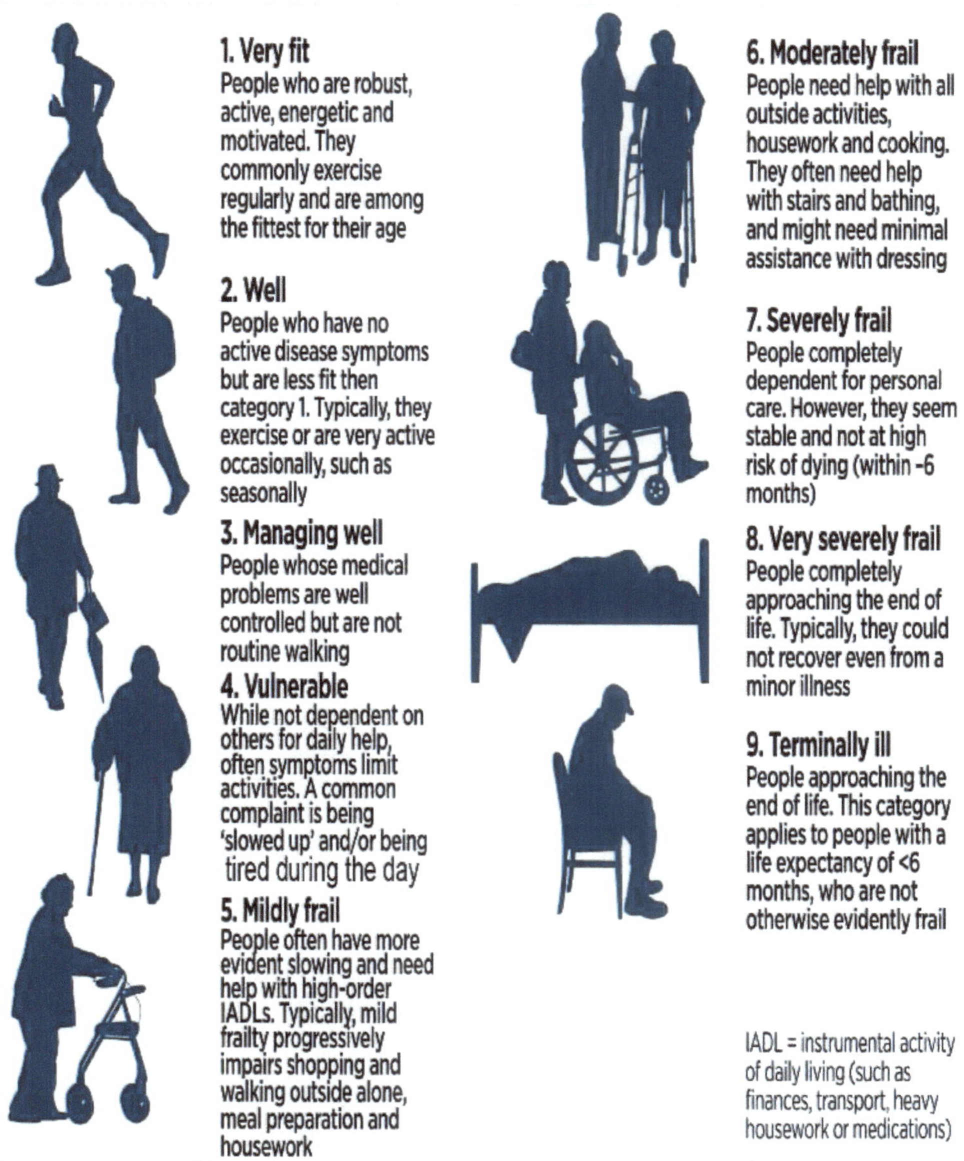

Fig. (1). Clinical Frailty Scale (CFS).

Advantages

1. **Simplicity and Accessibility**: The CFS is easy to understand and use, requiring minimal training for healthcare professionals, which facilitates widespread adoption in various clinical settings.
2. **Holistic Assessment**: It considers both physical and cognitive aspects of frailty, providing a comprehensive view of an individual's health status.
3. **Prognostic Value**: The CFS is associated with outcomes such as hospitalisation, institutionalisation, and mortality, aiding in risk stratification and care planning.
4. **Standardised Framework**: Offers a consistent method for evaluating frailty across different populations and settings, enhancing comparability in research and clinical practice.
5. **Guides Treatment Decisions**: Helps healthcare providers identify frail patients who may benefit from targeted interventions, rehabilitation, or palliative care approaches.

Disadvantages

1. **Subjectivity**: The CFS relies on clinical judgment, which can introduce variability in assessments based on the evaluator's perspective.
2. **Limited Depth**: While it provides a general categorisation of frailty, the CFS does not delve into specific underlying causes or contribute to a comprehensive geriatric assessment.
3. **Potential Cultural Sensitivity**: The scale may not fully account for cultural differences in health perceptions and responses, which could impact its applicability.
4. **Not Diagnostic**: The CFS is a screening tool and does not provide a definitive diagnosis or detail specific health issues that may require further evaluation.
5. **Ceiling Effect**: In very fit older adults, the scale may not capture subtle variations in frailty, possibly leading to under-identification of those at risk.

Psychometric Property

Inter-rater reliability = 0.74 [27]

CLINICAL CONSIDERATIONS, STRENGTHS, LIMITATIONS, AND EMERGING PERSPECTIVES

Assessment of older adults requires a multidimensional approach that extends beyond isolated physical performance measures. Ageing is often accompanied by a complex interplay of mobility limitations, balance impairment, cognitive decline, mood disorders, and frailty, all of which contribute to functional dependence and reduced quality of life [17, 18]. The scales included in this chapter, such as the Elderly Mobility Scale (EMS), Balance Outcome Measure for Elder Rehabilitation (BOOMER), Karnofsky Performance Scale (KPS), Geriatric Depression Scale (GDS), and Clinical Frailty Scale (CFS), reflect this multidomain perspective and are widely used across geriatric, neurological, and rehabilitation settings.

The **Elderly Mobility Scale (EMS)** is commonly employed to assess basic mobility tasks, including transfers, gait, and balance, in older adults. Its primary strength lies in its simplicity and clinical feasibility, making it particularly suitable for acute hospital settings and early rehabilitation phases. The EMS provides useful information regarding mobility-related assistance needs and discharge planning. However, its focus on basic tasks may limit sensitivity in higher-functioning older adults, leading to ceiling effects that reduce its usefulness for detecting subtle improvements during rehabilitation.

The **Balance Outcome Measure for Elder Rehabilitation (BOOMER)** integrates several balance-related tests into a composite score, allowing for a broader assessment of postural control. This approach is advantageous in identifying balance deficits that may not be apparent with a single test. BOOMER is especially relevant in inpatient rehabilitation and fall-risk assessment. Nevertheless, its administration requires familiarity with multiple component tests, and performance may be influenced by fatigue or comorbid musculoskeletal conditions, which are common in elderly populations.

The **Karnofsky Performance Scale (KPS)** provides a global measure of functional status and has been extensively used in medical and oncological populations. In geriatric practice, it offers a quick overview of overall independence and care needs. However, the scale is relatively coarse and lacks specificity regarding physical, cognitive, or psychosocial domains. Consequently, while the KPS is useful for broad functional categorisation, it should not be relied upon as a standalone assessment in comprehensive geriatric evaluation.

The **Geriatric Depression Scale (GDS)** addresses an often underrecognized but critically important aspect of elderly assessment—mood and psychological well-being. Depression in older adults frequently presents with somatic complaints or functional decline rather than overt emotional symptoms. The GDS is specifically designed to minimise the influence of physical illness on scoring, making it well-suited for this population. Despite its strengths, the GDS remains a screening tool rather than a diagnostic instrument and should be followed by clinical evaluation when scores indicate depressive symptoms [20].

The **Clinical Frailty Scale (CFS)** has gained increasing prominence as a concise and clinically intuitive measure of frailty. By categorising individuals based on functional ability, comorbidity burden, and dependency, the CFS supports risk stratification and prognostication. It has been widely adopted in acute care, geriatric medicine, and research settings. However, the scale relies on clinical judgment, which may introduce subjectivity, particularly among less experienced clinicians. Training and standardised interpretation are therefore essential to optimise reliability [21].

A key limitation across elderly assessment scales is the potential overlap between domains, which may increase assessment burden without necessarily providing additional clinically meaningful information. Additionally, performance on physical and balance measures may be influenced by acute illness, pain, or fear of falling, leading to underestimation of true functional capacity. These factors highlight the importance of interpreting scale scores within the broader clinical context rather than in isolation.

Recent developments in geriatric assessment have increasingly emphasized frailty-centered and technology-assisted approaches. Wearable activity monitors, digital gait analysis, and remote monitoring platforms are being explored to complement traditional scales and capture real-world function over extended periods. Such tools may enhance sensitivity to change and provide valuable insights into daily activity patterns, particularly in community-dwelling older adults. While these technologies are not yet universally implemented, they represent a promising adjunct to established clinical measures [22].

In clinical practice, the selection of elderly assessment scales should be guided by the care setting and assessment objective. Mobility-focused tools such as the EMS and BOOMER are particularly relevant in rehabilitation and fall-risk evaluation, while the GDS and CFS address psychological and frailty-related dimensions that strongly influence outcomes. An integrated assessment strategy that combines physical, psychological, and frailty measures offers the most comprehensive understanding of functional status in older adults (Table **6**).

Table 6. Commonly used scales for elderly assessment.

Scale	Primary Domain	Strengths	Limitations	Best Clinical Application
Elderly Mobility Scale (EMS)	Basic mobility and transfers	Simple, quick, suitable for acute care	Ceiling effects in high-functioning elderly	Inpatient and early rehabilitation
BOOMER	Balance and postural control	Multicomponent balance assessment	Requires multiple test administrations	Fall risk and balance assessment

(Table 6) cont.....

Scale	Primary Domain	Strengths	Limitations	Best Clinical Application
Karnofsky Performance Scale (KPS)	Global functional status	Rapid overview of independence	Lacks domain specificity	General functional categorisation
Geriatric Depression Scale (GDS)	Mood and depression	Minimises physical symptom bias	Screening only, not diagnostic	Psychological screening
Clinical Frailty Scale (CFS)	Frailty and vulnerability	Intuitive, prognostic value	Subjective judgment	Acute care and geriatric stratification

CONCLUSION

A comprehensive assessment of elderly individuals is essential for understanding the multifactorial impact of Ageing on physical, psychological, and functional health. Scales such as the Elderly Mobility Scale (EMS) and BOOMER provide valuable insights into mobility and balance, aiding in fall prevention and rehabilitation planning. The Karnofsky Performance Scale Index assists clinicians in evaluating overall performance status, while the Geriatric Depression Scale enables early detection and management of emotional distress. The Clinical Frailty Scale (CFS) further contributes to holistic geriatric evaluation by identifying vulnerability and guiding individualised care strategies. Together, these tools offer a structured approach for clinicians to assess, monitor, and improve the functional independence and quality of life of older adults. Ongoing research and clinical validation will continue to enhance the precision, applicability, and cultural adaptability of these assessment scales for the growing elderly population.

AI DISCLOSURE STATEMENT

During the preparation of this chapter, the authors used ChatGPT (OpenAI) as a support tool for language refinement, structural organisation, and clarification of ideas. All content generated with AI assistance was carefully reviewed, verified, and revised by the authors to ensure factual accuracy, originality, and consistency with the scientific literature. The authors take full responsibility for the integrity, interpretation, and final content of the published chapter.

ACKNOWLEDGEMENT

The authors wish to acknowledge the valuable contributions of geriatric clinicians, rehabilitation specialists, and researchers whose work has advanced the understanding and assessment of physical and psychological health in older adults. Their efforts continue to improve the quality of care, independence, and well-being of the elderly population.

REFERENCES

[1] Guo H, Liu Y, Yang R, Li X, Teng Y, Wei W, Zhang D. Relationship between biological ageing, premature mortality, life expectancy, and number of live births: a prospective cohort study of the UK women. BMC Public Health. 2025 Sep 30; 25(1): 3239. doi: 10.1186/s12889-025-24534-x. PMID: 41029623; PMCID: PMC12487170.

[2] GBD 2017 Disease and Injury Incidence and Prevalence Collaborators. Global, regional, and national incidence, prevalence, and years lived with disability for 354 diseases and injuries for 195 countries and territories, 1990-2017: a systematic analysis for the Global Burden of Disease Study 2017. Lancet. 2018 Nov 10;392(10159):1789-1858. doi: 10.1016/S0140-6736(18)32279-7. Epub 2018 Nov 8. Erratum in: Lancet. 2019 Jun 22; 393(10190): e44. doi: 10.1016/S0140-6736(19)31047-5. PMID: 30496104; PMCID: PMC6227754.

[3] Sherbiny AA. Influences on Skin and Intrinsic Aging: Biological, Environmental, and Therapeutic Insights. J Cosmet Dermatol. 2025 Feb; 24(2): e16688. doi: 10.1111/jocd.16688. Epub 2024 Nov 27. PMID: 39604792; PMCID: PMC11845971.

[4] Huang J, Pham VT, Fu S, Huang G, Liu YG, Zheng L. Mitophagy's impacts on cancer and neurodegenerative diseases: implications for future therapies. J Hematol Oncol. 2025 Aug 1; 18(1): 78. doi: 10.1186/s13045-025-01727-w. PMID: 40750884; PMCID: PMC12317492.

[5] Neller SA, Cloyes KG, Edelman LS, Wong B, Baines B, Towsley GL. Preparing for the future while living in the present: Older adults' experiences creating a legacy of values. Gerontologist 2023; 63(9): 1488-96.

[6] Social, Economic, and Demographic Changes among the Elderly. In: Gilford DM, Ed. The Ageing Population in the Twenty-First Century: Statistics for Health Policy. Washington (DC): National Academies Press (US) 2025; 9: pp. 560-890.

[7] Ishikawa M. Internalization of negative societal views on old age into self-perceptions of aging: exploring factors associated with self-directed ageism. Front Sociol. 2023 Nov 17; 8: 1291325. doi: 10.3389/fsoc.2023.1291325. PMID: 38045535; PMCID: PMC10691258.

[8] Ekwonye AU, Malek A, Farah I, Nguyen S, Chonyi T, Ponce-Diaz V, Hearst M. "Aging is beautiful and graceful:" Exploring college students' perceptions of aging, older adults, and future older selves. Educ Gerontol. 2023; 49(9): 803-816. doi: 10.1080/03601277.2022.2164642. Epub 2023 Jan 10. PMID: 37942281; PMCID: PMC10629836.

[9] Merchant RA, Aprahamian I, Woo J, Vellas B, Morley JE. Resilience And Successful Aging. J Nutr Health Aging 2022; 26(7): 652-6.
[http://dx.doi.org/10.1007/s12603-022-1818-4] [PMID: 35842754]

[10] Prosser L, Canby A. Further validation of the Elderly Mobility Scale for measurement of mobility of hospitalized elderly people. Clin Rehabil 1997; 11(4): 338-43.
[http://dx.doi.org/10.1177/026921559701100412] [PMID: 9408676]

[11] de Morton NA, Nolan J, O'Brien M, *et al.* A head-to-head comparison of the de Morton Mobility Index (DEMMI) and Elderly Mobility Scale (EMS) in an older acute medical population. Disabil Rehabil 2015; 37(20): 1881-7.
[http://dx.doi.org/10.3109/09638288.2014.982832] [PMID: 26292173]

[12] Tan JM, Halford GRJ, Lukin M, Kohler F. Recommendations from the ISPO lower-limb COMPASS: Patient-reported and performance-based outcome measures. Prosthet Orthot Int. 2023 Feb 1; 47(1): 13-25. doi: 10.1097/PXR.0000000000000197. Epub 2023 Jan 5. PMID: 36629556; PMCID: PMC9945573.

[13] de Melo TA, Silva Guimarães F, Lapa E Silva JR. The five times sit-to-stand test: safety, validity and reliability with critical care survivors's at ICU discharge. Arch Physiother. 2022 Dec 18;13(1):2. doi: 10.1186/s40945-022-00156-z. Erratum in: Arch Physiother. 2023 Mar 7; 13(1): 5. doi: 10.1186/s40945-023-00161-w. PMID: 36597159; PMCID: PMC9809000.

[14] Weber M, Van Ancum J, Bergquist R, *et al.* Concurrent validity and reliability of the Community Balance and Mobility scale in young-older adults. BMC Geriatr 2018; 18: 156. [http://dx.doi.org/10.1186/s12877-018-0845-9]

[15] Brown ZM, Gibbs JC, Adachi JD, *et al.* Score Distributions of the Balance Outcome Measure for Elder Rehabilitation (BOOMER) in Community-Dwelling Older Adults With Vertebral Fracture. J Geriatr Phys Ther 2019; 42(3): E87-93. [http://dx.doi.org/10.1519/JPT.0000000000000158] [PMID: 29210932]

[16] Kuys SS, Morrison G, Bew PG, Clarke J, Haines TP. Further Validation of the Balance Outcome Measure for Elder Rehabilitation. Arch Phys Med Rehabil 2011; 92(1): 101-5. [http://dx.doi.org/10.1016/j.apmr.2010.10.001] [PMID: 21187212]

[17] Haines T, Kuys SS, Morrison G, Clarke J, Bew P, McPhail S. Development and validation of the balance outcome measure for elder rehabilitation. Arch Phys Med Rehabil 2007; 88(12): 1614-21. [http://dx.doi.org/10.1016/j.apmr.2007.09.012] [PMID: 18047876]

[18] Mor V, Laliberte L, Morris JN, Wiemann M. The Karnofsky performance status scale: An examination of its reliability and validity in a research setting. Cancer 1984; 53(9): 2002-7. [http://dx.doi.org/10.1002/1097-0142(19840501)53:9<2002::AID-CNCR2820530933>3.0.CO;2-W] [PMID: 6704925]

[19] Crooks V, Waller S, Smith T, Hahn TJ. The use of the Karnofsky Performance Scale in determining outcomes and risk in geriatric outpatients. J Gerontol 1991; 46(4): M139-44. [http://dx.doi.org/10.1093/geronj/46.4.M139] [PMID: 2071835]

[20] Timmermann C. 'Just give me the best quality of life questionnaire': the Karnofsky scale and the history of quality of life measurements in cancer trials. Chronic Illn. 2013 Sep; 9(3): 179-90. doi: 10.1177/1742395312466903. Epub 2012 Dec 13. PMID: 23239756; PMCID: PMC3837542.

[21] Goto Y, Hino A, Hashimoto N. A comparative analysis of the modified Rankin Scale, Karnofsky Performance Status and Kurtzke expanded disability status scale in the perioperative management of patients with brainstem cavernous malformations. Clin Neurol Neurosurg 2021; 207: 106785. [http://dx.doi.org/10.1016/j.clineuro.2021.106785] [PMID: 34252689]

[22] Balsamo M, Cataldi F, Carlucci L, Padulo C, Fairfield B. Assessment of late-life depression *via* self-report measures: a review. Clin Interv Aging. 2018 Oct 16; 13: 2021-2044. doi: 10.2147/CIA.S178943. PMID: 30410319; PMCID: PMC6199213.

[23] Liwsrisakun C, Pothirat C, Chaiwong W, *et al.* Diagnostic ability of the Timed Up & Go test for balance impairment prediction in chronic obstructive pulmonary disease. J Thorac Dis. 2020 May; 12(5): 2406-2414. doi: 10.21037/jtd.2020.03.47. PMID: 32642146; PMCID: PMC7330337.

[24] Brañez-Condorena A, Soriano-Moreno DR, Navarro-Flores A, Solis-Chimoy B, Diaz-Barrera ME, Taype-Rondan A. Accuracy of the Geriatric Depression Scale (GDS)-4 and GDS-5 for the screening of depression among older adults: A systematic review and meta-analysis. PLoS One. 2021 Jul 1; 16(7): 0253899. doi: 10.1371/journal.pone.0253899. PMID: 34197527; PMCID: PMC8248624.

[25] Yesavage JA, Brink TL, Rose TL, *et al.* Development and validation of a geriatric depression screening scale: A preliminary report. J Psychiatr Res 1982-1983; 17(1): 37-49. [http://dx.doi.org/10.1016/0022-3956(82)90033-4] [PMID: 7183759]

[26] Rockwood K, Theou O. Using the Clinical Frailty Scale in Allocating Scarce Health Care Resources. Can Geriatr J. 2020 Sep 1; 23(3): 210-215. doi: 10.5770/cgj.23.463. PMID: 32904824; PMCID: PMC7458601.

[27] Cesari M, Prince M, Thiyagarajan JA, *et al*. Frailty: an emerging public health priority. J Am Med Dir Assoc 2018; 19(3): 185-92.
[PMID: 26805753]

CHAPTER 5

Scales for Ataxia

Yashleen Kaur Sandhu[1,2], **Anshu Sharma**[2,3], **Simranjeet Kaur**[2,4] and **Parveen Kumar**[4,*]

[1] *University School of Physiotherapy and Radiology, Rayat Bahra University, Mohali, Punjab, India*

[2] *Maharishi Markandeshwar Institute of Physiotherapy and Rehabilitation, Maharishi Markandeshwar (Deemed to be University), Mullana, Ambala, Haryana, India*

[3] *Department of Physiotherapy, School of Health Care and Allied Science, G.D. Goenka University, Sohna, Haryana, India*

[4] *Pal Physiotherapy and Rehabilitation Centre, Pal Healthcare, Ambala City, Haryana, India*

Abstract: Ataxia refers to impaired coordination of voluntary movements. Historically, the term also encompassed disturbances of gait, overall mobility, and even cardiac rhythm. The condition arises when sensory or motor pathways of the central or peripheral nervous system are affected. Accurate assessment is crucial to understanding the patient's current functional status. This chapter provides an overview of commonly used clinical tools for ataxia evaluation, focusing on the Scale for the Assessment and Rating of Ataxia (SARA), the Brief Ataxia Rating Scale (BARS), and the International Cooperative Ataxia Rating Scale (ICARS). Each section outlines the background, application methods, psychometric properties, and clinical indications for these instruments.

Keywords: Ataxia, Cerebellar ataxia, Gait, Psychometrics, Scale for the Assessment and Rating of Ataxia (SARA).

INTRODUCTION

Ataxia may result from diverse pathological processes, making the identification of the underlying cause essential. It is clinically defined by poor coordination and postural instability, most often linked to damage within the cerebellum and its associated neural pathways. Both hereditary and acquired forms exist. Pure manifestations of ataxia are uncommon in acquired disorders, where other neurological signs typically accompany the condition. With the expanding spect-

* **Corresponding author Parveen Kumar:** Pal Physiotherapy and Rehabilitation Centre, Pal Healthcare, Ambala City, Haryana, India; E-mail: parveen34134@gmail.com

Nidhi Sharma, Simranjeet Kaur & Parveen Kumar (Eds.)

rum of hereditary degenerative ataxias, clinical focus should remain on identifying potentially reversible or treatable forms, particularly those that may pose serious risks to the patient's health [1]. The pathophysiology of ataxia has not been fully elucidated. Research in this field frequently investigates voluntary limb movements in patients with cerebellar pathology or peripheral neuropathy.

The pathophysiology of ataxia has not been fully elucidated. Research in this field frequently investigates voluntary limb movements in patients with cerebellar pathology or peripheral neuropathy. In those with cerebellar lesions, abnormalities are often documented using advanced motion analysis. Findings typically include: (a) reduced amplitude and prolonged activation of agonist muscles, resulting in impaired acceleration, and (b) delayed activation of antagonist muscles, causing slowed or incomplete deceleration [2].

The following sections review clinical questionnaires designed to quantify ataxia severity.

SCALES FOR ASSESSMENT AND RATING OF ATAXIA (SARA)

Introduction

The Scale for the Assessment and Rating of Ataxia (SARA) was developed by Schmitz-Hübsch and colleagues in 2006 to provide a concise and reliable clinical measure for cerebellar ataxia, particularly in patients with spinocerebellar ataxia [3]. Beyond spinocerebellar ataxia, the scale has also been applied in other rare conditions, including lysosomal storage disorders, where it demonstrated acceptable responsiveness and clinical relevance [4]. It is a short, semi-quantitative tool that enables clinicians to evaluate the severity of symptoms and track disease progression over time [3].

Items

The scale consists of eight performance-based tasks:

- **Gait (0–8 points):** Evaluates walking ability and distance covered.
- **Stance (0–6 points):** Measures stability while standing.
- **Sitting (0–4 points):** Assesses the ability to maintain upright sitting posture without foot support.
- **Speech disturbance (0–6 points):** Examines clarity and fluency of speech during conversation.
- **Finger chase (0–4 points):** Tests for dysmetria by having the patient follow the examiner's finger.

- **Nose–finger test (0–4 points):** Measures tremor and accuracy in reaching a target.
- **Fast alternating hand movements (0–4 points):** Evaluates dysdiadochokinesia.
- **Heel–shin slide (0–4 points):** Assesses lower-limb coordination and balance.

Items 5 to 8 are performed bilaterally.

Administration

The scale is straightforward to use, requires no specialised training, and typically takes about 22 minutes to administer (average patient time: 14.2 ± 7.5 minutes; average control time: 7.2 ± 2.6 minutes).

Scoring and Interpretation

The maximum possible score is 40. A score of **0** indicates no impairment, while **40** reflects the most severe form of ataxia. The minimal detectable change is < 3.5 ($p < 0.0001$).

Indications

SARA applies to patients with spinocerebellar ataxia, ataxic stroke, and Friedreich's ataxia.

Translations

Validated versions of SARA exist in multiple languages:

- **Brazilian Portuguese:** excellent internal consistency ($\alpha = 0.94$) [3]
- **Chinese:** good reliability ($\alpha = 0.78$) and criterion validity (0.9) [4]
- **Korean (K-SARA):** very high inter-rater reliability (ICC = 0.985, $p < 0.001$) and test–retest reliability (ICC = 0.997, $p < 0.001$) [5]

PSYCHOMETRIC PROPERTIES

- **Reliability:**
    - Test–retest reliability: excellent (Spinocerebellar ataxia: ICC = 0.90; Friedreich's ataxia: ICC = 0.99) [6]
    - Inter-rater reliability: high (Spinocerebellar ataxia: ICC = 0.98; Friedreich's ataxia: ICC = 0.80) [6]
    - Internal consistency: strong (Spinocerebellar ataxia: ICC = 0.94; Friedreich's ataxia: ICC = 0.89) [6]

- **Validity:**
  - Correlates well with the Barthel Index ($r = -0.8$, $p < 0.0001$) [7]
  - Shows excellent construct validity compared with ICARS ($r = 0.953$) [8]
- **Floor/Ceiling Effects:**
  - Minimal floor effect reported at one-year follow-up (0.6%) [9].

Scoring Guidelines

1. Gait (0–8 points)
Patient walks safely along a wall, performs a half-turn, and walks in tandem (heel-to-toe).

- **0:** Normal, no errors (≤1 misstep in tandem).
- **1:** Slight difficulty, noticeable only in tandem walk.
- **2:** Clearly abnormal, tandem walking >10 steps is not possible.
- **3:** Considerable staggering, problems with turning, but no support.
- **4:** Marked staggering, needs occasional wall support.
- **5:** Requires one stick or light support from one arm.
- **6:** Needs two sticks, a stroller, or bilateral support to walk >10 m.
- **7:** Can walk <10 m only with strong support (two sticks, stroller, or helper).
- **8:** Unable to walk, even with support.

2. Stance (0–6 points)
Patient stands in a natural position, feet together, in a tandem stance (shoes off, eyes open). Three attempts allowed, best recorded.

- **0:** Holds tandem stance >10 s.
- **1:** Holds feet together >10 s, tandem not possible.
- **2:** Feet together >10 s, but with sway.
- **3:** Natural stance >10 s, cannot hold feet together.
- **4:** Natural stance >10 s only with intermittent support.
- **5:** Natural stance >10 s only with continuous one-arm support.
- **6:** Cannot maintain stance >10 s, even with support.

3. Sitting (0–4 points)
Patient sits on exam table, feet unsupported, arms outstretched, eyes open.

- **0:** Stable for >10 s.
- **1:** Slight sway.
- **2:** Constant sway, but >10 s without support.
- **3:** Maintains >10 s only with intermittent support.
- **4:** Needs continuous support to sit.

4. Speech Disturbance (0–6 points)
Conversational speech assessed.

- **0:** Normal.
- **1:** Slight irregularity.
- **2:** Speech impaired but intelligible.
- **3:** Some words are unclear.
- **4:** Many words are unclear.
- **5:** Only isolated words are intelligible.
- **6:** Anarthria or incomprehensible.

5. Finger Chase (0–4 Points, Right and Left)
Examiner makes 5 sudden pointing movements (30 cm apart, every 2 s); patient follows with the index finger. Last 3 movements scored.

- **0:** No error.
- **1:** Overshoot/undershoot <5 cm.
- **2:** Error <15 cm.
- **3:** Error > 15 cm.
- **4:** Unable to perform.

Score each side separately; final value = mean of right and left.

6. Nose–Finger Test (0–4 Points, Right and Left)
Patient alternates between nose and examiner's finger (90% arm reach). Kinetic tremor amplitude rated.

- **0:** No tremor.
- **1:** Tremor <2 cm.
- **2:** Tremor <5 cm.
- **3:** Tremor >5 cm.
- **4:** Cannot complete 5 movements.

Score each side separately; final value = mean of right and left.

7. Fast Alternating Hand Movements (0–4 Points, Right and Left)
Patient performs 10 rapid pronation–supination cycles on the thigh within 7 seconds.

- **0:** Smooth, completed <10 s.
- **1:** Slight irregularity, <10 s.
- **2:** Clear irregularity or interruptions, <10 s.

- **3:** Very irregular, requires >10 s.
- **4:** Unable to perform the task.

Score each side separately; final value = mean of right and left.

8. Heel–Shin Slide (0–4 Points, Right and Left)
Supine, patient places the heel on the opposite knee, slides down the shin to the ankle, and repeats 3 times.

- **0:** Smooth and accurate.
- **1:** Slightly abnormal, maintains shin contact.
- **2:** Deviates ≤3 times over 3 cycles.
- **3:** Deviates ≥4 times.
- **4:** Cannot perform the task.

Score each side separately; final value = mean of right and left.

BRIEF ATAXIA RATING SCALE (BARS)

Introduction

The Brief Ataxia Rating Scale (BARS) is a short, five-item clinical tool designed to measure the functional impact of cerebellar ataxia. It evaluates motor domains, including gait, limb coordination, speech, and eye movements, allowing clinicians to quantify deficits using a structured approach [10, 11]. Unlike longer assessments, BARS can be completed in a few minutes while still capturing essential neurological findings.

Items

The five domains assessed are:

- **Gait:** walking independence and stability.
- **Knee–tibia test:** quality of leg movement and intention tremor.
- **Finger–nose test:** accuracy and decomposition of upper limb movements.
- **Speech:** fluency and clarity of spoken language.
- **Eye movements:** presence of oculomotor disturbances.

Administration

The test requires approximately 5 minutes, making it more practical than several longer scales.

Scoring and Interpretation

The total possible score is **30**. Higher scores represent greater impairment. Severity is typically classified as mild, moderate, or severe functional loss.

Indications

This scale is suitable for patients presenting with ataxia or ataxia-like symptoms.

Translations

Validated versions are available in Brazilian Portuguese and Turkish [12, 13].

Psychometric Properties

- **Reliability:**
  - Test–retest reliability: ICC = 0.91 [11].
  - Inter-rater reliability: ICC = 0.91 [11].
  - Internal consistency: Cronbach's $\alpha = 0.90$ [11].
- **Validity:**
  - Factor analysis demonstrated high construct validity (0.952, $p < 0.0001$) [11].

Scoring Guidelines

Gait (0–8 Points)

- **0:** Walks normally.
- **1:** Walks normally, but is unable to complete a tandem gait.
- **2:** Walks independently, but gait is irregular.
- **3:** Ambulates independently, with marked staggering and problems turning.
- **4:** Cannot walk without using a wall or support for 10 m.
- **5:** Requires one stick or cane.
- **6:** Requires two sticks or a stroller.
- **7:** Needs one accompanying person.
- **8:** Unable to walk, even with one person assisting (wheelchair needed).

Knee–Tibia Test (0–4 Points, Right and Left)

Patient in the supine position moves the heel of one leg along the shin of the opposite leg.

- **0:** Smooth lowering of heel along shin.
- **1:** Movement decomposed into several phases, but without jerks.
- **2:** Jerky lowering along the axis.

- **3:** Jerky lowering with sideways deviation.
- **4:** Movement extremely disorganised or impossible.

Score both sides separately; final = mean of right and left.

Finger–Nose Test (0–4 Points, Right and Left)

Patient alternates between touching their nose and the examiner's finger, repeated 3 times.

- **0:** Smooth, accurate.
- **1:** Oscillating movement, no segmentation.
- **2:** Segmented into 2 phases and/or moderate dysmetria.
- **3:** Segmented into >2 phases and/or severe dysmetria.
- **4:** Unable to reach the nose accurately.

Score both sides separately; final = mean of right and left.

Speech (0–4 Points)

Evaluates conversational fluency and clarity.

- **0:** Normal.
- **1:** Slightly slowed or slurred.
- **2:** Moderately impaired but understandable.
- **3:** Severely slow and dysarthric.
- **4:** Speech absent or unintelligible.

Eye Movements (0–2 Points)

The examiner assesses pursuit and saccadic movements.

- **0:** Normal.
- **1:** Slight abnormality (mild slowing, saccadic intrusions, hypo/hypermetric saccades, or nystagmus).
- **2:** Prominent abnormality (marked slowing, frequent saccadic intrusions, or severe nystagmus).

Severity Classification (based on total score)

- **Mild:** ≤ 5.5
- **Minimal:** ≤ 10.0
- **Moderate:** ≤ 14.25
- **Severe:** ≥ 23

INTERNATIONAL COOPERATIVE ATAXIA RATING SCALE (ICARS)

Introduction

The International Cooperative Ataxia Rating Scale (ICARS), introduced by Trouillas *et al.* in 1997, is one of the earliest standardised instruments for quantifying ataxia [14]. It contains 19 items organised into four subscales, covering posture and gait, limb coordination, speech, and oculomotor control. Although comprehensive, ICARS is relatively lengthy, taking 15–20 minutes to complete, which can limit its routine clinical use. Nevertheless, it has been widely adopted in clinical research and therapeutic trials [15].

Domains

- Posture and Gait (34 points)
- Kinetic Functions (52 points)
- Speech (8 points)
- Oculomotor Disorders (6 points)

Administration

Typically requires between 15 and 20 minutes. Each item is scored on a scale from 0 (normal) to 4 or 5 (severe impairment), depending on the task. The maximum possible score is **100**, reflecting the most severe level of impairment.

Scoring and Interpretation

- **0:** Normal performance
- **100:** Maximum impairment

Higher total scores reflect more advanced functional decline.

Indications

Useful in both inherited and acquired ataxias, particularly in research contexts where a detailed functional profile is required.

Translations

Validated versions are available in Korean, Portuguese, and Chinese [16 - 18].

Psychometric Properties

- **Reliability**

Test-retest reliability: The scale exhibits excellent test-retest reliability with an ICC value of 0.97 [15]

Inter-rater reliability: The inter-rater reliability for all items in the scale is excellent, with an ICC of 0.95. Regarding individual domains, the inter-rater reliability is: Posture and Gait Disturbances, ICC = 0.96; Limb ataxia, ICC = 0.88; Dysarthria, ICC = 0.76; and Oculomotor Disorder, ICC = 0.87 [15].

- **Intra-rater reliability**: The intra-rater reliability of the complete scale is excellent, too, with the ICC value of 0.97. Regarding the individual domains, the intra-rater reliability is: Posture and Gait Disturbances, ICC = 0.93; Limb ataxia, ICC = 0.95; Dysarthria, ICC = 0.85; and Oculomotor Disorder, ICC = 0.81 [15].
- **Internal consistency**: The scale shows excellent internal consistency for Spinocerebellar Ataxia with Cronbach's alpha, α= 0.95; but a poor value of Cronbach's alpha for Friedreich's Ataxia, α= 0.69 [15].

- **Validity**

Criterion validity

The scale shows excellent correlation with the Barthel Index, r= 0.70 [15].

Construct Validity

The scale has good construct validity for non-specific ataxic patients as well, with a correlation coefficient, r=0.60 [16].

Detailed Administration and Scoring Instructions

The ICARS is a structured, observer-rated tool designed to quantify the severity of ataxia across **19 items** grouped into four domains: **Posture and Gait, Kinetic Functions, Speech, and Oculomotor Control**. The maximum score is **100 points**, with higher values reflecting greater impairment.

General Administration Guidelines

- **Environment:** Conduct assessments in a well-lit, quiet room with enough space for safe walking tasks. Provide stable furniture or rails for safety.
- **Patient Preparation:** Patients should remove shoes when performing stance, gait, and coordination tasks. Glasses or hearing aids may be used if needed.
- **Trial and Scoring:** Each task should be demonstrated once by the examiner. Patients may attempt up to two practice trials if unclear. Final scoring is based on the best of up to three valid attempts.
- **Bilateral Tasks:** For limb coordination tasks (finger–nose, finger chase, alternating hand movements, heel–shin), score each side separately. Record both values, then calculate the **mean of the right and left** for the final score.
- **Safety:** Always remain close to the patient during balance tasks to prevent falls. If external support is required, note this in the score.
- **Time Required:** Full administration usually takes **15–20 minutes**.

A. Posture and Gait (0–34 Points)

1. **Walking capacity (0–8):**
   - Ask the patient to walk 10 meters, turn around, and return.
   - Observe gait rhythm, stability, and use of aids.
   - Score 0 (normal) to 8 (unable to walk).
2. **Standing stance (0–6):**
   - Patient stands with feet together, arms at sides, eyes open.
   - Note sway, stability, and need for assistance.
   - Score 0 (stable) to 6 (unable to stand even with support).
3. **Sitting posture (0–4):**
   - Patient sits on a firm surface without foot support, arms extended forward.
   - Watch for postural sway or need for support.
   - Score 0 (stable) to 4 (cannot sit without continuous help).
4. **Tandem gait (0–8):**
   - Patient walks heel-to-toe in a straight line for 10 steps.
   - Count errors (loss of contact, stepping aside).
   - Score 0 (completes smoothly) to 8 (unable to attempt).
5. **Rising from chair (0–8):**
   - Patient rises from a standard chair without using arms.
   - Note speed, stability, and independence.
   - Score 0 (smoothly) to 8 (unable to rise).

B. Kinetic Functions (0–52 Points)

(All performed bilaterally, with mean recorded.)

1. **Finger–Nose Test (0–4 each side):**
   - Patient alternately touches their nose and the examiner's finger (arm at 90% length).
   - Observe tremor, accuracy, and dysmetria.
   - Score 0 (smooth) to 4 (cannot complete).
2. **Finger Chase Test (0–4 each side):**
   - Examiner moves finger quickly in unpredictable directions.
   - Patient tries to follow with their own finger.
   - Score based on distance of error: 0 (no error) to 4 (unable).
3. **Alternating Hand Movements (0–4 each side):**
   - The patient rapidly alternates pronation and supination on the thigh.
   - Assess rhythm, speed, and coordination.
   - Score 0 (smooth, <10 s) to 4 (unable to perform).
4. **Heel–Shin Slide (0–4 each side):**
   - Supine, patient places heel on opposite knee and slides it down the shin to the ankle.
   - Observe accuracy, tremor, and contact loss.
   - Score 0 (smooth) to 4 (cannot complete).

C. Speech (0–8 Points)

- Engage the patient in free conversation or ask them to read a prepared text.
- Evaluate fluency, articulation, and rhythm.
- Score 0 (normal) to 8 (anarthria or incomprehensible)

D. Oculomotor Control (0–6 Points)

1. Smooth pursuit (0–3):
   - Patient follows the examiner's finger as it moves slowly horizontally and vertically
   - Score 0 (normal) to 3 (severe impairment or failure).

2. Saccadic eye movement (0–3):
   - Patient looks back and forth between two fixed points.
   - Evaluate speed, accuracy, and initiation.
   - Score 0 (normal) to 3 (severe inaccuracy or absence).

Scoring Summary

- **Maximum score:** 100 points
- **Subscale maximums:** Posture/Gait = 34; Kinetic = 52; Speech = 8; Oculomotor = 6
- **Interpretation:**
  - **0:** No impairment

- **1–30:** Mild ataxia
- **31–60:** Moderate ataxia
- **61–100:** Severe ataxia

FRIEDREICH ATAXIA RATING SCALE (FARS)

Introduction

The Friedreich Ataxia Rating Scale (FARS) was developed specifically to capture the neurological manifestations of Friedreich's ataxia, though it has also been applied to other ataxic disorders [19]. Unlike more general ataxia scales, FARS emphasises functional outcomes, activities of daily living, and neurologic examination findings relevant to disease progression.

The instrument consists of several subscales:

- **Neurological Examination (0–117 Points)**
- **Functional Staging (0–6 points)**
- **Activities of Daily Living (0–36 points)**
- **Upright Stability (0–40 points)**

Administration

The assessment is conducted by a trained clinician. It typically requires 20–30 minutes, as it combines direct observation of motor and coordination tasks with structured patient interviews about daily activities.

Scoring and Interpretation

- **Neurological Examination:** Evaluates gait, limb coordination, speech, and sensory function. Higher scores indicate worse impairment.
- **Functional Staging:** Six levels, ranging from fully ambulatory (0) to wheelchair-bound.
- **Activities of Daily Living:** Patient self-report or caregiver input is used to assess independence in eating, dressing, hygiene, and mobility.
- **Upright Stability:** Patients perform balance tasks with increasing difficulty; scored from 0 (stable) to 40 (complete loss of upright function).

The total maximum score is **199**, reflecting the most severe disability.

Translations

Validated translations are available only in German [20].

Psychometric Properties

- **Reliability:** Test–retest ICC > 0.90 across subscales [19].
- **Validity:** Strong correlation with SARA and ICARS, as well as with patient-reported outcomes [19].
- **Sensitivity:** Well-suited for monitoring longitudinal change in Friedreich's ataxia progression.

Scoring Guidelines and Instructions

A. Neurological Examination (0–117 Points)

Includes tasks adapted from standard neurological exams:

- **Gait and posture:** Assessed during a 10-meter walk, tandem gait, and chair rise.
- **Upper limb coordination:** Finger–nose test, finger chase, rapid alternating hand movements. Each limb was scored separately; the mean was recorded.
- **Lower limb coordination:** Heel–shin slide, tapping, and foot placement tasks. Both sides scored; the mean was recorded.
- **Speech:** Conversational fluency and articulation.
- **Sensation:** Light touch and vibration sense in the upper and lower limbs.

Instructions

- Each item is scored on a 0–4 scale, where **0 = normal** and higher scores reflect worsening function.
- Examiner records performance and notes the need for assistance.
- For bilateral tests, the average right and left scores.

B. Functional Staging (0–6 Points)

Simple categorical rating of ambulation:

- **0:** Normal walking, no restriction.
- **1:** Slight difficulty, but no aid required.
- **2:** Walks independently short distances, may need support for long distances.
- **3:** Needs a single walking aid (stick or cane).
- **4:** Requires two aids for walking.
- **5:** Ambulates only with constant human assistance.
- **6:** Wheelchair-dependent.

C. Activities of Daily Living (0–36 Points)

Self-reported questionnaire covering independence in feeding, dressing, bathing, toileting, and mobility.

- **0:** Independent
- **1–2:** Slight assistance required
- **3–4:** Moderate assistance required
- **5–6:** Dependent in task

D. Upright Stability (0–40 Points)

Balance assessed progressively: standing with feet together, tandem stance, and one-leg stance, each with increasing challenge.

- **0:** Stable >10 seconds
- **1–2:** Minimal sway, maintains posture
- **3–4:** Marked sway, frequent corrections
- **5–6:** Unable to maintain without assistance
- **7–8:** Unable to attempt

Administration Notes

- Conduct in a safe environment, with the examiner standing nearby during gait and balance tasks.
- Allow rest breaks if fatigue develops.
- Patients who cannot attempt a task due to severity receive the maximum score for that item.
- Total score is the sum of all four domains (maximum 199).

Interpretation

- **0–50:** Mild functional loss
- **51–100:** Moderate impairment
- **101–150:** Severe disability
- **151–199:** Very severe, complete dependence

UNIFIED MULTIPLE SYSTEM ATROPHY RATING SCALE (UMSARS)

Introduction

The Unified Multiple System Atrophy Rating Scale (UMSARS) was created to provide a standardised tool for evaluating both functional capacity and motor performance in patients with multiple system atrophy (MSA). It helps clinicians monitor disease progression and has been widely used in clinical trials assessing therapeutic interventions [21].

UMSARS is structured into four parts:

- **Part I – Historical review (0–48 points)**
- **Part II – Motor examination (0–56 points)**
- **Part III – Autonomic function (optional)**
- **Part IV – Global disability (0–4 points)**

Administration

- **Part I:** Interview-based questionnaire on daily activities (feeding, dressing, hygiene, mobility, and autonomic symptoms such as bladder control).
- **Part II:** Neurological examination assessing motor skills, including speech, gait, limb coordination, and posture.
- **Part III:** Autonomic testing (blood pressure, bladder function, *etc.*), performed only when resources allow.
- **Part IV:** Clinician rates overall disability on a 0–4 scale.

The full evaluation typically requires **20–30 minutes**.

Scoring and Interpretation

- **Higher scores = greater disability.**
- **Total possible score (Parts I + II + IV) = 108 points.**
- Part III is descriptive and not included in the composite score.

Translations

Validated versions are available in Japanese only [22].

Psychometric Properties [21]

- **Reliability**

Inter-rater reliability: The interrater reliability of most of the UMSARS-I and -

II items, as well as of total UMSARS-I and -II sub scores, was substantial (κ= 0.6 – 0.8) to excellent (κ= 0.8).

Internal consistency: The scale shows good internal consistency with the value of Cronbach's alpha: $\alpha = 0.84$ for UMSARS-I and $\alpha = 0.90$ for UMSARS-II.

Validity: The scales depicts high correlation coefficient with other global disability measures, with the value of $r = 0.83$ ($p < 0.001$).

Scoring Guidelines and Instructions

Part I – Historical Review (0–48 Points)

Patient (or caregiver) answers 12 questions on daily living activities:

- Speech, swallowing, handwriting, cutting food, dressing, hygiene, turning in bed, walking, falling, orthostatic symptoms, bladder function, bowel function.
- Each item scored **0 (normal) to 4 (severe impairment/complete dependence)**.

Part II – Motor Examination (0–56 Points)

The clinician directly observes 14 motor functions:

- Speech, facial expression, tremor at rest, finger taps, hand movements, rapid alternating hand movements, leg agility, arising from chair, posture, gait, body bradykinesia, limb rigidity, and coordination tasks.
- Each scored **0 (normal) to 4 (most impaired)**.
- For bilateral limb tasks, score right and left separately, then average the two.

Part III – Autonomic Function (Descriptive, not scored)

Optional domain including:

- Measurement of orthostatic blood pressure drop.
- Assessment of urinary dysfunction (frequency, incontinence, retention).
- Evaluation of erectile dysfunction in males.
- Gastrointestinal motility (constipation, swallowing difficulties).

Part IV – Global Disability Scale (0–4 Points)

The clinician makes an overall judgment of the patient's disability:

- **0:** Minimal or no disability.
- **1:** Mild disability, independent.

- **2:** Moderate disability, requires occasional assistance.
- **3:** Severe disability, dependent on regular help.
- **4:** Very severe disability, bedridden or completely dependent.

Administration Notes

- **Interview Part I** before the motor exam. Caregivers may supplement patient answers if cognitive or speech difficulties interfere.
- **Safety:** During Part II tasks (especially gait and balance), the examiner should provide standby assistance.
- **Scoring:** Always record the best performance if multiple trials are attempted.
- **Monitoring:** Recommended at 6- or 12-month intervals in clinical settings and trials.

Interpretation

- **0–25:** Mild functional loss
- **26–50:** Moderate impairment
- **51–80:** Severe impairment
- **81–108:** Very severe disability

CLINICAL CONSIDERATIONS, STRENGTHS, LIMITATIONS, AND EMERGING PERSPECTIVES

Ataxia is a heterogeneous clinical syndrome characterised by impaired coordination of gait, limb movements, speech, and ocular control. It may arise from a wide range of etiologies, including degenerative, genetic, vascular, inflammatory, and metabolic disorders. Given this diversity, the assessment of ataxia requires tools that are not only reliable and sensitive but also capable of capturing both disease severity and progression over time. The scales included in this chapter, the Scale for the Assessment and Rating of Ataxia (SARA), the Brief Ataxia Rating Scale (BARS), the International Cooperative Ataxia Rating Scale (ICARS), and the Unified Multiple System Atrophy Rating Scale (UMSARS), represent different approaches to evaluating ataxic disorders in clinical and research contexts.

The Scale for the Assessment and Rating of Ataxia (SARA) has gained widespread acceptance due to its balance between comprehensiveness and feasibility. By focusing on key functional domains such as gait, stance, limb coordination, speech, and oculomotor control, SARA provides a practical overview of ataxia severity. Its relatively short administration time makes it suitable for both clinical practice and longitudinal follow-up. Importantly, SARA has demonstrated good responsiveness to change, which is essential for monitoring disease progression and treatment effects. Nevertheless, subtle impairments in early or very mild ataxia may not be adequately captured, and ceiling effects can occur in advanced disease stages.

The Brief Ataxia Rating Scale (BARS) was developed as a rapid, simplified alternative to longer assessment tools. Its streamlined format makes it particularly useful in busy clinical settings or when patient endurance is limited. While BARS offers good feasibility, its reduced number of items may limit sensitivity to small but clinically meaningful changes, especially in research settings where precise quantification is required. Consequently, BARS is best viewed as a screening or adjunct tool rather than a replacement for more comprehensive scales.

The International Cooperative Ataxia Rating Scale (ICARS) is one of the most detailed instruments available for ataxia assessment. It evaluates posture and gait, limb coordination, speech, and oculomotor function through a broad set of items. This depth allows for thorough characterisation of ataxic features and has made ICARS a preferred outcome measure in several research studies. However, the length and complexity of ICARS can be a significant drawback in routine clinical practice. Administration requires considerable time and examiner expertise, and inter-rater variability may increase if standardised training is not ensured. These factors have contributed to a gradual shift toward shorter scales such as SARA in many clinical settings.

The Unified Multiple System Atrophy Rating Scale (UMSARS) is a disease-specific instrument designed to assess the severity and progression of multiple system atrophy, a condition in which ataxia frequently coexists with Parkinsonism and autonomic dysfunction. UMSARS offers the advantage of capturing multiple disease domains within a single framework, thereby providing a comprehensive overview of functional status. However, its disease-specific nature limits generalizability to other ataxic disorders, and its broader focus may reduce sensitivity to isolated cerebellar features in non-MSA populations.

Across all ataxia scales, a common limitation is the challenge of capturing early disease changes and subtle progression. Many patients experience functional decline before marked changes in clinical scores become apparent. Additionally, performance-based assessments may be influenced by fatigue, motivation, and comorbid conditions, which can affect score reliability. These limitations highlight the importance of interpreting scale scores alongside clinical judgment and patient-reported outcomes [23].

Recent advances in ataxia assessment have increasingly emphasised objective and technology-assisted measures. Instrumented gait analysis, wearable inertial sensors, and digital coordination tasks are being explored to quantify movement variability, balance instability, and fine motor control with greater precision. These tools show promise in detecting early disease changes and providing continuous, real-world data that complement traditional clinical scales. While such technologies are currently more common in research settings, they are likely to play an expanding role in clinical trials and longitudinal disease monitoring [24, 25].

In clinical practice, the choice of ataxia assessment scale should be guided by the purpose of evaluation. For routine clinical monitoring and follow-up, SARA offers an efficient and reliable option. In research contexts that require detailed phenotyping, ICARS may offer greater granularity, albeit at the cost of feasibility. Disease-specific instruments, such as UMSARS, are most appropriate for assessing conditions like multiple system atrophy. A combined approach, integrating clinical scales with emerging objective measures, offers the most comprehensive strategy for assessing ataxia severity and progression (Table **1**).

Table 1. Commonly used scales for ataxia.

Scale	Domains Assessed	Key Strengths	Major Limitations	Best Clinical Use
SARA	Gait, stance, limb coordination, speech, eye movements	Time-efficient; responsive to change	Limited sensitivity in very early disease	Routine clinical monitoring and follow-up
BARS	Core ataxic features	Rapid and simple	Reduced sensitivity to subtle changes	Screening and bedside assessment
ICARS	Posture, gait, limb coordination, speech, oculomotor function	Comprehensive and detailed	Time-consuming; examiner dependent	Research and detailed phenotyping
UMSARS	Ataxia, Parkinsonism, autonomic dysfunction	Disease-specific; multidomain	Limited generalizability	Multiple system atrophy

SUMMARY AND CONCLUSION

A variety of rating instruments are available to assess ataxia, each designed with distinct purposes and patient groups in mind. The Scale for the Assessment and Rating of Ataxia (SARA) and the Brief Ataxia Rating Scale (BARS) are concise, practical, and well-suited for everyday clinical follow-up. The International Cooperative Ataxia Rating Scale (ICARS) provides a detailed evaluation across multiple domains, but its length can limit routine application. Disease-specific measures such as the Friedreich Ataxia Rating Scale (FARS) and the Unified Multiple System Atrophy Rating Scale (UMSARS) add value by capturing clinical features unique to those disorders, including functional staging, daily living skills, and autonomic dysfunction.

Overall, no single tool meets the needs of every context. For rapid outpatient use, shorter scales like SARA or BARS are most practical. For research trials or baseline characterisation, ICARS remains useful due to its comprehensive nature. FARS and UMSARS, meanwhile, are essential for monitoring progression in Friedreich's ataxia and multiple system atrophy, respectively.

Conclusion: The choice of scale should be guided by the specific clinical question, disease type, and intended use. Incorporating these validated instruments enhances diagnostic accuracy, enables reliable monitoring of disease progression, and provides standardised outcome measures for clinical research. Looking forward, the integration of emerging digital technologies with established scales may further refine ataxia assessment by improving sensitivity and reducing examiner variability.

AI DISCLOSURE STATEMENT

During the preparation of this chapter, the authors used ChatGPT (OpenAI) as a support tool for language refinement, structural organisation, and clarification of ideas. All content generated with AI assistance was carefully reviewed, verified, and revised by the authors to ensure factual accuracy, originality, and consistency with the scientific literature. The authors take full responsibility for the integrity, interpretation, and final content of the published chapter.

ACKNOWLEDGEMENT

The authors extend their gratitude to clinicians, neuroscientists, and rehabilitation specialists who have contributed to the research and validation of ataxia assessment tools. Their ongoing work has been instrumental in improving diagnostic precision, functional evaluation, and therapeutic outcomes for individuals with cerebellar and sensory ataxias.

REFERENCES

[1] de Silva RN, Vallortigara J, Greenfield J, Hunt B, Giunti P, Hadjivassiliou M. Diagnosis and management of progressive ataxia in adults. Pract Neurol 2019; 19(3): 196-207. [http://dx.doi.org/10.1136/practneurol-2018-002096] [PMID: 31048364]

[2] Manto M, Serrao M, Filippo Castiglia S. Neurophysiology of cerebellar ataxias and gait disorders. Clin Neurophysiol Pract 2023; 8: 143-60. [http://dx.doi.org/10.1016/j.cnp.2023.07.002] [PMID: 37593693]

[3] Schmitz-Hübsch T, du Montcel ST, Baliko L, *et al.* Scale for the assessment and rating of ataxia. Neurology 2006; 66(11): 1717-20. [http://dx.doi.org/10.1212/01.wnl.0000219042.60538.92] [PMID: 16769946]

[4] Park J, Bremova-Ertl T, Brands M, *et al.* Assessment of the reliability, responsiveness, and meaningfulness of the scale for the assessment and rating of ataxia (SARA) for lysosomal storage disorders. J Neurol. 2024; 271(10): 6888-6902. [http://dx.doi.org/10.1007/s00415-024-12664-y]

[5] Kim BR, Lee JY, Kim MJ, Jung H, Lee J. Korean version of the scale for the assessment and rating of ataxia in ataxic stroke patients. Ann Rehabil Med 2014; 38(6): 742-51. [http://dx.doi.org/10.5535/arm.2014.38.6.742] [PMID: 25566472]

[6] Milne SC, Roberts M, Ross HL, *et al.* Interrater reliability of the scale for the assessment and rating of ataxia, Berg Balance Scale, and functional independence measure motor domain in individuals with hereditary cerebellar ataxia. Arch Phys Med Rehabil 2023; 104(10): 1646-51. [http://dx.doi.org/10.1016/j.apmr.2023.05.003] [PMID: 37268274]

[7] Weyer A, Abele M, Schmitz-Hübsch T, *et al.* Reliability and validity of the scale for the assessment and rating of ataxia: A study in 64 ataxia patients. Mov Disord 2007; 22(11): 1633-7. [http://dx.doi.org/10.1002/mds.21544] [PMID: 17516493]

[8] Yabe I, Matsushima M, Soma H, Basri R, Sasaki H. Usefulness of the Scale for Assessment and Rating of Ataxia (SARA). J Neurol Sci 2008; 266(1-2): 164-6. [http://dx.doi.org/10.1016/j.jns.2007.09.021] [PMID: 17950753]

[9] Potashman M, Popoff E, Powell L, *et al.* Psychometric validation of the modified functional Scale for the Assessment and Rating of Ataxia (f-SARA) in patients with spinocerebellar ataxia. Cerebellum 2024; 23(5): 2095-108. [http://dx.doi.org/10.1007/s12311-024-01707-9] [PMID: 38865059]

[10] Schmahmann JD, Gardner R, MacMore J, Vangel MG. Development of a brief ataxia rating scale (BARS) based on a modified form of the ICARS. Mov Disord 2009; 24(12): 1820-8. [http://dx.doi.org/10.1002/mds.22681] [PMID: 19562773]

[11] Perez-Lloret S, van de Warrenburg B, Rossi M, *et al.* Assessment of Ataxia Rating Scales and Cerebellar Functional Tests: Critique and Recommendations. Mov Disord. 2021; 36(2): 283-297. [http://dx.doi.org/10.1002/mds.28313]

[12] Camargos S, Cardoso F, Maciel R, *et al.* Brief Ataxia Rating Scale: A Reliable Tool to Rate Ataxia in a Short Timeframe. Mov Disord Clin Pract. 2016; 3(6): 621-623. [http://dx.doi.org/10.1002/mdc3.12364]

[13] Acar Arslan E, Erden A, Dilber B, *et al.* Turkish version of Brief Ataxia Rating Scale. Disabil Rehabil. 2021; 43(17): 2497-2501. [http://dx.doi.org/10.1080/09638288.2019.1701101]

[14] Trouillas P, Takayanagi T, Hallett M, *et al.* International Cooperative Ataxia Rating Scale for pharmacological assessment of the cerebellar syndrome. J Neurol Sci 1997; 145(2): 205-11. [http://dx.doi.org/10.1016/S0022-510X(96)00231-6] [PMID: 9094050]

[15] Schmitz-Hübsch T, Tezenas du Montcel S, Baliko L, *et al.* Reliability and validity of the International Cooperative Ataxia Rating Scale: A study in 156 spinocerebellar ataxia patients. Mov Disord 2006; 21(5): 699-704. [http://dx.doi.org/10.1002/mds.20781] [PMID: 16450347]

[16] Park J, Cho JW, Youn J, *et al.* Validity and reliability of the Korean-translated version of the International Cooperative Ataxia Rating Scale in cerebellar ataxia. J Mov Disord 2023; 16(1): 86-90. [http://dx.doi.org/10.14802/jmd.22137] [PMID: 36537063]

[17] Maggi FA, Braga-Neto P, Chien HF, *et al.* Cross-cultural adaptation and validation of the International Cooperative Ataxia Rating Scale (ICARS) to Brazilian Portuguese. Arq Neuropsiquiatr 2018; 76(10): 674-84. [http://dx.doi.org/10.1590/0004-282x20180098] [PMID: 30427507]

[18] Salcı Y, Fil A, Keklicek H, *et al.* Validity and reliability of the International Cooperative Ataxia Rating Scale (ICARS) and the Scale for the Assessment and Rating of Ataxia (SARA) in multiple sclerosis patients with ataxia. Mult Scler Relat Disord 2017; 18: 135-40. [http://dx.doi.org/10.1016/j.msard.2017.09.032] [PMID: 29141795]

[19] Subramony SH, May W, Lynch D, *et al.* Measuring Friedreich ataxia: Interrater reliability of a

neurologic rating scale. Neurology 2005; 64(7): 1261-2.
[http://dx.doi.org/10.1212/01.WNL.0000156802.15466.79] [PMID: 15824358]

[20] Cook A, Giunti P. Friedreich's ataxia: clinical features, pathogenesis and management. Br Med Bull. 2017 Dec 1; 124(1): 19-30. doi: 10.1093/bmb/ldx034. PMID: 29053830; PMCID: PMC5862303.

[21] Wenning GK, Tison F, Seppi K, *et al.* Development and validation of the Unified Multiple System Atrophy Rating Scale (UMSARS). Mov Disord 2004; 19(12): 1391-402.
[http://dx.doi.org/10.1002/mds.20255] [PMID: 15452868]

[22] Chikada A, Mitsui J, Matsukawa T, *et al.* Reliability and validity of Japanese version of Unified Multiple System Atrophy Rating Scale. Neurol Clin Neurosci 2021; 9(2): 171-80.
[http://dx.doi.org/10.1111/ncn3.12477]

[23] Schöls L, Bauer P, Schmidt T, Schulte T, Riess O. Autosomal dominant cerebellar ataxias: clinical features, genetics, and pathogenesis. Lancet Neurol 2004; 3(5): 291-304.
[http://dx.doi.org/10.1016/S1474-4422(04)00737-9] [PMID: 15099544]

[24] Seemann J, Daghsen L, Cazier M, *et al.* Digital Gait Measures Capture 1-Year Progression in Early-Stage Spinocerebellar Ataxia Type 2. Mov Disord 2024; 39: 788-797.
[http://dx.doi.org/10.1002/mds.29757]

[25] Knudson KC, Gupta AS. Assessing Cerebellar Disorders with Wearable Inertial Sensor Data Using Time-Frequency and Autoregressive Hidden Markov Model Approaches. Sensors (Basel) 2022; 22(23): 9454.
[http://dx.doi.org/10.3390/s22239454] [PMID: 36502155]

CHAPTER 6

Scales for Parkinson's Disease

Yashleen Kaur Sandhu[1,2], **Nidhi Sharma**[2,3], **Anshu Sharma**[2,4] and **Parveen Kumar**[5,*]

[1] *University School of Physiotherapy and Radiology, Rayat Bahra University, Mohali-140301, Punjab, India*

[2] *Maharishi Markandeshwar Institute of Physiotherapy and Rehabilitation, Maharishi Markandeshwar (Deemed to be University), Mullana, Ambala, Haryana, India*

[3] *Department of Physiotherapy, Amity Institute of Health Allied Sciences, Amity University, Noida, Uttar Pradesh, India*

[4] *Department of Physiotherapy, School of Health Care and Allied Science, G.D. Goenka University, Sohna, Haryana, India*

[5] *Pal Physiotherapy and Rehabilitation Centre, Pal Healthcare, Ambala City, Haryana, India*

Abstract: Parkinson's disease is a progressive neurodegenerative disorder primarily affecting motor function due to the loss of dopamine-producing neurons in the substantia nigra of the brain. This reduction in dopamine leads to common symptoms such as tremors, bradykinesia (slowed movement), muscle rigidity, and impaired balance. The disease also affects non-motor functions, contributing to symptoms like cognitive decline, mood disorders, sleep disturbances, and changes in speech and handwriting. While the exact cause of Parkinson's remains unknown, it is believed to involve a combination of genetic and environmental factors. Diagnosis is typically clinical, based on symptom presentation and physical examination. Treatment focuses on managing symptoms, often with medications such as levodopa to increase dopamine levels or dopamine agonists to mimic its effects. In advanced cases, surgical interventions like deep brain stimulation (DBS) may be considered. Although there is no cure, ongoing research seeks to understand the disease mechanisms better and develop more effective therapies to improve the quality of life for those affected by Parkinson's disease.

Keywords: Bradykinesia, Cognitive decline, Impaired balance, Rigidity, Tremors.

* **Corresponding author Parveen Kumar:** Pal Physiotherapy and Rehabilitation Centre, Pal Healthcare, Ambala City, Haryana, India; E-mail: parveen34134@gmail.com

Nidhi Sharma, Simranjeet Kaur & Parveen Kumar (Eds.)

INTRODUCTION

Parkinson's disease (PD) is a progressive neurodegenerative disorder that impacts both motor and non-motor pathways within the basal ganglia. The loss of dopamine-producing neurons in the substantia nigra results in key motor symptoms of PD, including bradykinesia, muscle stiffness, resting tremors, and impaired postural reflexes. PD presents as a distinct clinical syndrome with various causes and symptom patterns. Its diagnosis relies solely on clinical evaluation, requiring the use of multiple assessment tools, such as scales and questionnaires, to determine the disease stage and related comorbidities [1].

Pathogenesis

A key pathological process in PD involves the misfolding and abnormal accumulation of α-synuclein, a presynaptic protein that assembles into toxic oligomers and fibrils. These aggregates lead to the development of Lewy bodies, the characteristic intracellular inclusions found in PD (1–3). The spread of α-synuclein pathology through interconnected brain regions supports the prion-like hypothesis, suggesting that misfolded proteins can trigger similar misfolding in adjacent healthy neurons. Other contributing mechanisms are mitochondrial dysfunction, particularly defects in Complex I of the electron transport chain, oxidative stress caused by excessive free radical accumulation, neuroinflammation driven by activated microglia releasing pro-inflammatory cytokines, Disruption of protein degradation systems, especially autophagy-lysosomal pathway dysfunction, and genetic influences, including mutations in the SNCA, LRRK2, PARK2, and GBA genes [2, 3].

Risk Factors

PD arises from a complex interaction between genetic susceptibility and environmental exposures. Established risk factors include [4]:

- Advancing Age: The most significant predictor of PD onset
- Exposure to environmental toxins, such as pesticides (*e.g.*, paraquat), herbicides, heavy metals, and certain industrial solvents.
- Recurrent head injuries: They elevate the risk of neurodegeneration.
- Genetic Predisposition: It involves both autosomal dominant and recessive mutations.
- Gender biases: Men show a higher incidence than women.

Note: Tobacco use and caffeine intake have been linked to a reduced risk of PD, though the biological mechanisms behind this protective effect remain unclear.

Symptom Spectrum (Non- Motor)

While PD is primarily defined by its motor manifestations, non-motor symptoms often emerge years before motor decline and profoundly affect quality of life. They are autonomic dysfunction, sensory disturbances, neuropsychiatric symptoms, sleep disturbances, and cognitive decline. Hyposmia and constipation are particularly notable, as they often represent the earliest detectable prodromal indicators of PD [2].

Treatment

PD treatment is tailored to disease stage, symptom profile, and patient characteristics. However, treatments primarily offer symptom control, as no therapy has yet demonstrated consistent disease-modifying effects. There are conservative treatment which included pharmacological management and physiotherapy regime and another line is the surgical treatment.

Pharmacological treatment: This includes Levodopa (the gold standard), Dopamine agonist (like ropinirole), MAO inhibitors (like selegiline), COMT inhibitors, and anticholinergic drugs [5].

Surgical Treatments: Deep Brain Stimulation (DBS) of the subthalamic nucleus or globus pallidus internus is reserved for advanced PD with medication-resistant motor fluctuations. Risks include infection, mood changes, and neuropsychiatric complications [2].

Critical Analysis and Integration of Advancement

PD rating scales are well-established and extensively validated; their use should be interpreted in light of recent advancements in PD research. These include developments in biomarker identification (such as α-synuclein seed amplification assays), trials exploring neuroprotective therapies, digital mobility assessment tools, and personalised treatment approaches. Adopting a more integrated and critical perspective enables clinicians and researchers to [3]:

- Recognise the strengths and limitations of existing assessment instruments
- Acknowledge the need for comprehensive, multidimensional evaluations given PD's clinical heterogeneity
- Understand how emerging technologies and imaging modalities can enhance traditional clinical scales.
- Anticipate how ongoing research may pave the way for earlier diagnosis and more tailored therapeutic strategies.

Comprehensive assessment of PD requires standardised scales that quantify symptom severity, functional limitations, disease staging, treatment complications, and fall risk. These scales are essential for diagnosis, monitoring disease progression, planning treatment, evaluating therapy outcomes, and predicting prognosis. The scales and questionnaires used to diagnose and predict the prognosis of this condition are listed below:

THE UNIFIED PARKINSON'S DISEASE RATING SCALE (UPDRS)

Introduction

The Unified Parkinson's Disease Rating Scale (UPDRS) is a measure that helps to evaluate the severity and progression of PD. It was developed in 1987 and revised in 2003 by the Movement Disorder Society. This scale is considered the gold standard for monitoring responses to medications used to reduce signs and symptoms of the disease [6].

No. of Items [7]

The scale consists of a total of 3 domains and 31 items, in addition to the H&Y staging scale and the S&E ADL scale, and one domain of any complications of therapy, which makes this scale as a total of 6-domain scale.

Domains:

I Mentation, Behaviour, and Mood
II Activities of Daily Living
III Motor Examination

Additional domain: Complications of Therapy (in the past week)

Additional scale:

- Hoehn and Yahr Staging scale
- Schwab and England Activities on Daily Living Scale

Scale Draft

4 Parts:

Part 1: Mentation, Behaviour, and Mood

Activities of Daily Living

Motor Examination

Part 2: Complications of Therapy (in the past week)

Part 3: Hoehn and Yahr Staging

Part 4: Schwab and England Activities on Daily Living Scale

List of Items [6]

1. Intellectual impairment
2. Thought disorder
3. Depression
4. Motivational initiative
5. Speech
6. Salivation
7. Swallowing
8. Handwriting
9. Cutting food
10. Dressing
11. Hygiene
12. Turning in bed
13. Falling
14. Freezing
15. Walking
16. Tremor
17. Sensory complaints
18. Speech
19. Facial expression
20. Tremor at rest
21. Action of postural tremor
22. Rigidity
23. Finger taps
24. Hand movements
25. Rapid alternating movements
26. Leg agility
27. Arising from the chair
28. Posture
29. Gait

30. Postural stability
31. Body bradykinesia

Scoring and Interpretation

Subscale I to III= ordinal scale of range 0-4; higher scores indicate more disability

Subscale IV= optional scale between yes and no.

Interpretation: the higher the score; severe the disability in a person suffering from PD

Indication

People with PD

Modified Unified Parkinson's Disease Rating Scale (MDS-UPDRS)

The Movement Disorder Society reviewed the original UPDRS and gave a revised version of this scale, named the Modified Unified Parkinson's Disease Rating Scale (MDS-UPDRS). This version was created in the year 2007. This new version included the non-motor activities of daily living as depicted in Table **1** [8].

Table 1. Unified Parkinson's Disease Rating Scale (UPDRS): Original with its modified version (MDS-UPDRS) [8].

Original UPDRS Item	MDS-UPDRS Item
Part I	
Intellectual impairment	Cognitive impairment
Though disorder	Hallucinations and psychosis
Depression	Depressed mood
Motivation/initiative	Anxious mood Apathy
	Features of dopamine dysregulation syndrome
Sleep disturbances	Nighttime sleep problem
Sleep disturbances	Daytime sleepiness
Sensory complaints related to Parkinsonism	Pain and other sensations
	Urinary problems
	Constipation problems

(Table 1) cont.....

Original UPDRS Item	MDS-UPDRS Item
Symptomatic orthostasis	Lightheadedness on standing
	Fatigue
Part II	
Speech	Speech
Salivation	Salivation and drooling
Swallowing	Chewing and swallowing
Cutting food and handling utensils	Eating tasks
Dressing	Dressing
Hygiene	Hygiene
Handwriting	Handwriting
	Doing hobbies and other activities
Turning in bed and adjusting bedclothes	Turning in bed
Tremor	Tremor
Walking	Walking and balance
Freezing when walking	Freezing
Falls	
Parts III	
Speech	Speech
Facial expression	Facial expression
Rigidity	Rigidity of the neck and four extremities
Finger taps	Finger taps
Hand movements	Hand movements
Pronation/supination	Pronation/supination
	Toe tapping
Leg agility	Leg agility
Arising from chair	Arising from chair
Gait	Gait
	Freezing of gait
Postural stability	Postural stability
Posture	Posture

(Table 1) cont.....

Original UPDRS Item	MDS-UPDRS Item
Body bradykinesia	Global spontaneity of movement
Action/postural tremor	Postural tremor of hand
Action/postural tremor	Kinetic tremor of the hand
	Rest tremor amplitude
	Constancy of rest tremors
Part IV	
Dyskinesia duration	Time spent with dyskinesia
	Functional impact of dyskinesias
Off duration	Time spent in the OFF state
	Functional impact of fluctuations
Offs predictable (yes/no) Offs unpredictable (yes/no) Offs sudden (yes/no)	Complexity of motor fluctuations
Presence of early morning dystonia (yes/no)	Painful OFF-state dystonia

Conceptual mapping of items from the original UPDRS to the MDS-UPDRS.

No. of Items

The scale is a total of 50- question assessment tool.

This scale includes 4 parts:

- Part I: Non-Motor Experiences of Daily Living
- Part II: Motor Experiences of Daily Living
- Part III: Motor Examination
- Part IV: Motor Complications
- Part V: Modified Hoehn and Yahr Staging scale
- Part VI: Modified Schwab and England Activities on Daily Living Scale

Administration

This scale requires a total of 30 minutes to be completed. But the timing may be adjusted based on the severity of the disease.

Scoring and Interpretation

Subscale I to III= ordinal scale of range 0-4; higher scores indicate more disability

Subscale IV = optional scale between yes and no.

Interpretation: The higher the score, the severe the disability in a person suffering from PD.

Once these IV parts are completed, the Hoehn and Yahr staging scale and the Schwab and England Activities of Daily Living Scale are administered.

Indication

People with PD.

Languages [9]

This scale is available in Arabic, Bulgarian, Chinese, Czech, Dutch, Estonian, French, German, Greek, Hebrew, Hindi, Hungarian, Italian, Japanese, Kazakh, Korean, Polish, Portuguese, Romanian, Russian, Slovak, Spanish, Swedish, Thai, and Turkish.

Psychometric Properties

- **Reliability**

Cross-sectional Reliability: The ICC value came out to be 0.92 [8].

Longitudinal Reliability: Longitudinal reliability was excellent with the ICC value of 0.92 [8].

Reliable factor structures for each part were obtained (comparative fit index > 0.90 for each part), which support the use of sum scores for each part in preference to a total score of all parts.

Internal consistency: The internal consistency of this scale was high, with Cronbach's range of α =0.79-0.93 [8]

- **Validity**

Concurrent validity: Pearson's Correlation coefficient with the original version of the scale came out to be high, with the value of 0.93 ($p < 0.0001$) [8]

HOEHN AND YAHR SCALE

Introduction

The Hoehn and Yahr Scale, devised by Margaret Hoehn and Melvin Yahr in 1967, is a widely utilised tool for evaluating the progression of Parkinson's disease. It delineates the severity of symptoms and degree of disability across stages ranging from 0 to 5. Originally delineating unilateral and bilateral involvement [10].

No. of Items [11]

The scale consists of a total of 5 items or 5 stages that depict the level and severity of PD in patients, as shown in Table **2**.

Table 2. The hoehn and yahr scale.

Stages	Description
1	Unilateral involvement, usually with minimal or no functional disability.
2	Bilateral or midline involvement without the impairment of balance.
3	Bilateral disease: mild to moderate disability with impaired postural reflexes; physically independent
4	Severely disabling disease; still able to walk or stand unassisted.
5	Confinement to bed or a wheelchair unless aided

Stage 1: Unilateral involvement is present.
Stage 2: Bilateral involvement occurs.
Stage 3: Advancement to postural instability.
Stage 4: Loss of physical independence.
Stage 5: This stage is wheelchair bound or bedridden.

Administration

This scale takes around 10 minutes to complete.

Scoring and interpretation

Scoring is based on the patient's history, and the stage is marked accordingly.

The stage marked provides a detailed overview of the condition and its associated dependency/ disability that the patient is suffering from.

Stage 1: Unilateral involvement with the percentage of difficulty.
Stage 2: Bilateral involvement without the association of impaired balance.
Stage 3: Bilateral involvement with the impairment of postural reflexes and a state of independence
Stage 4: Severe disability with maximal assistance

Stage 5: This stage is marked when a person is a wheelchair user, *i.e.*, maximum level of dependency.

Indication

The scale has been applied to the staging of Parkinson's disease-related functional impairment. It assists in characterising the disease's course through several phases, enabling us to gauge the severity of the situation.

Types of Parkinsonism this scale fulfils: Primary PD and Secondary PD

Languages: This scale is available in the English language.

Psychometric Properties

- **Reliability**

Intra-rater: The scale shows excellent intra-rater reliability with the value of the inter-class correlation coefficient: ICC= 0.99 [10]

Inter-rater: The scale shows excellent intra-rater reliability with the value of the inter-class correlation coefficient: ICC= 0.95 [10]

Bland-Altman plots: The plot shows a narrow confidence interval, and the mean difference is close to 0 [12].

- **Validity**

Construct validity: The construct validity of the scale was calculated using Spearman's rho correlation, which came out to be good the value ranging between 0.51 and 0.63 [10].

Content validity: The scale shows a good level of content validity with the value of 0.63 [12].

Specificity

The scale shows a specificity of 98%, which is excellent [12].

Modified Hoehn and Yahr Scale

Introduction: This scale was modified in the year 1983 by Larsen *et al.* The original scale has undergone modifications to incorporate additional stages, such as 1.5 and 2.5, for a more nuanced assessment. This scale, often utilised in conjunction with the Unified Parkinson's Disease Rating Scale, assists in precise diagnosis, treatment planning, and monitoring of Parkinson's disease advancements [13].

No. of Items

As shown in Table **3**, this scale has 7 items and includes 2 additional levels compared to the previous one.

Table 3. Modified hoehn and yahr scale.

Stages	Description
1	Unilateral involvement only
1.5	Unilateral and axial involvement
2	Bilateral involvement without impairment of balance
2.5	Mild bilateral disease with recovery on pull test
3	Mild to moderate bilateral disease; some postural instability; physically independent
4	Severe disability; still able to walk or stand unassisted
5	Wheelchair bound or bedridden unless aided

Stage 1: Unilateral involvement.
Stage 1.5: Axial involvement
Stage 2: Bilateral involvement.
Stage 2.5: Bilateral but recovery from pull
Stage 3: Postural instability.
Stage 4: Loss of physical independence.
Stage 5: This stage is wheelchair bound or bedridden.

Administration

This scale takes around 10 minutes to complete.

Scoring and Interpretation

The scoring is done based on the history provided by the patient, and the stage is marked accordingly.

- Stage 1.0: Symptoms are very mild; unilateral involvement only.
- Stage 1.5: Unilateral and axial involvement
- Stage 2: Bilateral involvement without the impairment of balance
- Stage 2.5: Mild bilateral disease with recovery on pull test

- Stage 3: Mild to moderate bilateral disease; some postural instability; physically independent
- Stage 4: Severe disability; still able to walk or stand unassisted.
- Stage 5: Wheelchair bound or bedridden unless aided.

The stage marked a detailed overview of the condition and its associated dependency/ disability that the patient is suffering from.

Indication

Patients with primary and secondary PD are administered this scale.

Languages

This scale is available in the English language.

TIMED UP AND GO TEST (TUG)

Introduction

The Timed Up and Go (TUG) test, published by Podsiadlo and Richardson in 1991, is an adaptation of the "Get Up and Go" test introduced by Mathias *et al.* in 1986. The TUG test incorporates a timing element to evaluate balance and functional mobility. It involves performing sequential motor tasks during walking and turning [14].

No. of items

The TUG test does not involve specific items. A person must get out of a chair (which should not be against a wall), walk three meters, turn around, walk back to the chair, and then sit down to score TUG. The scoring criteria and age-matched norms are displayed in Tables **4** and **5**, respectively.

Table 4. Scoring and interpretation [14].

Score	Interpretation
Less than 10 seconds	Completely independent (With or without walking aid for ambulation and transfers).
Less than 20 seconds	Independent for main transfers (With or without walking aid, independent for basic tub or shower transfers and able to climb most stairs and go outside alone).
More than 30 seconds	Requires assistance. Dependent on most activities)

Table 5. Age-matched norms [14].

Age (in Years)	Mean Time (in Seconds)
60-69	7.9 ± -0.9
70-79	7.7 ± -2.3
80-89	No device: 11.0 ± -2.2 With device: 19.9 ± -6.4
90-101	No device: 14.7 ± -7.9 With device: 19.9 ± -2.5

Timing begins when the verbal cue "go" is given and ends when the client returns to a seated position. The individual wears their usual footwear and may use their walking aid (cane/walker), with its use noted on the data collection form. No physical assistance is provided.

Administration

A practice trial is allowed to be versed with the test performance. This is done to avoid any errors or incorrect recordings. This test requires 1-2 minutes to administer.

Indications[15]

Patients with:

- Parkinson's disease
- Multiple sclerosis
- Vertigo
- Cerebellar disorders.
- Alzheimer's disease
- Hip fracture.
- Total Knee Arthroplasty
- Huntington disease

Languages

Not Applicable. This is a test that requires a verbal command and the recording of performance timings.

Psychometric Properties
Reliability
Test-retest reliability

In frail elderly patients, the test shows excellent test-retest reliability (ICC = 0.99) [14].
In community-dwelling older adults, the ICC value was 0.97, which is excellent [16].
In patients with Parkinson's disease, the ICC value ranged between 0.87 and 0.99 [17].
In a stroke patient, the ICC value was 0.95, showing excellent reliability [18].

Intra-rater reliability

The scale has an excellent ICC value depicting high intra-rater reliability; ICC= 0.99 [14].

Inter-rater reliability

The scale has an excellent level of inter-rater reliability with an ICC value of 0.99 [14].

Sensitivity

The scale has a high level of sensitivity, with the numeric values of 80% [19].

Specificity

The scale is highly specific with the numeric values of 87% [15].

BERG BALANCE SCALE (BBS)

Introduction

The Berg Balance Scale is a tool used to assess functional balance. Developed by Katherine Berg in 1989, it was originally designed to evaluate balance in older adults, with the initial group averaging 73 years of age. The scale measures both static and dynamic balance through fourteen mobility-related tasks. It was primarily used for stroke patients, but is now applied across various patient populations [20].

No. of Items

The ordinal scale consists of 14 items or tasks, each scored from 0 to 4 based on the level of functionality. These 14 items are categorised into 3 groups.

1. Sitting balance: Sitting unsupported
2. Standing balance: Standing unsupported
    - Standing with eyes closed
    - Standing with feet together
    - Standing with one foot in front
    - Standing on one foot
    - Turning to look behind
    - Retrieving an object from the floor
    - Reaching forward with an outstretched arm
3. Dynamic balance: Sitting to standing
    - Standing to sitting
    - Turning 360 degrees
    - Placing the alternate foot on the stool
    - Transfers

Administration

The administration of this scale requires around 15 to 20 minutes, and no specific training is required for this. The scale is administered on the adult and elderly population as well.

Equipment:

- Yardstick
- One standard chair with armrests
- One standard chair without armrests
- Footstool/step
- Stopwatch or wristwatch
- 15-foot walkway

Scoring and Interpretation: Total Score = 56

The scale has 5 points, ranging from 0 to 4, where 4 indicates the least problem, and 0 indicates the highest level of problem. The maximum score is 56, and the minimum is 0. The lower the score great the functional capacities [21, 22].

- A score of < 45 indicates a greater risk of falling.
- 41-56 = Low fall risk

- 21-40 = Medium fall risk
- 0 –20 = High fall risk

Indications

This scale can be administered to patients suffering from-

- Parkinson's disease
- Osteoarthritis
- Lower limb Amputation
- Vestibular problems
- Spinal cord injuries
- Multiple sclerosis
- Traumatic Brain Injuries
- Intellectual disabilities

Languages

This scale is available in multiple translations, such as Brazilian [23], Urdu [24], Russian [25], Arabic [26], Italian [27], Marathi [28], and Greek [29].

Psychometric Properties

- **Reliability**

Test-retest Reliability

The Test-retest reliability of this scale, when administered to TBI patients, was excellent, with ICC values of 0.99 [30].

When tested on older adults, the scale showed good test-retest reliability (ICC = 0.77) [31], and when tested on older adults living in nursing homes, it showed excellent test-retest reliability (ICC = 0.88) [32].

Inter-rater Reliability

The inter-rater reliability for this scale, when administered to community-dwelling older adults, was excellent, with an ICC of 0.98 [21].

The inter-rater reliability in older adults living in nursing homes was excellent, with an ICC of 0.993 [32].

Intra-rater reliability

The inter-rater reliability for this scale, when administered to community-dwelling older adults, was excellent, with an ICC of 0.98 [33].

• Validity

Criterion Validity

The validity of this scale, when compared with the dynamic gait index, was good, with a value of r=0.67 [34].

Construct Validity

The validity was excellent, with a value of r r= 0.95 [32].

Berg Balance Scale

1. SITTING TO STANDING

INSTRUCTIONS: Please stand up. Try not to use your hand for support.

( ) 4 able to stand without using hands and stabilise independently.
( ) 3 able to stand independently using a hand.
( ) 2 able to stand using hands after several tries.
( ) 1 needs minimal aid to stand or stabilise.
( ) 0 needs moderate or maximal assistance to stand.

1. STANDING UNSUPPORTED

INSTRUCTIONS: Please stand for two minutes without holding on.

( ) 4 able to stand safely for 2 minutes.
( ) 3 able to stand 2 minutes with supervision.
( ) 2 able to stand 30 seconds unsupported.
( ) 1 needs several tries to stand 30 seconds unsupported.
( ) 0 unable to stand 30 seconds unsupported.
If a subject is able to stand 2 minutes unsupported, score full points for sitting unsupported. Proceed to item #4

SITTING WITH BACK UNSUPPORTED BUT FEET SUPPORTED ON FLOOR OR ON A STOOL

INSTRUCTIONS: Please sit with arms folded for 2 minutes.

( ) 4 able to sit safely and securely for 2 minutes.
( ) 3 able to sit 2 minutes under supervision.
( ) 2 able to sit 30 seconds.
( ) 1 able to sit 10 seconds.
( ) 0 unable to sit without support 10 seconds.

STANDING TO SITTING

INSTRUCTIONS: Please sit down.

( ) 4 sits safely with minimal use of hands.
( ) 3 controls descent by using hands.
( ) 2 uses the back of the legs against the chair to control descent.
( ) 1 sits independently but has uncontrolled descent.
( ) 0 needs assistance to sit.

TRANSFERS

INSTRUCTIONS: Arrange chair(s) for pivot transfer. Ask the subject to transfer one way toward a seat with armrests and one way toward a seat without armrests. You may use two chairs (one with and one without armrests) or a bed and a chair.

( ) 4 able to transfer safely with minor use of hands.
( ) 3 able to transfer safely, definite need of hands.
( ) 2 able to transfer with verbal cuing and/or supervision.
( ) 1 needs one person to assist.
( ) 0 needs two people to assist or supervise for safety.

STANDING UNSUPPORTED WITH EYES CLOSED

INSTRUCTIONS: Please close your eyes and stand still for 10 seconds.

( ) 4 able to stand 10 seconds safely.
( ) 3 able to stand 10 seconds with supervision.
( ) 2 able to stand for 3 seconds.

( ) 1 unable to keep eyes closed for 3 seconds, but stays safely.
( ) 0 needs help to keep from falling.

STANDING UNSUPPORTED WITH FEET TOGETHER

INSTRUCTIONS: Place your feet together and stand without holding on.

( ) 4 able to place feet together independently and stand for 1 minute safely.
( ) 3 able to place feet together independently and stand 1 minute with supervision.
( ) 2 able to place feet together independently, but unable to hold for 30 seconds.
( ) 1 needs help to attain a position, but can stand 15 seconds with feet together.
( ) 0 needs help to attain a position and is unable to hold for 15 seconds.

REACHING FORWARD WITH OUTSTRETCHED ARM WHILE STANDING

INSTRUCTIONS: Lift arm to 90 degrees. Stretch out your fingers and reach forward as far as you can. (Examiner places a ruler at the end of fingertips when the arm is at 90 degrees. Fingers should not touch the ruler while reaching forward. The recorded measure is the distance forward that the fingers reach in the subject's most forward lean position. When possible, ask the subject to use both arms when reaching to avoid rotation of the trunk).

( ) 4 can reach forward confidently 25 cm (10 inches).
( ) 3 can reach forward 12 cm (5 inches).
( ) 2 can reach forward 5 cm (2 inches).
( ) 1 reaches forward but needs supervision.
( ) 0 loses balance while trying/requires external support.

PICK UP OBJECT FROM THE FLOOR FROM A STANDING POSITION

INSTRUCTIONS: Pick up the shoe/slipper, which is placed in front of your feet.

( ) 4 able to pick up a slipper safely and easily.
( ) 3 able to pick up a slipper but needs supervision.
( ) 2 unable to pick up but reaches 2-5 cm(1-2 inches) from slipper and keeps balance independently.

( ) 1 is unable to pick up and needs supervision while trying.
( ) 0 unable to try/needs assist to keep from losing balance or falling.

TURNING TO LOOK BEHIND OVER LEFT AND RIGHT SHOULDERS WHILE STANDING

INSTRUCTIONS: Turn to look directly behind you over toward the left shoulder. Repeat to the right. The examiner may pick an object directly behind the subject to encourage better twisting and turning.

( ) 4 looks behind from both sides, and weight shifts well.
( ) 3 looks behind one side, only the other side shows less weight shift.
( ) 2 turn sideways only, but maintain balance.
( ) 1 needs supervision when turning.
( ) 0 needs assistance to keep from losing balance or falling.

TURN 360 DEGREES

INSTRUCTIONS: Turn completely around in a full circle. Pause. Then turn a full circle in the other direction.

( ) 4 able to turn 360 degrees safely in 4 seconds or less.
( ) 3 able to turn 360 degrees safely, one side only 4 seconds or less.
( ) 2 able to turn 360 degrees safely but slowly.
( ) 1 needs close supervision or verbal cuing.
( ) 0 needs assistance while turning.

PLACE ALTERNATE FOOT ON STEP OR STOOL WHILE STANDING UNSUPPORTED

INSTRUCTIONS: Place each foot alternately on the step/stool. Continue until each foot has touched the step/stool four times.

( ) 4 able to stand independently and safely, and complete 8 steps in 20 seconds.
( ) 3 able to stand independently and complete 8 steps in > 20 seconds.
( ) 2 able to complete 4 steps without aid with supervision.
( ) 1 able to complete > 2 steps needs minimal assistance.
( ) 0 needs assistance to keep from falling/unable to try.

STANDING UNSUPPORTED ONE FOOT IN FRONT

INSTRUCTIONS: (DEMONSTRATE TO SUBJECT) Place one foot directly in front of the other. If you feel that you cannot place your foot directly in front, try to step far enough ahead that the heel of your forward foot is ahead of the toes of the other foot. (To score 3 points, the length of the step should exceed the length of the other foot, and the width of the stance should approximate the subject's normal stride width.)

( ) 4 able to place foot tandem independently and hold for 30 seconds.
( ) 3 able to place foot ahead independently and hold for 30 seconds.
( ) 2 able to take a small step independently and hold for 30 seconds.
( ) 1 needs help to step, but can hold for 15 seconds.
( ) 0 loses balance while stepping or standing.

STANDING ON ONE LEG

INSTRUCTIONS: Stand on one leg as long as you can without holding on.

( ) 4 able to lift leg independently and hold for> 10 seconds
( ) 3 able to lift leg independently and hold for 5-10 seconds
( ) 2 able to lift leg independently and hold for≥ 3 seconds
( ) 1 tries to lift the leg, unable to hold for 3 seconds, but remains standing independently.
( ) 0 unable to try and needs assistance to prevent a fall
TOTAL SCORE: ______ / 56

FUNCTIONAL REACH TEST (FRT)

Introduction

The Functional Reach test (FRT) was developed in 1990 by Pamela Duncan and colleagues. This is a single-task, dynamic assessment designed to help predict fall risk in older adults. This test evaluates both the stability margin and balance capability during a functional activity. The FRT clinical measure of balance is calculated as the difference between an individual's arm length and their maximum forward reach while maintaining a fixed base of support [35].

No. of Items

FRT evaluates a patient's stability by measuring the farthest distance they can reach forward while maintaining a fixed standing position. The patient must be able to stand unsupported for at least 30 seconds and flex their shoulder to at least 90 degrees.

Procedure

The patient is asked to stand close to, but not touching, a wall, positioning the arm nearest the wall at 90 degrees of shoulder flexion with the fist closed. The assessor records the starting position at the third metacarpal head on the yardstick. The patient is then instructed to reach forward as far as possible without lifting their feet from the ground. The position of the third metacarpal is recorded again. The reach distance is calculated as the difference between the starting and ending positions, typically measured in inches. Three trials are performed, and the average of the last two is recorded as shown in Table **6** [36].

Table 6. Functional Reach Test (FRT).

<table>
<tr><th colspan="2">NAME:</th><th colspan="2">Date:</th></tr>
<tr><td>Trails:</td><td>1</td><td>2</td><td>3</td></tr>
<tr><td>Recordings:</td><td></td><td></td><td></td></tr>
</table>

Administration

The scale takes 4-5 minutes to complete, and no prior training is required to perform this scale.

Scoring and interpretation

The normative value for the Functional Reach Test (FRT) is 26.6 cm (approximately 10.5 inches) for older adults living in the community and 15.4 cm for those not living in the community, as described in Table **7** [37].

Table 7. Age-specific normative values.

Age (in Years)	Men (Dist. in Inches)	Women (Dist. in Inches)
20-40	16.7 ± 1.9	14.6 ± 2.2
41-69	14.9 ± 2.2	13.8 ± 2.2
70-87	13.2 ± 1.6	10.5 ± 3.5

The readings are noted as [38]:

- **10"/25 cm or greater:** Low risk of falls
- **6"/15cm to 10"/25cm** . The risk of falling is twice as great as normal.
- **6"/15cm or less**. The risk of falling is four times greater than normal
- **Unwilling to reach:** Risk of falling is much greater (eight times) than normal.

The cut-off scores for FRT are as follows:

For Community Dwelling Elderly

- FRT < 7 inches:
- Unable to leave the neighbourhood without help
- Limited in mobility skills
- Most restricted in ADLs

Frail Elderly Patients: FRT< 18.5 cm indicates fall risk [39].

Indications

This scale can be administered to the patients of:

- Parkinson's disease
- People suffering from movement disorders
- SCI
- Stroke recovery
- Vestibular disorders
- Older Adults and Geriatric care people

Languages

Since this outcome measure involves only demonstration and instruction, with recordings as the sole documentation, translation is neither necessary nor available. The procedure is explained verbally, eliminating any language barriers.

Psychometric properties

- **Reliability**

The test-retest reliability of this scale is excellent, with an ICC of 0.89 [39].

The inter-rater reliability for asymptomatic adults was ICC = 0.99 [40], and for Community-Dwelling Elderly, ICC = 0.98 [41]. For Frail Elderly Patients, the ICC was 0.97, indicating excellent reliability [39].

The Intra-rater reliability for asymptomatic adults was excellent, with an ICC of 0.90 [40], and for Frail Elderly Patients, it was ICC = 0.92 [42].

- **Validity**

Criterion Validity of the scale showed a good correlation (r r= 0.76) [39].

The sensitivity of this scale was 76%, and the specificity was 46% [43].

MODIFIED FUNCTIONAL REACH TEST (MFRT)

Introduction

The Modified Functional Reach Test (mFRT) is a clinical assessment tool used to evaluate a patient's balance and functional mobility in a seated position. The original version involved only a standing component, but this includes a seated variation as well.

The mFRT was designed specifically for individuals with spinal cord injuries (SCI). Anyone with 90 degrees of shoulder flexion should be able to perform this test. The test simulates functional movements needed in daily life. It can differentiate between individuals with abdominal and back extensor function (*e.g.*, those with high tetraplegia or high paraplegia *versus* low paraplegia), though it cannot distinguish between individuals with higher-level lesions [44].

No. of Items

There are no specific items. The task is performed in 3 directions: a) Forward reach, b) Lateral reach to the left, and c) Lateral reach to the right, as shown in Table **8**. The patient is taught about the procedure; if required, a demonstration is provided, and then asked to perform the test.

Table 8. Modified Functional Reach Test (mFRT).

Direction	Trail 1	Trail 2	Trail 3
Forward reach			
Lateral reach to the left			
Lateral reach to the right			

Procedure

The patient is seated in a chair with hips, knees, and ankles bent at 90 degrees. The arm is raised to 90 degrees with the fist closed. The patient then reaches forward as far as they can without losing balance, moving at a comfortable pace.

The maximum reach distance is recorded. For reference, the ulnar styloid process is considered [45].

Administration

The scale can be completed in just 4-5 minutes and does not require any prior training for its administration. A 15-second break is provided before proceeding to the next trial. Table **9** presents the scoring and interpretation, where the average score across all three trials is considered, and results are provided.

Table 9. Scoring and interpretation [46].

Direction	Normative Values (in cm)
Forward reach	34.05 ± 9.03 cm
Lateral reach to the left	18.2 ± 5.26 cm
Lateral reach to the right	17.32 ± 5.21 cm

Indications

The enlisted category is targeting population for this test:

- Parkinson's disease
- Spinal cord injury
- Stroke recovery
- Vestibular disorders
- Older adults and geriatric care.

Languages

This outcome measure relies solely on demonstration and verbal instruction, with recordings serving as the only form of documentation. Therefore, translation is not required or provided, as the procedure is explained verbally, removing any language barriers.

Psychometric Properties

• Reliability

The test-retest reliability of this scale is excellent, with an ICC of 0.94 [47].

The inter-rater reliability for the scale, when calculated, was ICC = 0.89, which was excellent [46].

• Validity

Criterion Validity, when calculated, was adequate, with numeric values ranging from 0.58 to 0.60 across all test directions ($p<0.05$) [42].

Face validity of this test came out to be high, with the value of $r=0.71$ [46].

PARKINSON'S DISEASE QUESTIONNAIRE – 39 (PDQ-39)

Introduction

The PDQ-39 is a self-report questionnaire consisting of 39 items, which evaluates health-related quality of life specific to Parkinson's disease over the past month [44]. It measures how frequently patients encounter challenges across eight dimensions of quality of life. Additionally, it examines the effects of Parkinson's disease on various aspects of functioning and well-being [48, 49].

No. of Items [49]

The PDQ-39 consists of 39 items organised into eight distinct areas, each addressing specific domains of health and well-being:

1. Mobility (10 items, 1-10)
2. Activities of Daily Living (6 items, 11-16)
3. Emotional Well-being (6 items, 17-22)
4. Stigma (4 items, 23-26)
5. Social Support (3 items, 27-29)
6. Cognitions (4 items, 30-33)
7. Communication (3 items, 34-36)
8. Bodily Discomfort (3 items, 37-39)

Respondents indicate how often they experience difficulties in these domains over the past month, using a five-point Likert scale from "0 = never" to "4 = always or cannot do at all".

Administration: Requires 10-20 minutes.

Scoring and Interpretation

Each dimension's total score ranges from 0 (no difficulty) to 100 (constant difficulty), with lower scores indicating a better quality of life. The score for each dimension is calculated by summing the scores of all items within that dimension, dividing by the maximum possible score for those items, and then multiplying by 100. The overall score can be summarised using the Parkinson's Disease Summary Index (PDSI) or the PDQ-39 Summary Index (PDQ-39 SI), which is derived by summing the total scores across all dimensions and dividing by 8 [50, 51].

Populations

- Parkinson's Disease
- Non-Specific Patient Population [52]
- Movement and Gait Disorders [53]

Languages

- Korean [54]
- Standard Chinese [55]
- Persian [56]
- French [49]
- Swedish

PDQ- 39 Questionnaire [6]

Due to having Parkinson's disease, how often during the last month have you....

1. Had difficulty doing the leisure activities that you would like to do?
2. Had difficulty looking after your home, *e.g.*, DIY, housework, cooking?
3. Had difficulty carrying bags of shopping?
4. Had problems walking half a mile?
5. Had problems walking 100 yards?
6. Had problems getting around the house as easily as you would like?
7. Had difficulty getting around in public?
8. Needed someone else to accompany you when you went out?
9. Felt frightened or worried about falling over in public?
10. Been confined to the house more than you would like?
11. Had difficulty washing yourself?
12. Had difficulty dressing yourself?

13. Had problems doing up your shoe laces?
14. Had problems writing clearly?
15. Had difficulty cutting up your food?
16. Had difficulty holding a drink without spilling it?
17. Felt depressed?
18. Felt isolated and lonely?
19. Felt weepy or tearful?
20. Felt angry or bitter?
21. Felt anxious?
22. Felt worried about your future?
23. Felt you had to conceal your Parkinson's from people?
24. Avoided situations that involve eating or drinking in public?
25. Felt embarrassed in public due to having Parkinson's disease?
26. Felt worried by other people's reaction to you?
27. Had problems with your close personal relationships?
28. Lacked support in the ways you need from your spouse or partner?
29. Lacked support in the ways you need from your family or close friends?
30. Unexpectedly fallen asleep during the day?
31. Had problems with your concentration, *e.g.*, when reading or watching TV?
32. Felt your memory was bad?
33. Had distressing dreams or hallucinations?
34. Had difficulty with your speech?
35. Felt unable to communicate with people properly?
36. Felt ignored by people?
37. Had painful muscle cramps or spasms?
38. Had aches and pains in your joints or body?
39. Felt unpleasantly hot or cold?

Psychometric Properties

• Reliability

Intra-rater: Studies have reported ICC values for the PDQ-39 ranging from 0.47 to 0.96, indicating varying levels of reliability across its different domains [57 - 59].

Inter-rater: Studies have reported ICC values ranging from 0.81 to 0.91, indicating high levels of reliability across its various dimensions [60, 61].

Internal Consistency: The Cronbach's alpha for the PDQ-39 has been reported to range from 0.66 to 0.98 across its various dimensions [62, 63].

• Validity

Construct validity: The PDQ-39 has demonstrated strong construct validity by effectively discriminating between different stages of Parkinson's disease. Studies have shown that scores on the PDQ-39 increase with disease progression, indicating that it can accurately reflect the worsening quality of life associated with more advanced stages of Parkinson's disease [64, 65].

Content validity: Items for the PDQ-39 were developed based on in-depth interviews with patients, prioritising their experiences over existing clinical scales. While this approach enhances the questionnaire's relevance, it has been noted to lack coverage in certain important areas, such as transfers, nighttime sleep issues, sexuality, self-image, and role functioning [66].

PARKINSON'S DISEASE QUESTIONNAIRE - 8

Introduction

The PDQ-8 is a short-form version that includes only 8 items, each selected from one of the eight dimensions of the PDQ-39. The PDQ-8 was developed to reduce respondent burden and is ideal for settings where time is limited or a quicker assessment is needed [67].

No. of Items

One question from each of the eight domains of the PDQ-39—mobility, activities of daily living, emotional well-being, stigma, social support, cognition, communication, and bodily discomfort—was selected based on its strong correlation with the overall domain score [49, 68].

Administration: It typically takes about 5 to 10 minutes to complete [68].

Scoring and Interpretation

Each question is scored on a scale from 0 to 4, where:

0 = Never
1 = Occasionally
2 = Sometimes
3 = Often
4 = Always or cannot do at all

The total score is calculated by summing the individual scores, with higher scores indicating poorer quality of life. The total score is then divided by the maximum possible score and expressed as a percentage out of 100.

Populations: Parkinson's Disease

Languages: The PDQ-8 is available in over 80 languages [69, 70].

PDQ- 8 Questionnaire

Due to having Parkinson's disease, how often during the last month have you…

1. Had difficulty getting around in public?
2. Had difficulty dressing yourself?
3. Felt depressed?
4. Had problems with your close personal relationships?
5. Had problems with your concentration, *e.g.*, when reading or watching TV?
6. Felt unable to communicate with people properly?
7. Had painful muscle cramps or spasms?
8. Felt embarrassed in public due to having Parkinson's disease?

Psychometric Properties

- **Reliability**

Intra-rater / Inter-rater: There is a significant correlation between the summary scores of the PDQ-8 and the PDQ-39, with a correlation coefficient of $r=0.93$ ($P<0.001$) [68].

Internal Consistency: The PDQ-8 demonstrates acceptable internal consistency, with a Cronbach's α of 0.80 and item-scale correlation coefficients ranging from 0.56 to 0.72 [68].

- **Validity**

The PDQ-8 demonstrates strong convergent and concurrent validity [70].

FREEZING OF GAIT QUESTIONNAIRE (FOG-Q)

Introduction

Developed by Giladi *et al.* [71], the FOG-Q consists of 6 items that quantify the frequency and severity of freezing episodes experienced by patients. The updated version, called the New Freezing of Gait Questionnaire (NFOG-Q), comprises 9 items and aims to improve upon the FOG-Q by providing a more comprehensive assessment of FOG. It includes questions about the patient's experience over the past month, focusing on the impact of freezing on daily activities and mobility [72].

No. of Items

This 6-item questionnaire includes four items that evaluate the severity of FOG and two items that assess gait. Respondents use a 5-point interval scale for each item. The total score can range from 0 to 24, with higher scores indicating more severe FOG. It is recommended to complete the questionnaire during the "on" phase or when the patient is in their best state.

Administration

It takes about 5- 10 minutes

Scoring and Interpretation

The scoring system consists of 6 items, each rated on a scale from 0 to 4, where 0 indicates the absence of symptoms and 4 the most severe stage of FOG. The total score can range from 0 to 24, with higher scores indicating more severe freezing episodes.

Populations: Parkinson's Disease

Languages

- Portuguese
- Spanish
- Swedish [73]
- Chinese [74]

Freezing of Gait Questionnaire (FOGQ)

1. During your worst state—Do you walk:
    1. Normally
    2. Almost normally—somewhat slow
    3. Slow but fully independent
    4. Need assistance or a walking aid
    5. Unable to walk
2. Are your gait difficulties affecting your daily activities and independence?
    1. Not at all

   2. Mildly
   3. Moderately
   4. Severely
   5. Unable to walk
3. Do you feel that your feet get glued to the floor while walking, making a turn, or when trying to initiate walking (freezing)?
   1. Never
   2. Very rarely—about once a month
   3. Rarely—about once a week
   4. Often—about once a day
   5. Always—whenever walking
4. How long is your longest freezing episode?
   1. Never happened
   2. 1–2 s
   3. 3–10 s
   4. 11–30 s
   5. Unable to walk for more than 30 s
5. How long is your typical start hesitation episode (freezing when initiating the first step)?
   1. None
   2. Takes longer than 1 s to start walking
   3. Takes longer than 3 s to start walking
   4. Takes longer than 10 s to start walking
   5. Takes longer than 30 s to start walking
6. How long is your typical turning hesitation: (freezing when turning)
   1. None
   2. Resume turning in 1–2 s
   3. Resume turning in 3–10 s
   4. Resume turning in 11–30 s
   5. Unable to resume turning for more than 30 s

Psychometric Properties

• Reliability

Intra-rater / Inter-rater: Good to excellent inter-rater reliability [70, 74].

Internal Consistency: High internal consistency (Cronbach's alpha ranging from 0.94 to 0.95) [28].

• **Validity**

Criterion validity: Strong positive correlation between the Thai version of the FOGQ and MDS-UPDRS item 2.13 (r = 0.81) and moderate correlations with other relevant measures like the Timed Up and Go test (TUG) (r = 0.42-0.60) and the Falls Efficacy Scale-International (FES-I) [75].

Content validity: High CVI scores for the FOGQ [74].

CLINICAL CONSIDERATIONS, STRENGTHS, LIMITATIONS, AND EMERGING PERSPECTIVES

Parkinson's disease (PD) is a progressive neurodegenerative disorder characterised by a complex combination of motor and non-motor manifestations. While cardinal motor features such as bradykinesia, rigidity, tremor, and postural instability remain central to diagnosis and staging, non-motor symptoms, including cognitive impairment, mood disorders, autonomic dysfunction, sleep disturbances, and reduced quality of life, often contribute equally, if not more significantly, to overall disease burden. Consequently, a comprehensive assessment of Parkinson's disease requires the use of multiple, complementary scales that address impairment, activity limitations, participation, and patient-reported outcomes.

The Unified Parkinson's Disease Rating Scale (UPDRS) remains the cornerstone for clinical and research assessment of Parkinson's disease. Its multidimensional structure allows evaluation of mentation, activities of daily living, motor function, and treatment-related complications. One of the major strengths of the UPDRS is its ability to provide a standardised framework for tracking disease progression over time. However, its comprehensive nature also represents a practical limitation. Administration can be time-consuming, and inter-rater variability may occur without adequate training. Additionally, while motor aspects are well represented, non-motor symptoms may still be underemphasized, particularly in earlier versions of the scale.

The Hoehn and Yahr Scale provides a simple, intuitive method for staging disease severity, primarily based on motor involvement and postural instability. Its ease of use makes it valuable for rapid clinical communication and broad categorisation of disease stage. Nevertheless, the scale provides only a coarse representation of disease progression and does not account for symptom asymmetry, non-motor manifestations, or functional impact. As a result, it is best used as a supplementary staging tool rather than as a standalone outcome measure.

Functional mobility and balance assessments such as the Timed Up and Go (TUG) test, Berg Balance Scale (BBS), and Functional Reach Test (FRT) address important aspects of postural control and fall risk in Parkinson's disease. These tools are particularly relevant in rehabilitation settings, where balance impairment and gait dysfunction are major contributors to disability. While these measures are practical and widely validated, they may demonstrate ceiling effects in early disease and reduced sensitivity to subtle gait abnormalities. Performance may also be influenced by medication state ("on" *versus* "off"), highlighting the importance of standardised testing conditions.

Patient-reported outcome measures such as the Parkinson's Disease Questionnaire–39 (PDQ-39) and its abbreviated version, PDQ-8, provide valuable insight into the subjective impact of the disease on quality of life. These instruments capture dimensions that are not readily assessed through clinician-rated motor scales, including emotional well-being, social participation, and stigma. However, responses may be influenced by mood, cognitive status, and cultural factors. Therefore, quality-of-life measures should be interpreted alongside objective clinical findings rather than in isolation.

The Freezing of Gait Questionnaire (FOG-Q) addresses a specific but highly disabling feature of Parkinson's disease. Freezing of gait is often episodic and difficult to observe during brief clinical encounters. The FOG-Q allows systematic assessment of frequency and severity from the patient's perspective. Nonetheless, recall bias and variability in symptom presentation may affect accuracy, and objective gait analysis may be required for detailed evaluation.

A key challenge across Parkinson's disease assessment scales is the dynamic and fluctuating nature of symptoms. Motor performance can vary significantly depending on medication timing, fatigue, and environmental context. As a result, single-point assessments may not fully reflect daily functional status. This limitation has driven increasing interest in continuous and real-world monitoring approaches.

Recent advancements in Parkinson's disease assessment have focused on technology-enabled tools, including wearable sensors, smartphone-based applications, and digital biomarkers. These technologies allow objective quantification of gait, tremor, bradykinesia, and activity levels in natural environments. Digital adaptations of established scales and remote assessment platforms have also gained relevance, particularly for long-term monitoring and telemedicine. While these innovations show promise in enhancing sensitivity and ecological validity, they currently serve as complementary tools rather than replacements for established clinical scales [76, 77].

In practice, the selection of assessment tools should be guided by disease stage, clinical objective, and care setting. The UPDRS remains essential for comprehensive evaluation and research applications, whereas staging scales and functional tests are particularly useful for clinical monitoring and rehabilitation planning. Patient-reported measures add critical insight into quality of life and symptom burden. An integrated assessment approach that combines clinician-rated scales, functional tests, and patient-reported outcomes provides the most comprehensive understanding of Parkinson's disease progression and treatment response. A comparative summary of commonly used assessment scales in Parkinson's disease, including their primary domain, strengths, limitations, and best clinical applications, is presented in Table **10.**

Table 10. A comparative summary of commonly used scales in Parkinson's disease.

Scale	Primary Domain	Strengths	Limitations	Best Clinical Application
UPDRS	Motor, ADL, complications	Comprehensive; longitudinal tracking	Time-consuming; training required	Clinical trials and detailed assessment
Hoehn and Yahr	Disease staging	Simple, rapid classification	Lacks functional and non-motor detail	Broad disease staging
TUG	Functional mobility	Quick; fall-risk screening	Influenced by the medication state	Rehabilitation and mobility assessment
BBS	Balance	Well validated; widely used	Ceiling effects in early PD	Balance and fall-risk evaluation
PDQ-39 / PDQ-8	Quality of life	Patient-centered; multidimensional	Subjective; mood influenced	Outcome evaluation and QoL assessment
FOG-Q	Freezing of Gait	Targets episodic symptoms	Recall Bias	Gait dysfunction assessment

CONCLUSION

This chapter provides a comprehensive overview of the various questionnaires and tests used to assess Parkinson's disease, each serving as an essential tool for evaluating symptoms, functional abilities, and quality of life in individuals with PD. It enables early detection of changes in motor function, cognitive health, balance, and other critical areas, allowing clinicians to tailor treatment and track disease progression effectively. By systematically incorporating these assessments into patient care, healthcare providers can enhance the management and understanding of Parkinson's disease, ultimately improving patient outcomes and supporting personalised care. This compilation of tools serves as a foundation for ongoing clinical evaluation and research, fostering a more precise approach to diagnosing and treating PD.

AI DISCLOSURE STATEMENT

During the preparation of this chapter, the authors used ChatGPT (OpenAI) as a support tool for language refinement, structural organisation, and clarification of ideas. All content generated with AI assistance was carefully reviewed, verified, and revised by the authors to ensure factual accuracy, originality, and consistency with the scientific literature. The authors take full responsibility for the integrity, interpretation, and final content of the published chapter.

ACKNOWLEDGEMENT

The authors sincerely acknowledge the contributions of neurologists, movement disorder specialists, and researchers whose work has advanced the understanding and clinical assessment of Parkinson's disease. Their efforts in developing and validating standardised scales have greatly improved diagnostic precision, therapeutic monitoring, and overall patient care in Parkinson's disease management.

REFERENCES

[1] Bloem BR, Okun MS, Klein C. Parkinson's disease. Lancet 2021; 397(10291): 2284-303. [http://dx.doi.org/10.1016/S0140-6736(21)00218-X] [PMID: 33848468]

[2] Saba RA, Maia DP, Cardoso FEC, *et al.* Guidelines for Parkinson's disease treatment: consensus from the Movement Disorders Scientific Department of the Brazilian Academy of Neurology - motor symptoms. Arq Neuropsiquiatr 2022; 80(3): 316-29. [http://dx.doi.org/10.1590/0004-282x-anp-2021-0219] [PMID: 35319667]

[3] Stebbins GT, Goetz CG, Burn DJ, Jankovic J, Khoo TK, Tilley BC. How to identify tremor dominant and postural instability/gait difficulty groups with the movement disorder society unified Parkinson's disease rating scale: comparison with the unified Parkinson's disease rating scale. Mov Disord. 2013; 28(5): 668-670. [http://dx.doi.org/10.1002/mds.25383]

[4] Atterling Brolin K, Schaeffer E, Kuri A, *et al.* Environmental Risk Factors for Parkinson's Disease: A Critical Review and Policy Implications. Mov Disord 2025; 40(2): 204-21. [http://dx.doi.org/10.1002/mds.30067] [PMID: 39601461]

[5] Höglinger G, Bähr M, Becktepe J, *et al.* Diagnosis and treatment of Parkinson´s disease (guideline of the German Society for Neurology). Neurological Research and Practice 2024; 6(1): 30. [http://dx.doi.org/10.1186/s42466-024-00325-4] [PMID: 38845028]

[6] Martínez-Martín P, Gil-Nagel A, Gracia LM, Gómez JB, Martínez-Sarriés J, Bermejo F. Unified Parkinson's disease rating scale characteristics and structure. Mov Disord 1994; 9(1): 76-83. [http://dx.doi.org/10.1002/mds.870090112] [PMID: 8139608]

[7] https://www.apta.org/patient-care/evidence-based-practice-resources/test-measures/unfied-parkinsons-disease-rating-scale-updrs-movement-disorders-society-mds-modified-unified-parkinsons-disease-rating-scale-mds-updrs

[8] Goetz CG, Tilley BC, Shaftman SR, *et al.* Movement Disorder Society-sponsored revision of the Unified Parkinson's Disease Rating Scale (MDS-UPDRS): Scale presentation and clinimetric testing results. Mov Disord 2008; 23(15): 2129-70. [http://dx.doi.org/10.1002/mds.22340] [PMID: 19025984]

[9] https://www.movementdisorders.org/MDS/MDS-Rating-Scales/MDS-Unified-Parkinsons-Di-ease-Rating-Scale-MDS-UPDRS.htm

[10] Hoehn MM, Yahr MD. Parkinsonism: onset, progression, and mortality. Neurology 1967; 17(5): 427-42.
[http://dx.doi.org/10.1212/WNL.17.5.427] [PMID: 6067254]

[11] Dallaire M, Houde-Thibeault A, Bouchard-Tremblay J, *et al.* Impact of frailty and sex-related differences on postural control and gait in older adults with Parkinson's Disease. Exp Gerontol 2024; 186: 112360.
[http://dx.doi.org/10.1016/j.exger.2024.112360] [PMID: 38215954]

[12] Verheyden G, Kampshoff CS, Burnett ME, *et al.* Psychometric properties of 3 functional mobility tests for people with Parkinson disease. Phys Ther 2014; 94(2): 230-9.
[http://dx.doi.org/10.2522/ptj.20130141] [PMID: 24231225]

[13] Goetz CG, Poewe W, Rascol O, *et al.* Movement Disorder Society Task Force report on the Hoehn and Yahr staging scale: status and recommendations. Mov Disord 2004; 19(9): 1020-8.
[http://dx.doi.org/10.1002/mds.20213] [PMID: 15372591]

[14] Podsiadlo D, Richardson S. The timed "Up & Go": a test of basic functional mobility for frail elderly persons. J Am Geriatr Soc 1991; 39(2): 142-8.
[http://dx.doi.org/10.1111/j.1532-5415.1991.tb01616.x] [PMID: 1991946]

[15] Shumway-Cook A, Brauer S, Woollacott M. Predicting the probability for falls in community-dwelling older adults using the Timed Up & Go Test. Phys Ther 2000; 80(9): 896-903.
[http://dx.doi.org/10.1093/ptj/80.9.896] [PMID: 10960937]

[16] Steffen TM, Hacker TA, Mollinger L. Age- and gender-related test performance in community-dwelling elderly people: Six-Minute Walk Test, Berg Balance Scale, Timed Up & Go Test, and gait speeds. Phys Ther 2002; 82(2): 128-37.
[http://dx.doi.org/10.1093/ptj/82.2.128] [PMID: 11856064]

[17] Morris S, Morris ME, Iansek R. Reliability of measurements obtained with the Timed "Up & Go" test in people with Parkinson disease. Phys Ther 2001; 81(2): 810-8.
[http://dx.doi.org/10.1093/ptj/81.2.810] [PMID: 11175678]

[18] Lexell J, Flansbjer U-B, Holmbäck AM, Downham D, Patten C. Reliability of gait performance tests in men and women with hemiparesis after stroke. J Rehabil Med 2005; 37(2): 75-82.
[http://dx.doi.org/10.1080/16501970410017215] [PMID: 15788341]

[19] Whitney SL, Marchetti GF, Schade A, Wrisley DM. The sensitivity and specificity of the Timed "Up & Go" and the dynamic gait index for self-reported falls in persons with vestibular disorders. J Vestib Res 2004; 14(5): 397-409.
[http://dx.doi.org/10.3233/VES-2004-14506] [PMID: 15598995]

[20] Berg KO, Wood-Dauphinee SL, Williams JI, Maki B. Measuring balance in the elderly: validation of an instrument. Can J Public Health 1992; 83 (Suppl. 2): S7-S11. https://www.ncbi.nlm.nih.gov/books/NBK574518/
[PMID: 1468055]

[21] Berg KO, Wood-Dauphinee SL, Williams JI, Maki B. Measuring balance in the elderly: validation of an instrument. Can J Public Health. 1992;83 Suppl 2: S7-S11.

[22] Lusardi MM, Pellecchia GL, Schulman M. Functional Performance in Community Living Older Adults. J Geriatr Phys Ther 2003; 26(3): 14-22.
[http://dx.doi.org/10.1519/00139143-200312000-00003]

[23] Miyamoto ST, Lombardi Junior I, Berg KO, Ramos LR, Natour J. Brazilian version of the Berg balance scale. Braz J Med Biol Res. 2004 Sep; 37(9): 1411-21. doi: 10.1590/s0100-879x2004000900017. Epub 2004 Aug 24. PMID: 15334208).

[24] Kashif M, Ahmad A, Bandpei MAM, Gilani SA, Iram H, Farooq M. Psychometric properties of the Urdu translation of the Berg balance scale in people with Parkinson's disease. Int J Environ Res Public Health 2022; 19(4): 2346.
[http://dx.doi.org/10.3390/ijerph19042346] [PMID: 35206533]

[25] Miyata K, Tamura S, Kobayashi S, Takeda R, Iwamoto H. Berg Balance Scale is a Valid Measure for Plan Interventions and for Assessing Changes in Postural Balance in Patients with Stroke. J Rehabil Med. 2022;54:jrm00359. Published 2022 Dec 9.
[http://dx.doi.org/10.2340/jrm.v54.4443]

[26] El-Gilany AH, Hatata ES, Aayob NS, Refaat R. Validation of the Arabic version of the Berg Balance Scale (A-BBS) among elderly residents in a rural community. Middle East J Age Ageing 2012; 9: 3-7.

[27] Ottonello M, Ferriero G, Benevolo E, Sessarego P, Dughi D. Psychometric evaluation of the Italian version of the Berg Balance Scale in rehabilitation inpatients. Eur J Phys Rehabil Med 2003; 39(4): 181.

[28] Miyata K, Tamura S, Kobayashi S, Takeda R, Iwamoto H. Berg Balance Scale is a Valid Measure for Plan Interventions and for Assessing Changes in Postural Balance in Patients with Stroke. J Rehabil Med. 2022;54:jrm00359. Published 2022 Dec 9.
[http://dx.doi.org/10.2340/jrm.v54.4443]

[29] Blum L, Korner-Bitensky N. Usefulness of the Berg Balance Scale in stroke rehabilitation: a systematic review. Phys Ther. 2008;88(5):559-566.
[http://dx.doi.org/10.2522/ptj.20070205]

[30] Newstead AH, Hinman MR, Tomberlin JA. Reliability of the Berg Balance Scale and balance master limits of stability tests for individuals with brain injury. J Neurol Phys Ther 2005; 29(1): 18-23.
[http://dx.doi.org/10.1097/01.NPT.0000282258.74325.cf] [PMID: 16386157]

[31] Holbein-Jenny MA, Billek-Sawhney B, Beckman E, Smith T. Balance in Personal Care Home Residents. J Geriatr Phys Ther 2005; 28(2): 48-53.
[http://dx.doi.org/10.1519/00139143-200508000-00003] [PMID: 16236228]

[32] Viveiro LAP, Gomes GCV, Bacha JMR, *et al.* Reliability, Validity, and Ability to Identity Fall Status of the Berg Balance Scale, Balance Evaluation Systems Test (BESTest), Mini-BESTest, and Brief-BESTest in Older Adults Who Live in Nursing Homes. J Geriatr Phys Ther 2019; 42(4): E45-54.
[http://dx.doi.org/10.1519/JPT.0000000000000215] [PMID: 30407272]

[33] Berg K, Wood-Dauphinee S, Williams JI. The Balance Scale: reliability assessment with elderly residents and patients with an acute stroke. J Rehabil Med 1995; 27(1): 27-36.
[http://dx.doi.org/10.2340/1650197719952736] [PMID: 7792547]

[34] Shumway-Cook A, Baldwin M, Polissar NL, Gruber W. Predicting the probability for falls in community-dwelling older adults. Phys Ther 1997; 77(8): 812-9.
[http://dx.doi.org/10.1093/ptj/77.8.812] [PMID: 9256869]

[35] Duncan PW, Weiner DK, Chandler J, Studenski S. Functional reach: a new clinical measure of balance. J Gerontol 1990; 45(6): M192-7.
[http://dx.doi.org/10.1093/geronj/45.6.M192] [PMID: 2229941]

[36] Billek-Sawhney B, Gay J. The functional reach test: Are 3 trials necessary? Top Geriatr Rehabil 2005; 21(2): 144-8.
[http://dx.doi.org/10.1097/00013614-200504000-00010]

[37] Rosa MV, Perracini MR, Ricci NA. Usefulness, assessment and normative data of the Functional Reach Test in older adults: A systematic review and meta-analysis. Arch Gerontol Geriatr 2019; 81: 149-70.
[http://dx.doi.org/10.1016/j.archger.2018.11.015] [PMID: 30593986]

[38] Wernick-Robinson M, Krebs DE, Giorgetti MM. Functional reach: Does it really measure dynamic balance? Arch Phys Med Rehabil 1999; 80(3): 262-9.

[http://dx.doi.org/10.1016/S0003-9993(99)90136-3] [PMID: 10084433]

[39] Weiner DK, Duncan PW, Chandler J, Studenski SA. Functional reach: a marker of physical frailty. J Am Geriatr Soc 1992; 40(3): 203-7. [http://dx.doi.org/10.1111/j.1532-5415.1992.tb02068.x] [PMID: 1538035]

[40] Bennie S, Bruner K, Dizon A, Fritz H, Goodman B, Peterson S. Measurements of Balance: Comparison of the Timed "Up and Go" Test and Functional Reach Test with the Berg Balance Scale. J Phys Ther Sci 2003; 15(2): 93-7. [http://dx.doi.org/10.1589/jpts.15.93]

[41] Thomas JI, Lane JV. A pilot study to explore the predictive validity of 4 measures of falls risk in frail elderly patients. Arch Phys Med Rehabil 2005; 86(8): 1636-40. [http://dx.doi.org/10.1016/j.apmr.2005.03.004] [PMID: 16084819]

[42] Thomas JI, Lane JV. A pilot study to explore the predictive validity of 4 measures of falls risk in frail elderly patients. Arch Phys Med Rehabil 2005; 86(8): 1636-40. [http://dx.doi.org/10.1016/j.apmr.2005.03.004] [PMID: 16084819]

[43] Eagle DJ, Salama S, Whitman D, Evans LA, Ho E, Olde J. Comparison of three instruments in predicting accidental falls in selected inpatients in a general teaching hospital. J Gerontol Nurs 1999; 25(7): 40-5. [http://dx.doi.org/10.3928/0098-9134-19990701-14] [PMID: 10476130]

[44] Lynch SM, Leahy P, Barker SP. Reliability of Measurements Obtained With a Modified Functional Reach Test in Subjects With Spinal Cord Injury, Physical Therapy 1998; 78(2): 128-33. [PMID: 10.1093/ptj/78.2.128]

[45] Katz-Leurer M, Fisher I, Neeb M, Schwartz I, Carmeli E. Reliability and validity of the modified functional reach test at the sub-acute stage post-stroke. Disabil Rehabil 2009; 31(3): 243-8. [http://dx.doi.org/10.1080/09638280801927830] [PMID: 18608433]

[46] Outermans JC, van Peppen RPS, Wittink H, Takken T, Kwakkel G. Effects of a high-intensity task-oriented training on gait performance early after stroke: a pilot study. Clin Rehabil 2010; 24(11): 979-87. [http://dx.doi.org/10.1177/0269215509360647] [PMID: 20719820]

[47] Katz-Leurer M, Fisher I, Neeb M, Schwartz I, Carmeli E. Reliability and validity of the modified functional reach test at the sub-acute stage post-stroke. Disabil Rehabil 2009; 31(3): 243-8. [http://dx.doi.org/10.1080/09638280801927830] [PMID: 18608433]

[48] Hagell P, Nilsson MH. The 39-item Parkinson's Disease Questionnaire (PDQ-39): is it a unidimensional construct? Ther Adv Neurol Disord 2009; 2(4): 205-14. [http://dx.doi.org/10.1177/1756285609103726] [PMID: 21179529]

[49] Hagell P, Nygren C. The 39 item Parkinson's disease questionnaire (PDQ-39) revisited: implications for evidence based medicine. J Neurol Neurosurg Psychiatry 2007; 78(11): 1191-8. [http://dx.doi.org/10.1136/jnnp.2006.111161] [PMID: 17442762]

[50] Peto V, Jenkinson C, Fitzpatrick R, Greenhall R. The development and validation of a short measure of functioning and well being for individuals with Parkinson's disease. Qual Life Res. 1995;4(3):241-248. [http://dx.doi.org/10.1007/BF02260863]

[51] Jenkinson C, Fitzpatrick R, Peto V, Greenhall R, Hyman N. The Parkinson's Disease Questionnaire (PDQ-39): development and validation of a Parkinson's disease summary index score. Age Ageing 1997; 26(5): 353-7. [http://dx.doi.org/10.1093/ageing/26.5.353] [PMID: 9351479]

[52] Peto V, Jenkinson C, Fitzpatrick R. Determining minimally important differences for the PDQ-39 Parkinson's disease questionnaire. Age Ageing 2001; 30(4): 299-302. [http://dx.doi.org/10.1093/ageing/30.4.299] [PMID: 11509307]

[53] Schrag A, Jenkinson C, Selai C, Mathias C, Quinn N. Testing the validity of the PDQ-39 in patients with MSA. Parkinsonism Relat Disord 2007; 13(3): 152-6. [http://dx.doi.org/10.1016/j.parkreldis.2006.08.008] [PMID: 17070089]

[54] Kwon DY, Kim JW, Ma HI, *et al.* Translation and validation of the korean version of the 39-item Parkinson's disease questionnaire. J Clin Neurol 2013; 9(1): 26-31. [http://dx.doi.org/10.3988/jcn.2013.9.1.26] [PMID: 23346157]

[55] Tsang KL, Chi I, Ho SL, Lou VW, Lee TMC, Chu LW. Translation and validation of the standard Chinese version of PDQ-39: A quality-of-life measure for patients with Parkinson's disease. Mov Disord 2002; 17(5): 1036-40. [http://dx.doi.org/10.1002/mds.10249] [PMID: 12360555]

[56] Dehghan A, Ghaem H, Borhani-Haghighi A, Safari-Faramani R, Moosazadeh M, Gholami A. Evaluation of Reliability and Validity of PDQ-39: Questionnaire in Iranian Patients With Parkinson's Disease. Zahedan J Res Med Sci 2016; 18(3): 1-6. [http://dx.doi.org/10.17795/zjrms-6245]

[57] Luo N, Tan LC, Li SC, Soh LK, Thumboo J. Validity and reliability of the Chinese (Singapore) version of the Parkinson's Disease Questionnaire (PDQ-39). Qual Life Res. 2005; 14(1): 273-279. doi:10.1007/s11136-004-2654-1

[58] Martínez-Martín P, Serrano-Dueñas M, Vaca-Baquero V. Psychometric characteristics of the Parkinson's disease questionnaire (PDQ-39)—Ecuadorian version. Parkinsonism Relat Disord 2005; 11(5): 297-304. [http://dx.doi.org/10.1016/j.parkreldis.2005.02.003] [PMID: 15886043]

[59] Damiano AM, Snyder C, Strausser B, Willian MK. A review of health-related quality-of-life concepts and measures for Parkinson's disease. Qual Life Res. 1999; 8(3): 235-243. doi:10.1023/a:1008823222574

[60] Fleming A, Cook KF, Nelson ND, Lai EC. Proxy reports in Parkinson's disease: Caregiver and patient self-reports of quality of life and physical activity. Mov Disord 2005; 20(11): 1462-8. [http://dx.doi.org/10.1002/mds.20592] [PMID: 16028212]

[61] Nojomi M, Mostafavian Z, Shahidi GA, Jenkinson C. Quality of life in patients with Parkinson's disease: Translation and psychometric evaluation of the Iranian version of PDQ-39. J Res Med Sci. 2010; 15(2): 63-69.

[62] Stathis P, Papadopoulos G. Evaluation and validation of a patient-reported quality-of-life questionnaire for Parkinson's disease. J Patient Rep Outcomes. 2022; 6(1): 17. Published 2022 Mar 2. doi:10.1186/s41687-022-00427-0

[63] Jesus-Ribeiro J, Vieira E, Ferreira P, Januário C, Freire A. Reliability and Validity of 39-Item Parkinson's Disease Questionnaire and Parkinson's Disease Quality of Life Questionnaire. Acta Med Port 2017; 30(5): 395-401. [http://dx.doi.org/10.20344/amp.8202] [PMID: 28865504]

[64] Jenkinson C, Fitzpatrick R, Norquist J, Findley L, Hughes K. Cross-cultural evaluation of the Parkinson's Disease Questionnaire: tests of data quality, score reliability, response rate, and scaling assumptions in the United States, Canada, Japan, Italy, and Spain. J Clin Epidemiol 2003; 56(9): 843-7. [http://dx.doi.org/10.1016/S0895-4356(03)00148-3] [PMID: 14505768]

[65] Marinus J, Ramaker C, van Hilten JJ, Stiggelbout AM. Health related quality of life in Parkinson's disease: a systematic review of disease specific instruments. J Neurol Neurosurg Psychiatry 2002; 72(2): 241-8. [http://dx.doi.org/10.1136/jnnp.72.2.241] [PMID: 11796776]

[66] Haapaniemi TH, Sotaniemi KA, Sintonen H, Taimela E. The generic 15D instrument is valid and feasible for measuring health related quality of life in Parkinson's disease. J Neurol Neurosurg

Psychiatry 2004; 75(7): 976-83.
[http://dx.doi.org/10.1136/jnnp.2003.015693] [PMID: 15201353]

[67] Peto V, Jenkinson C, Fitzpatrick R. PDQ-39: a review of the development, validation and application of a Parkinson's disease quality of life questionnaire and its associated measures. J Neurol 1998; 245(S1) (Suppl. 1): S10-4.
[http://dx.doi.org/10.1007/PL00007730] [PMID: 9617716]

[68] Chen K, Yang YJ, Liu FT, *et al.* Evaluation of PDQ-8 and its relationship with PDQ-39 in China: a three-year longitudinal study. Health Qual Life Outcomes 2017; 15(1): 170.
[http://dx.doi.org/10.1186/s12955-017-0742-5] [PMID: 28838316]

[69] Kahraman T, Genç A, Söke F, GÖz E, Çolakoğlu BD, Keskįnoğlu P. Validity and Reliability of the Turkish Version of the 8-Item Parkinson's Disease Questionnaire. Noro Psikiyatr Ars. 2018; 55(4): 337-340. doi:10.5152/npa.2017.19343

[70] Huang TT, Hsu HY, Wang BH, Chen KH. Quality of life in Parkinson's disease patients: validation of the Short-Form Eight-item Parkinson's Disease Questionnaire (PDQ-8) in Taiwan. Qual Life Res. 2011; 20(4): 499-505. doi:10.1007/s11136-010-9777-3

[71] Giladi N, Shabtai H, Simon ES, Biran S, Tal J, Korczyn AD. Construction of freezing of gait questionnaire for patients with Parkinsonism. Parkinsonism Relat Disord 2000; 6(3): 165-70.
[http://dx.doi.org/10.1016/S1353-8020(99)00062-0] [PMID: 10817956]

[72] Hulzinga F, Nieuwboer A, Dijkstra BW, *et al.* The New Freezing of Gait Questionnaire: Unsuitable as an Outcome in Clinical Trials? Mov Disord Clin Pract (Hoboken) 2020; 7(2): 199-205.
[http://dx.doi.org/10.1002/mdc3.12893] [PMID: 32071940]

[73] Nilsson MH, Hagell P. Freezing of Gait Questionnaire: validity and reliability of the Swedish version. Acta Neurol Scand 2009; 120(5): 331-4.
[http://dx.doi.org/10.1111/j.1600-0404.2009.01175.x] [PMID: 19456303]

[74] Tao P, Shao X, Zhuang J, *et al.* Translation, Cultural Adaptation, and Reliability and Validity Testing of a Chinese Version of the Freezing of Gait Questionnaire (FOGQ-CH). Front Neurol 2021; 12: 760398.
[http://dx.doi.org/10.3389/fneur.2021.760398] [PMID: 34887830]

[75] Taweekitikul A, Tanvijit P, Tantisuvanitchkul P, *et al.* Validity and Reliability of the Thai Version of the Freezing of Gait Questionnaire in Individuals With Parkinson's disease. Ann Rehabil Med 2023; 47(1): 45-51.
[http://dx.doi.org/10.5535/arm.22149] [PMID: 36792053]

[76] Polvorinos-Fernández C, Sigcha L, Borzì L, *et al.* Evaluating Motor Symptoms in Parkinson's Disease Through Wearable Sensors: A Systematic Review of Digital Biomarkers. Appl Sci (Basel) 2024; 14(22): 10189.
[http://dx.doi.org/10.3390/app142210189]

[77] Li X, Chen C, Pan T, *et al.* Trends and hotspots in non-motor symptoms of Parkinson's disease: a 10-year bibliometric analysis. Front Aging Neurosci 2024; 16: 1335550.
[http://dx.doi.org/10.3389/fnagi.2024.1335550] [PMID: 38298610]

CHAPTER 7

Scales and Questionnaires to Assess Neuropathy

Sidharth Bansal[1], **Parveen Kumar**[2] and **Nidhi Sharma**[3,4,*]

[1] *Department of Physiotherapy, School of Allied Medical Sciences, Lovely Professional University, Phagwara, Punjab, India*

[2] *Pal Physiotherapy and Rehabilitation Centre, Pal Healthcare, Ambala City, Haryana, India*

[3] *Department of Physiotherapy, Amity Institute of Health Allied Sciences, Amity University, Noida, Uttar Pradesh, India*

[4] *Maharishi Markandeshwar Institute of Physiotherapy and Rehabilitation, Maharishi Markandeshwar (Deemed to be University), Mullana, Ambala, Haryana, India*

Abstract: This chapter provides an in-depth review of six widely used scales for assessing neuropathy, including their interpretation, intended population, administration, and psychometric properties. The chapter covers the Leeds Assessment of Neuropathic Symptoms and Signs (LANSS), Douleur Neuropathique 4 (DN4), Neuropathic Pain Questionnaire (NPQ), Overall Neuropathy Limitation Scale (ONLS), the Veterans Affairs Neuropathy Scale (VANS), and Utah Early Neuropathy Scale (UENS). Each scale is critically analysed for its clinical utility, with a focus on its target populations, such as patients with diabetic neuropathy, chemotherapy-induced neuropathy, or other neuropathic conditions. Practical details on the administration process, including time requirements and scoring methods, are discussed. Additionally, the chapter highlights the psychometric properties of each scale, such as validity, reliability, and sensitivity to change, providing clinicians and researchers with a comprehensive guide for selecting appropriate tools for neuropathy assessment in diverse patient populations.

Keywords: Neuropathy, Outcome measures, Peripheral neuropathy, Questionnaire, Scales.

INTRODUCTION

Peripheral neuropathy encompasses a variety of conditions involving damage to the peripheral nervous system and is one of the most prevalent neurological disorders. The peripheral nervous system is one of the most prevalent neurological disorders [1, 2]. It affects approximately 77 out of every 100,000 pe-

* **Corresponding author Nidhi Sharma:** Department of Physiotherapy, Amity Institute of Health Allied Sciences, Amity University, Noida, Uttar Pradesh, India; E-mail: sharmanidhiphysio@gmail.com

ople annually and occurs in 1-12% of the general population, with the prevalence rising to as high as 30% among older adults [2]. Peripheral neuropathy is most frequently observed in individuals with diabetes mellitus, Human Immunodeficiency Virus (HIV) infection, and dysproteinemic disorders, as well as in patients undergoing chemotherapy or radiotherapy [1]. The primary care physician faces three key challenges when managing patients with peripheral neuropathy: first, quickly screening asymptomatic patients (in under 2 minutes) for neuropathy, particularly when they have conditions like diabetes where neuropathy is common, second, clinically assessing patients with neuropathy symptoms to decide who needs specialist referral and what tests are suitable for those who do not, and third, managing the symptoms of painful peripheral neuropathy effectively [1]. These challenges highlight the need for specific tools and questionnaires to assist caregivers in evaluating the severity of symptoms and ensuring appropriate care is provided. Additionally, these tools can be valuable for quantifying symptoms for research purposes, contributing to a better understanding of peripheral neuropathy and its management.

DOULEUR NEUROPATHIQUE 4 (DN4)

Douleur Neuropathique 4 (DN4) was developed to evaluate sensory descriptors and symptoms of neuropathic pain (NP) besides sensory examination. DN4 has been extensively used in a variety of NP conditions with varied aetiology. The questionnaire was originally written in French, but the same team of developers immediately translated it into English. Since 2005, the scale has become increasingly popular due to its clarity and convenience. Neuropathic pain caused by central and peripheral lesions is usually evaluated using this approach [3].

Description

The questionnaire consists of four questions with 10 items. Questions 1 and 2 discuss the characteristics and symptoms associated with pain. They are marked based on an interview with the person. Questions 3 and 4 are marked based on a physical examination that assesses the perception of the stimulus and aggravating factors, as shown in Table **1**.

Table 1. Douleur neuropathique 4 questionnaire.

Interview with the patient		
Question 1: Does the pain have one or more of the following characteristics?		
1. Burning	○ Yes	○ No
2. Painful cold	○ Yes	○ No

(Table 1) cont.....

Interview with the patient		
3. Electric shocks	○ Yes	○ No
Question 2: Is the pain associated with one or more of the following symptoms in the same area?		
4. Tingling	○ Yes	○ No
5. Pins and needles	○ Yes	○ No
6. Numbness	○ Yes	○ No
7. Itching	○ Yes	○ No
Examination of the patient		
Question 3: Is the pain located in an area where the physical examination may reveal one or more of the following characteristics?		
8. Hypoesthesia to touch	○ Yes	○ No
9. Hypoesthesia to prick	○ Yes	○ No
Question 4: In the painful area, can the pain be caused or increased by:		
10. Brushing?	○ Yes	○ No

Note: Please complete this questionnaire by ticking one answer for each item.

Administration

It is a clinician-administered outcome measure and takes about 5 minutes to complete.

Scoring and Interpretation [3]

- Score 1 for each Yes answer
- Score 0 for each No answer
- If the score is 4 or higher, the pain is most likely neuropathic.
- If the score is less than 4, the pain is unlikely to be neuropathic.

Intended Population

Conditions that often have Neuropathic Pain [3]

1. Complex Regional Pain Syndrome (CRPS) Type 1
2. Lumbar or Cervical Radiculopathy
3. Brachial Plexus Injury
4. Peripheral Neuropathies
5. Central Nervous System Lesions (Stroke, Traumatic Brain Injury, Multiple Sclerosis)
6. Polyneuropathies

Psychometric Properties [4]

Reliability

Inter-Rater Agreement Coefficient: 0.80 (0.71–0.89)

Test-Retest Intra-Class Correlation Coefficient: 0.95 (0.92–0.97)

Sensitivity

The DN4 questionnaire has a very good sensitivity 83%.

Specificity

It has a specificity of 90%.

THE VETERANS AFFAIRS NEUROPATHY SCALE (VANS)

In telemedicine settings, the VA Neuropathy Scale (VANS) is a useful clinical evaluation tool for diagnosing and monitoring the extent of peripheral neuropathy. It is a standardised peripheral neuropathy evaluation tool that is similar to an in-person neuromuscular exam. Based on previously validated neuropathy assessment scales, it was amended for use in clinical tele-neurology settings [5].

Description

The VANS assesses six domains: balance, gait, knee reflexes, foot inspection, pinprick testing, and vibration. It is an assessment-based evaluation tool, so proper equipment and expertise are required (Table **2**, Fig. **1**).

Table 2. The veterans affairs neuropathy scale.

Domain	Item	Scoring Criteria	Obtained Score
Balance	**Romberg**	0=Normal 1=Abnormal	
Gait	**Casual Gait**	0=Normal 1=Abnormal	
	Heel Walk	0=Normal 1=Abnormal	
	Tandem Walk	0=Normal 1=Abnormal	
Knee Reflexes	**Left Knee Reflex**	0=Normal or Brisk 1=Absent or Depressed	

(Table 2) cont.....

Domain	Item	Scoring Criteria	Obtained Score	
	Right Knee Reflex	0=Normal or Brisk 1=Absent or Depressed		
Foot Inspection	**Left Foot Inspection**	0=Normal 2=Ulcers, skin fissures		
	Right Foot Inspection	0=Normal 2=Ulcers, skin fissures		
Vibration	**Left Toe Vibration**	0=Normal 1=Decreased 2=Absent		
	Right Toe Vibration	0=Normal 1=Decreased 2=Absent		
	Left Knee Vibration	0=Normal 1=Decreased 2=Absent		
	Right Knee Vibration	0=Normal 1=Decreased 2=Absent		
Pinprick testing Fig. **1** **(Segments of Pinprick testing)**	**Left Pinprick**	0=Normal 1=Reduced 2=Absent	Region 8	-
			Region 7	-
			Region 6	-
			Region 5	-
			Region 4	-
			Region 3	-
			Region 2	-
			Region 1	-
	Right Pinprick	0=Normal 1=Reduced 2=Absent	Region 8	-
			Region 7	-
			Region 6	-
			Region 5	-
			Region 4	-
			Region 3	-
			Region 2	-
			Region 1	-
Total Score				

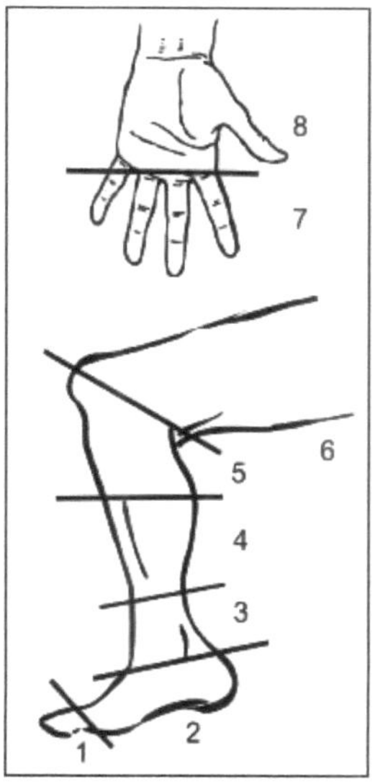

Fig. (1). Segments of pinprick testing.

Administration

It is a clinician-administered outcome measure and takes about 6-7 minutes to complete.

Scoring and Interpretation [5]

VANS scores can range from 0 to 50, with the examiner awarding points for anomalies attributed to distal symmetric peripheral neuropathy. Score 0 signifies no abnormalities, and 50 signifies the worst possible situation.

Intended Population

1. Inflammatory Neuropathies
2. Diabetic Large-fibre Neuropathy
3. Sensory Neuropathies
4. Lumbar Radiculopathy
5. Other neuropathies with motor weakness and balance disturbances

Psychometric Properties [5]

Reliability

Inter-rater reliability: ICC = 0.89

Intra-rater reliability: ICC = 0.90-0.95

Specificity: 91%

Sensitivity: 98%

OVERALL NEUROPATHY LIMITATION SCALE (ONLS)

The Overall Disability Sum Score (ODSS) was modified to a small degree, and a new peripheral neuropathy activity measure, the overall neuropathy limitation scale (ONLS), was introduced. The Overall Disability Sum Score (ODSS) was the initial scale developed to assess the constraints of patients with immune-mediated peripheral neuropathies. It was based on Guy's Neurological Disability Scale, intended to evaluate disability in patients with multiple sclerosis [6].

Description

Within ONLS, two separate scales for arm and leg assessment measure limitations in everyday activities of the upper and lower limbs. It is also compatible with measuring peripheral neurological damage and treatment response. The extensively used Hughes' functional grading scale (f score) and the Rankin scale, which focus primarily on mobility and exclude relevant data on arm function, are less comprehensive in their concepts if compared to ONLS. Additionally, the ONLS optimised the monitoring of overall loss of strength as well as sensory deficits that result in disability [7].

Administration

It is a clinician-administered outcome measure delivered in an interview mode. It takes about 6-7 minutes to complete (Table **3**).

Table 3. Overall neuropathy limitation scale.

Instructions: The examiner should question and observe the patient to determine the answers to the following questions. Note should be made of any other disorder other than peripheral neuropathy that limits function.			
Arm Scale			
Does the patient have any symptoms in their hands or arms, *e.g*, tingling, numbness, or weakness? (If no, go to the legs section)	**Yes**	**No**	
Is the patient affected in their ability to:	**Not affected**	**Affected but not prevented**	**Prevented**
Wash and brush their hair.			
Turn a key in a lock.			

(Table 3) cont.....

Use a knife and fork together (or spoon, if a knife and fork are not used)			
Do or undo buttons or zips.			
Dress the upper part of their body, excluding buttons or zips.			
If all these functions are prevented, can the patient make purposeful movements with their hand or arms?	**Yes**	**No**	**Not Applicable**
Leg Scale			
	Yes	**No**	**Not Applicable**
Does the patient have difficulty running or climbing stairs?			
Does the patient have difficulty walking?			
Does their gait look abnormal?			
How do they mobilise for about 10 meters (*i.e.*, 33 feet)?			
• Without aid			
• With one stick, a crutch, or by holding onto someone's arm			
• With two sticks or crutches, or one stick or crutch, holding onto someone's arm or frame.			
• With a wheelchair.			
• If they use a wheelchair, can they stand and walk 1 meter with the help of one person?			
If they cannot walk as above, are they able to make some purposeful movements of their legs, *e.g.*, reposition their legs in bed?			
Does the patient use ankle foot orthoses/braces (if yes, please indicate right or left)			

Scoring and Interpretation [6, 7]

Scores range from 0 to 5 for the arm scale and 0 to 7 for the leg scale. A score of 0 denotes no functional limitations (the highest possible score on the scale) while scores of 5 or 7 indicate no specific movements (the lowest possible score on the scale). The overall score is calculated by summing the individual scores; a total score of 0 indicates no disability, and 12 indicates maximum disability.

Arms Grade Score

0 = Normal

1 = Minor symptoms in one or both arms, but not affecting any of the functions listed

2 = Disability in one or both arms affecting but not preventing any of the functions listed
3 = Disability in one or both arms, preventing at least one but not all functions listed
4 = Disability in both arms, preventing all functions listed, but purposeful movement is still possible
5 = Disability in both arms, preventing all purposeful movements

Legs Grade Score

0 = Walking/climbing stairs/ running not affected
1 = walking/climbing stairs/ running is affected, but the gait does not look abnormal
2 = walks independently, but gait looks abnormal
3 = requires unilateral support to walk 10 meters (stick, single crutch, one arm)
4 = requires bilateral support to walk 10 meters (sticks, crutches, crutch and arm, frame)
5 = requires a wheelchair to travel 10 meters, but can stand and walk 1 meter with the help of one person
6 = restricted to wheelchair, unable to stand and walk 1 meter with the help of one person, but able to make some purposeful leg movements
7 = restricted to a wheelchair or bed most of the day, unable to make any purposeful movements

Overall Neuropathy Limitation Scale Score

Arm scale score (0 to 5) + Leg scale score (0 to 7) [**Range** – 0 (No Disability) to 12 (Maximum Disability)]

Intended Population

1. Multiple Sclerosis
2. Polyneuropathies
3. Gullian-Barré Syndrome
4. Chronic Inflammatory Demyelinating Polyneuropathy (CIDP)
5. Paraprotien-associated Demyelinating Neuropathy

Psychometric Properties [7]

Reliability

Inter-rater reliability: ICC = 0.97

Internal consistency: Cronbach's alpha = 0.59

Validity

Construct Validity: r = 0.97

Floor and ceiling effect

Total = 3

Upper limb = 24

Lower limb = 13

Responsiveness

0.88 (0.8 to 0.95)

UTAH EARLY NEUROPATHY SCALE (UENS)

The Utah Early Neuropathy Scale (UENS) was created with the purpose of identifying and measuring acute small-fibre sensory neuropathy as well as detecting subtle differences in sensory distribution and intensity. It is observed that the UENS is more sensitive in detecting neuropathy than NIS-LL and MDNS, and shows a good correlation with them. It is a research-oriented scale specifically designed to meet the requirements of clinical assessment in trials of early-stage neuropathy [8].

Description

UENS is a scale that primarily focuses on the lower extremity and the area below the knee. It is a 42-point scale in which 24 points are allotted to a concise anatomical tracking of sensory loss to pinprick in the lower leg and foot. The remaining 24 points include the assessment of motor function, large-fibre sensation (vibration time, joint position sense), allodynia/hyperaesthesia, and deep tendon reflexes (Table **4**).

Table 4. The utah early neuropathy scale.

Motor Examination	**Left**	**Right**
0 Normal		
2 Weak		
Great Toe Extension		
Total both sides (out of 4)		

(Table 4) cont.....

Pin Sensations 0 Normal	**Left**	**Right**
1 For each segment with reduced sensations		
2 For each segment with absent sensation		
Total both sides (out of 24)		
Allodynia/Hyperaesthesia	**Left**	**Right**
0 Normal		
1 If present in the toes or the foot		
Total both sides (out of 2)		
Large Fibre Sensation	**Left Right**	
0 Normal 1 Diminished 2 Absent		
Great toe vibration		
Time	s	s
Great toe joint position		
Total both sides (out of 24)		
Deep Tendon Reflexes	**Left Right**	
0 normal 1 diminished 2 absent		
Ankle		
Total of both sides (out of 4)		
Total Score (out of 42)		

Intended Population

1. Sensory Polyneuropathies
2. Mild-moderate Diabetic Neuropathy
3. Chronic Cervical or Lumbar Radiculopathies
4. Small fibre neuropathies
5. Other milder neuropathies

Administration

It is an assessment-based clinical evaluation tool that requires precision. The UENS takes approximately three minutes and requires a number 2 safety pin and a regular 128 Hz tuning fork. Before commencing the test, the patient's name, study number, and visit have been noted for each patient.

To test pin sensation, start by establishing what a normal sharp sensation feels like on an unaffected area of the skin. Once this baseline is set, use the pin to touch the dorsal surface of the foot and leg, beginning at the great toe and moving centripetally in 1-2 cm increments. Ask the patient to indicate when they first feel "any sharpness" and again when the pin feels "as sharp as expected." Repeat this process to confirm these levels. On each side, score 2 points for each region where the patient feels no sharpness, and 1 additional point for each region where the sharpness is less than expected. Only distal sensory loss is scored. For example, if a person reports no pin sensation up to the mid-foot dorsum (4 points) and reduced sensation up to the low ankle (1 point) on both sides, they would score a total of 10 points for this portion of the UENS (Fig. **2**) [8].

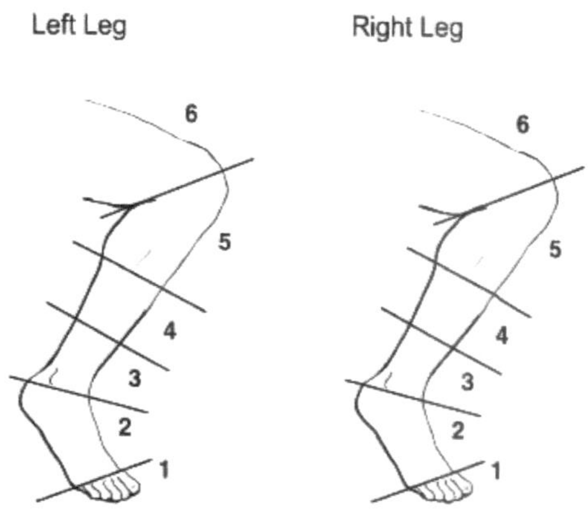

Fig. (2). Segments for pin sensation reporting.

For vibration testing, first familiarise the patient with the sensation of vibration, distinct from that of pressure. Then place a maximally vibrating tuning fork on the dorsum of the great toe at the distal interphalangeal joint. Vibration extinction in less than 10 seconds is considered "diminished," while "absent" means the patient cannot detect the vibration at all. The motor examination focuses on dorsiflexion of the great toe, with other aspects performed as typically done in a neurological examination [8].

Scoring and Interpretation [8]

Scoring varies for different components of the scale. For the motor component, a score of 0 indicates a normal response, while a score of 2 indicates a weak response. For pin sensation, 0 is given for normal sensation, 1 for reduced sensation, and 2 for absent sensation. For allodynia, 0 is given for normal sensation, and 1 if allodynia is present in the foot or toes. For large fibre sensations and deep tendon reflexes, 0 indicates a normal response, 1 indicates a diminished response, and 2 indicates an absent response. Each component is tested bilaterally, with the total score reaching up to 42.

Psychometric Properties [8]

Reliability: Inter-rater Reliability: 0.94

Sensitivity: 92%

LEEDS ASSESSMENT OF NEUROPATHIC SYMPTOMS AND SIGNS (LANSS)

An assessment tool designed to evaluate and categorise pain is the Leeds Assessment of Neuropathic Symptoms and Signs (LANSS) pain scale. Its primary purpose is to establish whether pain is primarily caused by nerve damage. This is the only instrument that has been scientifically proven to distinguish between nociceptive and neuropathic pain. It helps clinicians evaluate the intensity or sources of pain [9].

Description

It is a clear, concise bedside test performed in two stages. *i.e.*, a quick clinical evaluation and a patient-completed questionnaire. It includes a 7-item pain scale with items for sensory examination and descriptors of sensory experience.

As an adjunct to the original LANSS pain scale, a modified S-LANSS (self-report LANSS) is also available for patients to utilise in the absence of a healthcare professional.

Intended Population

1. Human Immuno-Deficiency Virus (HIV)
2. Cancer
3. Diabetic Neuropathy
4. Phantom Limb Pain
5. Peripheral Neuropathy
6. Chronic Low Back Pain
7. Complex Regional Pain Syndrome

Administration

Out of the 7 items on the scale, 5 are interview-based symptom-related items, and the other 2 are examination-based items.

Leeds Assessment of Neuropathic Symptoms and Signs (LANSS)

A. Pain Questionnaire

- Think about how your pain has felt over the last week.
- Please say whether any of the descriptions match your pain exactly.

1. Does your pain feel like strange, unpleasant sensations in your skin?

Words like pricking, tingling, pins, and needles might describe these sensations.

a. NO – My pain doesn't really feel like this .... (0)

b. YES – I get these sensations quite a lot .... (5)

2. Does your pain make the skin in the painful area look different from normal?

Words like mottled or looking more red or pink might describe the appearance.

a. NO – My pain doesn't affect the colour of my skin .... (0)

b. YES – I've noticed that the pain does make my skin look different from normal .... (5)

3. Does your pain make the affected skin abnormally sensitive to touch?

Getting unpleasant sensations when lightly stroking the skin, or getting pain when wearing tight clothes, might

Describe the abnormal sensitivity.

a. NO – My pain does not make my skin abnormally sensitive in that area .... (0)

b. YES – My skin seems abnormally sensitive to touch in that area .... (3)

4. Does your pain come on suddenly and in bursts for no apparent reason when you're still?

Words like electric shocks, jumping, and bursting describe these sensations.

a. NO – My pain doesn't really feel like this .... (0)

b. YES – I get these sensations quite a lot .... (2)

5. Does your pain feel as if the skin temperature in the painful area has changed abnormally?

Words like hot and burning describe these sensations.

a. NO – I don't really get these sensations .... (0)

b. YES – I get these sensations quite a lot .... (1)

B. SENSORY TESTING

Skin sensitivity can be examined by comparing the painful area with a contralateral or adjacent non-painful area for the presence of allodynia and an altered pin-prick threshold (PPT).

Allodynia

Examine the response to lightly stroking cotton wool across the non-painful area and then the painful area. If normal sensations are experienced in the non-painful site, but pain or unpleasant sensations (tingling, nausea) are experienced in the painful area when stroking, allodynia is present.

a. NO – Normal sensations in both areas.. (0)
b. YES – Allodynia in the painful area only.. (5)

Altered Pin-prick Threshold

Determine the pin-prick threshold by comparing the response to a 23-gauge (blue) needle mounted inside a 2ml syringe barrel placed gently onto the skin in non-painful and then painful areas.

If a sharp pin prick is felt in the non-painful area, but a different sensation is experienced in the painful area, *e.g*, none/blunt only (raised PPT) or a very painful sensation (lowered PPT), an altered PPT is present.

If a pinprick is not felt in either area, mount the syringe onto the needle to increase the weight and repeat.

a. NO – Equal sensation in both areas.. (0)
b. YES – Altered PPT in painful area.. (3)

SCORING

Add values in parentheses for sensory description and examination findings to obtain an overall score.

Total Score (Maximum 24)

Scoring and Interpretation [9]

A maximum of 24 points will be assigned to the patient's current condition. On this scale, a result of 12 or higher supports the diagnosis of neuropathic pain. Neuropathic pain is less likely to be present in scores under 12.

The LANSS has indeed been found to be very precise and result-oriented in its evaluations. However, a patient with a score below 12 on the scale, according to experts, still has a remote chance of also having neuropathic pain. A patient who receives a score of more than 12 may not also be experiencing neuropathic pain.

Psychometric Properties [10]

Specificity: 80-94%

Sensitivity: 82-91%

NEUROPATHIC PAIN QUESTIONNAIRE (NPQ)

Following the formulation and application of the McGill Pain Questionnaire, LANSS, and neuropathic pain scale, it was sometimes realized that a new pain evaluation tool was needed to differentiate between various types of pain. Hence, the development of a neuropathic pain questionnaire (NPQ) clinically helped to distinguish between neuropathic and non-neuropathic pain [11].

NPQ is not sensitive to differentiate between dynamic and static mechanical hyperalgesia [11].

Description

NPQ is a 12-item scale that helps to differentiate neuropathic pain, in which 10 items assess the sensory perception of pain and the remaining 2 assess the effects of pain.

Using a systematic approach, it was found that out of the 12 NPQ items, only 3- tingling pain, numbness, and increased pain due to touch were considered significant predictors. Based on these items, the authors devised a concise version of the NPQ.

Intended Population

1. Complex Regional Pain Syndrome 1 (CRPS) and Causalgia
2. Lumbar or Cervical Radiculopathy
3. Brachial Plexus Injury
4. Peripheral Neuropathies
5. Polyneuropathies
6. Trigeminal Neuralgia

Administration

It is a clinician-administered outcome measure based on the interview mode. It takes about 10 minutes to complete.

Neuropathic Pain Questionnaire (NPQ) (Table 5a)

Table 5a. Neuropathic Pain Questionnaire (NPQ) details.

1.	**Burning Pain**			
	0..................................100		Please rate your usual pain:	....
	No Burning Pain	Worst Burning Pain Imaginable		
2.	**Over-sensitive to touch**			
	0..................................100		Please rate your usual pain:	....
	No Oversensitivity	Worst Oversensitivity Imaginable		
3.	**Shooting Pain**			
	0..................................100		Please rate your usual pain:	....
	No Shooting Pain	Worst Shooting Pain Imaginable		
4.	**Numbness**			
	0..................................100		Please rate your usual pain:	....
	No Numbness	Worst Numbness Imaginable		
5.	**Electric Pain**			
	0..................................100		Please rate your usual pain:	....
	No Electric Pain	Worst Electric Pain Imaginable		
6.	**Tingling Pain**			

(Table 5a) cont.....

<table>
<tr><td>1.</td><td colspan="2">Burning Pain</td><td></td><td></td></tr>
<tr><td></td><td colspan="2">0………………………………100</td><td rowspan="2">Please rate your usual pain:</td><td rowspan="2">…………</td></tr>
<tr><td></td><td>No Tingling Pain</td><td>Worst Tingling Pain Imaginable</td></tr>
<tr><td>7.</td><td colspan="2">Squeezing Pain</td><td></td><td></td></tr>
<tr><td></td><td colspan="2">0………………………………100</td><td rowspan="2">Please rate your usual pain:</td><td rowspan="2">…………</td></tr>
<tr><td></td><td>No Squeezing Pain</td><td>Worst Squeezing Pain Imaginable</td></tr>
<tr><td>8.</td><td colspan="2">Freezing Pain</td><td></td><td></td></tr>
<tr><td></td><td colspan="2">0………………………………100</td><td rowspan="2">Please rate your usual pain:</td><td rowspan="2">…………</td></tr>
<tr><td></td><td>No Freezing Pain</td><td>Worst Freezing Pain Imaginable</td></tr>
<tr><td>9.</td><td colspan="2">How unpleasant is your usual pain?</td><td></td><td></td></tr>
<tr><td></td><td colspan="2">0………………………………100</td><td rowspan="2">Please rate your usual pain:</td><td rowspan="2">…………</td></tr>
<tr><td></td><td>Most Unpleasant Pain Imaginable</td><td>Worst Unpleasant Pain Imaginable</td></tr>
<tr><td>10.</td><td colspan="2">How Overwhelming is your usual pain?</td><td></td><td></td></tr>
<tr><td></td><td colspan="2">0………………………………100</td><td rowspan="2">Please rate your usual pain:</td><td rowspan="2">…………</td></tr>
<tr><td></td><td>Most Overwhelming Pain Imaginable</td><td>Worst Overwhelming Pain Imaginable</td></tr>
<tr><td>11.</td><td colspan="2">Increased pain due to touch</td><td></td><td></td></tr>
<tr><td></td><td colspan="2">0………………………………100</td><td rowspan="2">Please rate your usual pain:</td><td rowspan="2">…………</td></tr>
<tr><td></td><td>No Increase at all</td><td>Greatest Increase Imaginable</td></tr>
<tr><td>12.</td><td colspan="2">Increased pain due to weather changes</td><td></td><td></td></tr>
<tr><td></td><td colspan="2">0………………………………100</td><td rowspan="2">Please rate your usual pain:</td><td rowspan="2">…………</td></tr>
<tr><td></td><td>No Increase at all</td><td>Greatest Increase Imaginable</td></tr>
</table>

To assess and treat your pain problem, we need to thoroughly understand just exactly what type of pain you have, and how it may not change over time. You may have only one site of pain, or you may have more than one.

Please name the site of pain that is most severe or disturbing for you (*e.g.*, arm, foot, *etc*):

For all of the following questions, please rate your pain at the site you just listed.

Please use the space below to describe your pain in your own words:

Please use the items below to rate your pain as it usually feels. Indicate a number that represents your pain on each scale. For example, if you have no burning pain, you would rate the first item "0". If you have the worst burning pain imaginable, you would rate it "100". If neither of those fits your pain because it is in between, choose a number that fits your pain.

Scoring Worksheet (Table 5b)

Table 5b. Scoring sheet.

S. No.	Component	Score		Coefficient		Product
1.	Burning Pain	....	X	0.006	=	....
2.	Overly Sensitive to touch	....	X	0.005	=	....
3.	Shooting Pain	....	X	0.005	=	....
4.	Numbness	....	X	0.020	=	....
5.	Electric Pain	....	X	-0.008	=	....
6.	Tingling Pain	....	X	0.010	=	....
7.	Squeezing Pain	....	X	-0.004	=	....
8.	Freezing Pain	....	X	0.004	=	....
9.	How unpleasant is usual pain?	....	X	0.006	=	....
10.	How overwhelming is usual pain?	....	X	-0.003	=	....
11.	Increased pain due to touch	....	X	0.006	=	....
12.	Increased pain due to weather changes	....	X	-0.005	=	....
	Constant					-1.408
	TOTAL DISCRIMINANT FUNCTION SCORE					....

Instructions: For each of the twelve items below, copy the subject's score into the first column. Multiply by the coefficient in the second column, and write the product in the third column. Total all the figures in the third column, including the constant. The resulting total represents the discriminant function score.

Subjects with scores below 0 are predicted to have non-neuropathic pain, while those with scores at or above 0 are predicted to have neuropathic pain.

Check one of the following boxes:

Discriminant Function Score <u>Below</u> 0: .... Predicts Non-neuropathic Pain

Discriminant Function Score <u>at or above</u> 0: .... Predicts Non-neuropathic

Pain

Scoring and interpretation

Pain is rated based on how it usually feels using the provided items. For each scale, the patient should indicate a number representing their pain level. If they feel no pain, they will rate the first item as "0." If they are experiencing the most excruciating pain, they will rate it as "100." If their pain intensity falls somewhere in between, they should choose a number that best reflects that level [11].

Take note of the subject's score for each of the twelve items listed. Multiply the product by the coefficient in the second column and write it in the third column. Add up all of the numbers in the third column, including the constant. The sum of the results represents the discriminant function score [11].

Subjects with scores less than 0 are expected to have non-neuropathic pain, while those with scores equal to or greater than 0 are expected to have neuropathic pain [11].

Psychometric Properties [11]

Specificity: 74.4%

Sensitivity: 66.6%

Accuracy: 71.4%

CLINICAL CONSIDERATIONS, STRENGTHS, LIMITATIONS, AND EMERGING PERSPECTIVES

Peripheral neuropathies represent a broad spectrum of disorders that affect the peripheral nervous system, leading to varied combinations of sensory loss, neuropathic pain, motor weakness, and autonomic dysfunction. Because of this heterogeneity, assessment must be multimodal: clinician-administered neurological tests, objective measures (nerve conduction studies, quantitative sensory testing), and patient-reported outcome measures (PROMs) all contribute complementary information. Choosing the appropriate combination of tools depends on the clinical question—screening, diagnostic characterization, monitoring progression, or evaluating treatment response.

Clinician-rated instruments such as the Veterans Affairs Neuropathy Scale (VANS) and Overall Neuropathy Limitations Scale (ONLS) provide structured approaches to measuring impairment and activity limitations. These scales are useful in clinical practice and research because they standardize neurological examination and functional assessment. However, clinician scales can under-represent subjective symptoms (notably neuropathic pain and paresthesia) and may be insensitive to small-fiber involvement, which often produces prominent symptoms with little change on large-fiber testing.

Patient-reported instruments address this shortfall by capturing symptom burden directly from the patient's perspective. Measures such as the Treatment-Induced Neuropathy Assessment Scale (TNAS) focus on symptom severity and functional interference, and have been psychometrically evaluated for use in chemotherapy-related neuropathy and other treatment-induced neuropathies [12]. Systematic evaluations of PROMs for chemotherapy-induced peripheral neuropathy (CIPN) have shown that PROMs frequently outperform clinician-rated scales in sensitivity to symptom onset and change over time, although instrument selection must be matched to the intended use and population [13].

A central limitation across commonly used measures is insufficient coverage of small-fiber and autonomic neuropathies. Many routine scales and clinical tests target large-fiber dysfunction (*e.g.*, vibration, muscle strength, reflexes), while small-fiber neuropathies (pain, thermal sensitivity, autonomic symptoms) often require specialized tests such as intraepidermal nerve fiber density or quantitative sensory testing. Integrating PROMs that specifically query small-fiber symptoms is therefore essential when small-fiber involvement is suspected.

Responsiveness and minimal clinically important difference (MCID) remain practical concerns. Some scales demonstrate good reliability but uncertain responsiveness in short clinical trials or early disease. This is particularly relevant in trials of disease-modifying therapies or neuroprotective agents, where sensitive outcome measures are needed to detect modest but meaningful change.

Emerging technologies offer promising ways to fill existing gaps. Wearable inertial sensors and remote activity monitors enable objective quantification of gait variability, step parameters, and daily mobility patterns, which can reflect functional impairment related to neuropathy and may be sensitive to progression or intervention effects [14]. In addition, novel sensory neuroprostheses and targeted peripheral neuromodulation approaches are being piloted to restore sensation or reduce neuropathic pain; early studies suggest these can produce measurable functional gains and symptom relief, although larger trials are needed [15].

Pragmatically, a tiered assessment strategy is recommended:

- Screening (primary care/diabetes clinics): brief PROM + focused exam (*e.g.*, MNSI or simple questionnaire + monofilament/vibration screening).
- Diagnostic characterization (specialist clinics): detailed neurological exam, nerve conduction studies, and targeted PROMs (*e.g.*, TNAS for treatment-related neuropathy).
- Monitoring/outcomes (trials & rehab): Combine objective functional measures (gait metrics from IMUs), validated PROMs, and clinician-rated functional scales to capture both symptom and performance change.

By aligning instrument selection with the clinical goal and by combining subjective, objective, and instrumented measures, clinicians and researchers can obtain a richer, more reliable picture of peripheral neuropathy and its impact (Table **6**).

Table 6. Comparative summary of commonly used neuropathy assessment scales.

Scale / Tool	Primary Domain Assessed	Key Strengths	Major Limitations	Most Appropriate Clinical Use
Michigan Neuropathy Screening Instrument (MNSI)	Screening (symptoms + signs)	Quick; feasible in outpatient and diabetes clinics	Limited sensitivity to early small-fiber neuropathy	Initial screening for diabetes and general practice
Neuropathy Disability Score (NDS)	Large-fiber sensory and reflex impairment	Simple bedside scoring; widely used in research	Insensitive to pain and autonomic symptoms	Disease severity grading in clinical studies
Overall Neuropathy Limitations Scale (ONLS)	Functional limitations (upper & lower limbs)	Links impairment to daily function	Less sensitive to subtle progression	Monitoring disability in chronic neuropathies
Veterans Affairs Neuropathy Scale (VANS)	Motor, sensory, reflex impairment	Structured neurological exam; reproducible	Examiner-dependent; limited symptom capture	Specialist neurological assessment
Treatment-Induced Neuropathy Assessment Scale (TNAS)	Patient-reported symptoms & interference	Sensitive to early change; patient-centered	Subjective; influenced by mood and cognition	Chemotherapy-induced and treatment-related neuropathy
Numeric Rating Scale / Pain Scales	Neuropathic pain severity	Easy to administer; responsive	Pain-specific; ignores motor and sensory loss	Symptom monitoring and analgesic response

(Table 6) cont.....

Scale / Tool	Primary Domain Assessed	Key Strengths	Major Limitations	Most Appropriate Clinical Use
Quantitative Sensory Testing (QST)	Sensory thresholds (small & large fibers)	Objective; detects small-fiber dysfunction	Time-consuming; equipment dependent	Diagnostic clarification and research
Wearable sensor-based gait metrics	Functional mobility in daily life	Objective; continuous monitoring	Limited standardization; data interpretation challenges	Emerging outcome measures in trials and rehabilitation

CONCLUSION

In summary, this chapter offers a comprehensive synthesis of the most commonly used neuropathy assessment scales, emphasising their clinical applicability, psychometric robustness, and suitability for various patient populations. By critically examining the LANSS, DN4, NPQ, ONLS, VANS, and UENS, it underscores the importance of selecting tools based on the specific neuropathic condition, assessment context, and desired outcome measures. Understanding the strengths and limitations of each scale enables clinicians and researchers to make informed decisions that enhance diagnostic accuracy, facilitate treatment monitoring, and promote evidence-based practice in neuropathy management. Ultimately, the thoughtful application of these validated instruments can contribute to more precise evaluation and improved patient-centred care in the field of neurology and rehabilitation.

AI DISCLOSURE STATEMENT

During the preparation of this chapter, the authors used ChatGPT (OpenAI) as a support tool for language refinement, structural organisation, and clarification of ideas. All content generated with AI assistance was carefully reviewed, verified, and revised by the authors to ensure factual accuracy, originality, and consistency with the scientific literature. The authors take full responsibility for the integrity, interpretation, and final content of the published chapter.

ACKNOWLEDGEMENT

The authors express their profound gratitude to the Maharishi Markandeshwar Institute of Physiotherapy and Rehabilitation, Maharishi Markandeshwar (Deemed to be University), Mullana-Ambala, Haryana, for fostering an encouraging academic and research environment and providing the essential resources that supported the preparation of this chapter. They also acknowledge the valuable contributions of healthcare professionals and rehabilitation specialists, whose ongoing dedication to developing and refining neuropathy assessment methods continues to inspire advancements in both research and clinical practice.

REFERENCES

[1] Watson JC, Dyck PJB. Peripheral Neuropathy: A Practical Approach to Diagnosis and Symptom Management. Mayo Clin Proc 2015; 90(7): 940-51. [http://dx.doi.org/10.1016/j.mayocp.2015.05.004] [PMID: 26141332]

[2] Lehmann HC, Wunderlich G, Fink GR, Sommer C. Diagnosis of peripheral neuropathy. Neurological Research and Practice 2020; 2(1): 20. [http://dx.doi.org/10.1186/s42466-020-00064-2] [PMID: 33324924]

[3] Bouhassira D, Attal N, Alchaar H, *et al.* Comparison of pain syndromes associated with nervous or somatic lesions and development of a new neuropathic pain diagnostic questionnaire (DN4). Pain 2005; 114(1): 29-36. [http://dx.doi.org/10.1016/j.pain.2004.12.010] [PMID: 15733628]

[4] Spallone V, Morganti R, D'Amato C, Greco C, Cacciotti L, Marfia GA. Validation of DN4 as a screening tool for neuropathic pain in painful diabetic polyneuropathy. Diabet Med 2012; 29(5): 578-85. [http://dx.doi.org/10.1111/j.1464-5491.2011.03500.x] [PMID: 22023377]

[5] Wilson AM, Ong MK, Saliba D, Jamal NI. The veterans affairs neuropathy scale: a reliable, remote polyneuropathy exam. Front Neurol 2019; 10: 1050. [http://dx.doi.org/10.3389/fneur.2019.01050] [PMID: 31736844]

[6] Graham RC, Hughes RA. A modified peripheral neuropathy scale: the Overall Neuropathy Limitations Scale. J Neurol Neurosurg Psychiatry 2006; 77(8): 973-6. [http://dx.doi.org/10.1136/jnnp.2005.081547] [PMID: 16574730]

[7] Merkies ISJ, Schmitz PI, van der Meché FG, Samijn JP, van Doorn PA. Clinimetric evaluation of a new overall disability scale in immune mediated polyneuropathies. J Neurol Neurosurg Psychiatry 2002; 72(5): 596-601. [http://dx.doi.org/10.1136/jnnp.72.5.596] [PMID: 11971045]

[8] Singleton JR, Bixby B, Russell JW, *et al.* The Utah Early Neuropathy Scale: a sensitive clinical scale for early sensory predominant neuropathy. J Peripher Nerv Syst 2008; 13(3): 218-27. [http://dx.doi.org/10.1111/j.1529-8027.2008.00180.x] [PMID: 18844788]

[9] Bennett M. The LANSS Pain Scale: the Leeds assessment of neuropathic symptoms and signs. Pain. 2001; 92(1-2): 147-157. [http://dx.doi.org/10.1016/s0304-3959(00)00482-6]

[10] Bennett MI, Attal N, Backonja MM, *et al.* Using screening tools to identify neuropathic pain. Pain 2007; 127(3): 199-203. [http://dx.doi.org/10.1016/j.pain.2006.10.034] [PMID: 17182186]

[11] Krause SJ, Backonja MM. Development of a neuropathic pain questionnaire. Clin J Pain 2003; 19(5): 306-14. [http://dx.doi.org/10.1097/00002508-200309000-00004] [PMID: 12966256]

[12] Mendoza TR, Williams LA, Shi Q, *et al.* The Treatment-induced Neuropathy Assessment Scale (TNAS): a psychometric update following qualitative enrichment. J Patient Rep Outcomes 2020; 4(1): 15. [http://dx.doi.org/10.1186/s41687-020-0180-8] [PMID: 32076879]

[13] Li T, Park SB, Battaglini E, *et al.* Assessing chemotherapy-induced peripheral neuropathy with patient

reported outcome measures: a systematic review of measurement properties and considerations for future use. Qual Life Res 2022; 31(11): 3091-107.
[http://dx.doi.org/10.1007/s11136-022-03154-7] [PMID: 35596913]

[14] Talha M, Hussain L, Ullah A, Khan A. A survey of peripheral neuropathy diagnosis using intelligent and wearable systems. Technologies (Basel) 2023; 11(6): 163.
[http://dx.doi.org/10.3390/technologies11060163]

[15] Gozzi N, Chee L, Odermatt I, *et al*. Wearable non-invasive neuroprosthesis for targeted sensory restoration in neuropathy. Nat Commun. 2024; 15(1): 10840. Published 2024 Dec 30. doi:10.1038/s41467-024-55152-7

CHAPTER 8

Scales to Assess Spinal Cord Injury

Jayshankar Choudhary[1], **Sukhpal Singh**[1] and **Akanksha Saxena**[1,*]

[1] *Maharishi Markandeshwar Institute of Physiotherapy and Rehabilitation, Maharishi Markandeshwar (Deemed to be University), Mullana, Ambala, Haryana, India*

Abstract: Spinal cord injury (SCI) is a serious condition caused by trauma, disease, or degeneration of the spine, leading to a loss of motor and sensory function below the level of the injury. This damage disrupts communication between the brain and the rest of the body, often resulting in paralysis, sensory loss, and dysfunction of autonomic functions. The extent and location of the injury largely determine the severity of the impact, ranging from minor impairments to complete loss of movement and sensation. Spinal cord injury symptoms include paralysis, sensory loss, bladder/bowel dysfunction, sexual impairment, respiratory issues, chronic pain, and autonomic problems such as low blood pressure and temperature regulation difficulties. Severity varies by injury level. So, accurate assessment and re-assessment are necessary for rehabilitation and for measuring progress. This chapter covers key spinal cord injury (SCI) assessment scales: the ASIA Impairment Scale for determining motor and sensory impairment levels, the Spinal Cord Independence Measure (SCIM) for evaluating functional independence in daily activities, and the Spinal Cord Assessment Tool for Spastic Reflexes (SCATS) for assessing spasticity and reflex severity in SCI patients. Additionally, the Balance Error Scoring System (BESS) is used to assess balance, while the Mini-Balance Evaluation System Test (Mini-BESTest) measures balance and mobility. The SCI Spasticity Evaluation Tool (SCISET) assesses spasticity, and gait and ambulation are evaluated using the Walking Index for SCI (WISCI). WISCI also assesses hand function. Other important tools include the SCI-QOL, which measures the overall quality of life in SCI patients, and the SCI Pain. Lastly, the Spinal Cord Injury Functional Ambulation Inventory (SCIFAI) is used for assessing walking and functional ambulation.

Keywords: Chronic pain, Functional status, Muscle spasticity, Paralysis, Quality of life, Spinal cord injuries.

INTRODUCTION

Spinal cord injury (SCI) is a serious condition resulting from damage to the spinal cord, often caused by accidents like car crashes. While trauma is the most comm-

* **Corresponding author Akanksha Saxena:** Maharishi Markandeshwar Institute of Physiotherapy and Rehabilitation, Maharishi Markandeshwar (Deemed to be University), Mullana-Ambala (Haryana), India;
E-mail: akankshasaxena623@gmail.com

Nidhi Sharma, Simranjeet Kaur & Parveen Kumar (Eds.)

on cause, other factors like cancer and tuberculosis can also lead to SCI. The damage can cause permanent disability, affecting movement, sensation, and even breathing. Injuries to the upper part of the spinal cord can be particularly dangerous, as they may impact vital functions like heart and lung activity, requiring immediate medical attention. Many scales have been designed to comprehensively evaluate various aspects of SCI, such as motor function, sensory perception, and overall well-being [1, 2]. These scales offer valuable insights for healthcare professionals, enabling them to tailor treatment plans and monitor patient progress. By contributing to a deeper understanding of SCI, these tools can play a vital role in improving outcomes and enhancing the lives of individuals affected by this condition.

AMERICAN SPINAL INJURY ASSOCIATION IMPAIRMENT SCALE (ASIA)

Introduction

The American Spinal Injury Association created the International Standards for Neurological Classification of Spinal Injury, a grading and classification system used in the treatment of patients with spinal cord injuries that helps practitioners identify neurologic levels of injury. It is a standardised, careful, detailed documentation of spinal cord injuries that guides further radiographic assessment and treatment and determines whether injuries are complete or incomplete [3].

Description

The AISA examination consists of three examinations, as shown in Fig. (**1**), which are:

1. Myotomal examination is a Motor Examination
2. Dermatomal examination is a Sensory Examination
3. Anorectal Examination

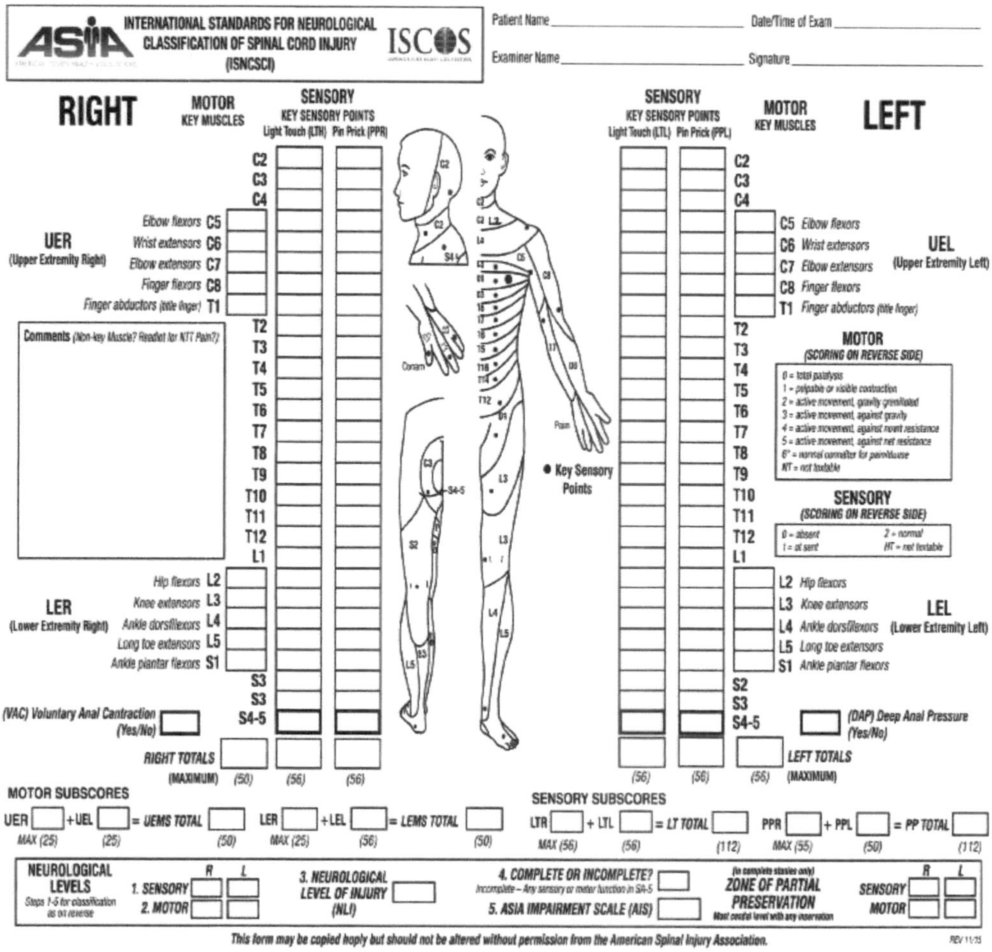

INTERNATIONAL STANDARDS FOR NEUROLOGICAL CLASSIFICATION OF SPINAL CORD INJURY (ISNCSCI)

Patient Name ____ Date/Time of Exam ____

Examiner Name ____ Signature ____

RIGHT — MOTOR KEY MUSCLES — SENSORY KEY SENSORY POINTS Light Touch (LTR) Pin Prick (PPR)

SENSORY KEY SENSORY POINTS Light Touch (LTL) Pin Prick (PPL) — MOTOR KEY MUSCLES — LEFT

C2, C3, C4

UER (Upper Extremity Right): Elbow flexors C5; Wrist extensors C6; Elbow extensors C7; Finger flexors C8; Finger abductors (little finger) T1

UEL (Upper Extremity Left): C5 Elbow flexors; C6 Wrist extensors; C7 Elbow extensors; C8 Finger flexors; T1 Finger abductors (little finger)

Comments (Non-key Muscle? Reason for NT? Pain?)

T2, T3, T4, T5, T6, T7, T8, T9, T10, T11, T12, L1

MOTOR (SCORING ON REVERSE SIDE)
0 = total paralysis
1 = palpable or visible contraction
2 = active movement, gravity eliminated
3 = active movement, against gravity
4 = active movement, against some resistance
5 = active movement, against full resistance
5* = normal corrected for pain/disuse
NT = not testable

SENSORY (SCORING ON REVERSE SIDE)
0 = absent 2 = normal
1 = altered NT = not testable

● Key Sensory Points

LER (Lower Extremity Right): Hip flexors L2; Knee extensors L3; Ankle dorsiflexors L4; Long toe extensors L5; Ankle plantar flexors S1

LEL (Lower Extremity Left): L2 Hip flexors; L3 Knee extensors; L4 Ankle dorsiflexors; L5 Long toe extensors; S1 Ankle plantar flexors

S2, S3, S4-5

(VAC) Voluntary Anal Contraction (Yes/No)

(DAP) Deep Anal Pressure (Yes/No)

RIGHT TOTALS (MAXIMUM) (50) (56) (56)

LEFT TOTALS (MAXIMUM) (56) (56) (50)

MOTOR SUBSCORES

UER ☐ + UEL ☐ = UEMS TOTAL ☐ MAX (25) (25) (50)

LER ☐ + LEL ☐ = LEMS TOTAL ☐ MAX (25) (25) (50)

SENSORY SUBSCORES

LTR ☐ + LTL ☐ = LT TOTAL ☐ MAX (56) (56) (112)

PPR ☐ + PPL ☐ = PP TOTAL ☐ MAX (56) (56) (112)

NEUROLOGICAL LEVELS (Steps 1-5 for classification as on reverse) R L — 1. SENSORY 2. MOTOR

3. NEUROLOGICAL LEVEL OF INJURY (NLI)

4. COMPLETE OR INCOMPLETE? (Incomplete = Any sensory or motor function in S4-5)

5. ASIA IMPAIRMENT SCALE (AIS)

ZONE OF PARTIAL PRESERVATION (In complete injuries only) (Most caudal level with any innervation) R L — SENSORY MOTOR

This form may be copied freely but should not be altered without permission from the American Spinal Injury Association.

REV 11/15

Fig. (1). American spinal injury association impairment scale.

The sensory evaluation assesses the light touch (usually a cotton piece) and pinprick (usually a clean safety pin) sensations bilaterally on 28 distinct dermatomes. Every aspect of the examination is documented for every dermatome and laterality. A score of 0 indicates no sensation, a grade of 1 indicates diminished or changed sensation, and a grade of 2 indicates normal experience. A typical unilateral sensory examination has 28 dermatomes, or 112 total points, each of which has 2/2 points for gentle touch and 2/2 points for pinprick. A bilateral sensory evaluation with a total score of 224 indicates full normalcy. A score of 0 is assigned for the inability to differentiate between light touch and pinprick sensation.

Five distinct muscle groups representing the primary cervical and lumbar myotomes in the upper extremities and five distinct muscle groups in the lower extremities are graded as part of the motor assessment. A six-point universal scale is used to grade motor strength (0–5). Bilateral measurements of motor strength are made for every muscle group. A healthy person can have a maximum bilateral motor score of 100, with 50 points awarded for each right upper and lower extremities myotome that scores 5/5, and an additional 50 points for the left.

To ascertain the extent of the damage and assess whether spinal shock is present, the anorectal examination is crucial. The ability to perceive deep anal pressure and to constrict voluntarily is assessed digitally in the external anal sphincter. Both are assigned a binary grade, with 0 denoting absence and 1 denoting presence. Squeezing the glans penis or clitoris causes a palpable contraction of the internal and external anal sphincters, which is how the bulbocavernosus reflex is evaluated during digital rectal examination. An indwelling urinary catheter tug may also trigger the reflex [3, 4].

Scoring [5]

For Motor:

Grade 1 = Complete impairment, with no motor or sensory function below the injury level

Grade 2 = Incomplete impairment, with sensory function but no motor function below the neurologic level, and some sensation in sacral segments S4 and S5

Grade 3 = Incomplete impairment, with motor function below the neurologic level, and most key muscles below that level having a muscle grade of less than 3

Grade 4 = Incomplete impairment, with motor function below the neurologic level, and most key muscles below that level having a muscle grade of greater than or equal to 3

Grade 5 = Normal sensory and motor function

For Sensory:

Grade 0 = Absent
Grade 1 = Altered
Grade 2 = Normal
NT = Not Testable

Training Required

Healthcare professionals administering the American Spinal Injury Association impairment scale (ASIA), as shown in Fig. (**1**), should have training in the interpretation of the measures. Training includes understanding the scoring system and ensuring that patients comprehend the questionnaire adequately [6, 7].

Psychometric Properties [4, 8]

Intra-rater reliability = 0.98

Inter-rater reliability = 0.99

ASIA scores demonstrated a very significant connection, with intraclass and Pearson correlation values above 0.96 and P<0.01 for the total motor, light touch, and pinprick scores [4, 8].

SPINAL CORD INDEPENDENCE MEASURE (SCIM)

Introduction

Spinal Cord Independent Measure is a disability scale that was developed to address the ability of SCI patients to perform basic activities of daily living independently. It examines breathing and sphincter control, self-care (feeding, grooming, bathing, and dressing), and a patient's mobility (bed and transfers, indoors and outdoors) as given in Fig. (**2a-d**). Additionally, physicians can use the SCIM to help determine therapy goals and objectives for patients with SCIs [6, 9].

ICF Domain

Body Functions

Activities and Participation

Body Structures

Spinal Cord Independence Measure (SCIM)

Self-Care DATE / / / / / /

1. Feeding (cutting, opening containers, pouring, bringing food to mouth, holding cup with fluid)
0. Needs parenteral, gastrostomy, or fully assisted oral feeding
1. Needs partial assistance for eating and/or drinking, or for wearing adaptive devices
2. Eats independently; needs adaptive devices or assistance only for cutting food and/or pouring and/or opening containers
3. Eats and drinks independently; does not require assistance or adaptive devices

2. Bathing (soaping, washing, drying body and head, manipulating water tap). **A-upper body; B-lower body**
A. 0. Requires total assistance
1. Requires partial assistance
2. Washes independently with adaptive devices or in a specific setting (*e.g.*, bars, chair)
3. Washes independently; does not require adaptive devices or specific setting (not customary for healthy people) (adss)

B. 0. Requires total assistance
1. Requires partial assistance
2. Washes independently with adaptive devices or in a specific setting (adss)
3. Washes independently; does not require adaptive devices (adss) or specific setting

3. Dressing (clothes, shoes, permanent orthoses: dressing, wearing, undressing). **A-upper body; B-lower body**
A. 0. Requires total assistance
1. Requires partial assistance with clothes without buttons, zippers or laces (cwobzl)
2. Independent with cwobzl; requires adaptive devices and/or specific settings (adss)
3. Independent with cwobzl; does not require adss; needs assistance or adss only for bzl
4. Dresses (any cloth) independently, does not require adaptive devices or specific setting

B. 0. Requires total assistance
1. Requires partial assistance with clothes without buttons, zipps or laces (cwobzl)
2. Independent with cwobzl; requires adaptive devices and/or specific settings (adss)
3. Independent with cwobzl without adss; needs assistance or adss only for bzl
4. Dresses (any cloth) independently, does not require adaptive devices or specific setting

4. Grooming (washing hands and face, brushing teeth, combing hair, shaving, applying makeup)
0. Requires total assistance
1. Requires partial assistance
2. Grooms independently with adaptive devices
3. Grooms independently without adaptive devices

SUBTOTAL (0-20)

Fig. (2a). Self-care activities assessment of the SCIM scale.

Respiration and Sphincter Management

5. Respiration
0. Requires tracheal tube (TT) and permanent or intermittent assisted ventilation (IAV)
2. Breathes independently with TT; requires oxygen, much assistance in coughing or TT management
4. Breathes independently with TT; requires little assistance in coughing or TT management
6. Breathes independently without TT; requires oxygen, much assistance in coughing, a mask (e.g., peep) or IAV (bipap)
8. Breathes independently without TT; requires little assistance or stimulation for coughing
10. Breathes independently without assistance or device

6. Sphincter Management - Bladder
0. Indwelling catheter
3. Residual urine volume (RUV) > 100cc; no regular catheterization or assisted intermittent catheterization
6. RUV < 100cc or intermittent self-catheterization; needs assistance for applying drainage instrument
9. Intermittent self-catheterization; uses external drainage instrument; does not need assistance for applying
11. Intermittent self-catheterization; continent between catheterizations; does not use external drainage instrument
11. RUV < 100cc; needs only external urine drainage; no assistance is required for drainage
13. RUV < 100cc; continent; doesnot use external drainage instrument

7. Sphincter Management - Bowel
0. Irregular timing or very low frequency (less than once in 3 days) of bowel movements
5. Regular timing, but requires assistance (*e.g.*, for applying suppository); rare accidents (less than twice a month)
8. Regular bowel movements, without assistance; rare accidents (less than twice a month)
10. Regular bowel movements, without assistance; no accidents

8. Use of Toilet (perineal hygiene, adjustment of clothes before/after, use of napkins or diapers).
0. Requires total assistance
1. Requires partial assistance; does not clean self
2. Requires partial assistance; cleans self independently
4. Uses toilet independently in all tasks but needs adaptive devices or special setting (*e.g.*, bars)
5. Uses toilet independently; does not require adaptive devices or special setting)

SUBTOTAL (0-40)

Fig. (2b). Respiratory and sphincter management of SCIM scale.

Mobility (room and toilet) DATE \ \ \ \ \ \ \

9. Mobility in Bed and Action to Prevent Pressure Sores

0. Needs assistance in all activities: turning upper body in bed, turning lower body in bed, sitting up in bed, doing push-ups in wheelchair, with or without adaptive devices, but not with electric aids
2. Performs one of the activities without assistance
4. Performs two or three of the activities without assistance
6. Performs all the bed mobility and pressure release activities independently

10. Transfers: bed-wheelchair (locking wheelchair, lifting footrests, removing and adjusting arm rests, transferring, lifting feet).

0. Requires total assistance
1. Needs partial assistance and/or supervision, and/or adaptive devices (*e.g.*, sliding board)
2. Independent (or does not require wheelchair)

11. Transfers: wheelchair-toilet-tub (if uses toilet wheelchair: transfers to and from; if uses regular wheelchair: locking wheelchair, lifting footrests, removing and adjusting armrests, transferring, lifting feet)

0. Requires total assistance
1. Needs partial assistance and/or supervision, and/or adaptive devices (*e.g.*, grab-bars)
2. Independent (or does not require wheelchair)

Mobility (indoors and outdoors, on even surface)

12. Mobility Indoors

0. Requires total assistance
1. Needs electric wheelchair or partial assistance to operate manual wheelchair
2. Moves independently in manual wheelchair
3. Requires supervision while walking (with or without devices)
4. Walks with a walking frame or crutches (swing)
5. Walks with crutches or two canes (reciprocal walking)
6. Walks with one cane
7. Needs leg orthosis only
8. Walks without walking aids

Fig. (2c). Mobility assessment of the SCIM scale.

13. Mobility for Moderate Distances (10-100 meters)

0. Requires total assistance
1. Needs electric wheelchair or partial assistance to operate manual wheelchair
2. Moves independently in manual wheelchair
3. Requires supervision while walking (with or without devices)
4. Walks with a walking frame or crutches (swing)
5. Walks with cratches or two canes (reciprocal walking)
6. Walks with one cane
7. Needs leg orthosis only
8. Walks without walking aids

14. Mobility Outdoors (more than 100 meters)

0. Requires total assistance
1. Needs electric wheelchair or partial assistance to operate manual wheelchair
2. Moves independently in manual wheelchair
3. Requires supervision while walking (with or without devices)
4. Walks with a walking frame or crutches (swing)
5. Walks with cratches or two canes (reciprocal waking)
6. Walks with one cane
7. Needs leg orthosis only
8. Walks without walking aids

15. Stair Management

0. Unable to ascend or descend stairs
1. Ascends and descends at least 3 steps with support or supervision of another person
2. Ascends and descends at least 3 steps with support of handrail and/or crutch or cane
3. Ascends and descends at least 3 steps without any support or supervision

16. Transfers: wheelchair-car (approaching car, locking wheelchair, removing arm- and footrests, transferring to and from car, bringing wheelchair into and out of car)

0. Requires total assistance
1. Needs partial assistance and/or supervision and/or adaptive devices
2. Transfers independent; does not require adaptive devices (or does not require wheelchair)

17. Transfers: ground-wheelchair

0. Requires assistance
1. Transfers independent with or without adaptive devices (or does not require wheelchair)

SUBTOTAL (0-40)

TOTAL SCIM SCORE (0-100)

Fig. (2d). Mobility assessment of the SCIM scale.

Number of Items

17

Equipment Needed

There is no need for any type of equipment to perform this outcome measure.

Completion Time

It takes approximately 30-40 mins.

Scoring

The total score is 100

1. Self-care: 0-20
2. Respiration: 0-40
3. Mobility: 0-40

Language

1. English
2. Brazilian
3. Greek
4. Spanish
5. Thai
6. Turkish

Training Required

Healthcare professionals administering the Spinal Cord Independence Measure (SCIM) should have training in interpreting the measures. Training includesunderstanding the scoring system and ensuring patients adequately comprehend the questionnaire.

Psychometric Properties

Reliability: 0.94, Validity: 0.790 [9]

Spinal Cord Independence Measure (SCIM)

SPINAL CORD ASSESSMENT TOOL FOR SPASTIC REFLEXES (SCATS)

Introduction

The Spinal Cord Assessment Tool for Spastic Reflexes (SCATS) is used to measure spastic reflexes in individuals with spinal cord injury. It was developed in response to the demand for a standardised, simple clinical measure that encompasses the primary spastic reaction in the SCI population [10].

ICF Domain

Body Functions
Activities and Participation
Body Structures

Number of Items

3

Equipment needed

Equipment to quantitatively measure joint angle changes.

Scoring

The SCATS, as shown in Fig. (**3**), is separated into 3 subscales.

1. Clonus
2. Flexor spasms
3. Extensor spasms

- SCATS clonus is measured by rapid passive dorsiflexion.

The degree of spasm is rated between 0 (no spasm) and 3 (severe spasm lasting longer than 10 seconds).

- SCATS flexor spasm is measured by applying a pinprick stimulus to the medial arch with the knee and hip extended straight.

The degree of spasm is rated between 0 (no spasm) and 3 (severe spasm, 30 degrees of knee and hip flexion).

- SCATS extensor spasm is measured by extending the hip and knee joints from the fully extended position at 90 and 110 degrees.

The degree of spasm is rated between 0 (no spasm) and 3 (severe spasm, longer than 10 seconds).

Patient name: ____________________

Date: ____________________

R	L	
	SCATS: Clonus	
0	0	no reaction
1	1	Mild <3 secs
2	2	3< Moderate <10 secs
3	3	Severe > 10 secs
	SCATS: *flexor spasms.*	
0	0	no reaction
1	1	less than 10° of excursion in flexion at the knee and hip or extension of the great toe
2	2	moderate, 10° to 30° of flexion at the knee and hip
3	3	severe, 30° or greater of knee and hip flexion.
	SCATS: *extensor spasms*	
0	0	no reaction
1	1	Mild <3 secs
2	2	3secs < Moderate <10 secs
3	3	Severe > 10 secs

Fig. (3). Spinal cord assessment tool for spastic reflexes (SCATS).

Training Required

Training is required

Psychometric Properties [10, 11]

Reliability

- High Test-Retest kappa coefficient:$\kappa = 0.614 \pm 0.08 - 1.000 \pm 0.08$
- High Inter-rater kappa coefficient:$\kappa = 0.669 \pm 1.000$ ($P < .01$)

Validity

- High correlation of SCATS extensor scores with Ashworth hip flexors:$r = 0.98$
- High correlation of SCATS extensor scores with Ashworth knee flexors:$r = 0.88$
- High correlation of SCATS extensor scores with Ashworth ankle plantar flexors:$r = 0.61$

BALANCE ERROR SCORING SYSTEM (BESS)

The Balance Error Scoring System is a brief, easily administered, cost-effective, and objective method of assessing static postural stability. It is often used in the population of athletes with the Assessment and Management of Concussion or mild traumatic brain injury. Information obtained from this clinical balance tool can be used to assist clinicians in making return-to-play decisions following mild head injury. The BESS can be performed in nearly any environment and takes approximately 10 minutes to conduct [12, 13].

Description

Intended Population: Can be used with people who have problems with balance and postural stability, *e.g.*, functional ankle instability, and people with diseases affecting the vestibular system and/or brain, *e.g.* Sport-related concussion, stroke, Parkinson's disease, multiple sclerosis, traumatic brain injury, blast exposure in the military. Blunt trauma to the head can cause persistent problems with dizziness and balance [12, 13].

Equipment Required

- Foam pad
- Stopwatch
- An assistant to act as a spotter

- BESS testing protocol (instructions to be read to the subject during testing)
- BESS scorecard

Administration

The balance testing consists of three stances on two different surfaces. The three stances are the double-leg stance, single-leg stance, and tandem stance. The two different surfaces include both a firm (ground) surface and a foam surface.

The athlete will stand with hands on hips and eyes closed, maintaining a consistent foot position for each stance. Shoes should not be worn.

In the double-leg stance, the feet are flat on the testing surface, approximately pelvic width apart.

In the single-leg stance position, the athlete is to stand on the non-dominant leg with the contralateral limb held at approximately 20° of hip flexion, 45° of knee flexion, and neutral in the frontal plane.

In the tandem stance, one foot is placed in front of the other with the heel of the anterior foot touching the toe of the posterior foot. The athlete's non-dominant leg is in the posterior position. The athlete's kicking preference should determine leg dominance.

Scoring

Twenty seconds are allotted to the trial. Count the number of mistakes made when in the correct position. Only once the candidate has taken the correct testing position should the examiner start counting errors. Only one error is counted if several happen at once. 10 mistakes can occur for a single condition.

A number ranging from 0 to 60 indicates better balance and fewer faults. To determine the overall score (out of 60), the number of errors in each trial is summed. The normal scores are presented in Table **1** [12] and the score card of BESS in Fig. (**4**).

Score Card

Balance Error Scoring System (BESS)
(Guskiewicz)

Balance Error Scoring System – Types of Errors
1. Hands lifted off iliac crest 2. Opening eyes 3. Step, stumble, or fall 4. Moving hip into > 30 degrees abduction 5. Lifting forefoot or heel 6. Remaining out of test position >5 sec
The BESS is calculated by adding one error point for each error during the 6 20-second tests.

SCORE CARD: (# errors)	FIRM Surface	FOAM Surface
Double Leg Stance (feet together)		
Single Leg Stance (non-dominant foot)		
Tandem Stance (non-dom foot in back)		
Total Scores:		
BESS TOTAL:		

Fig. (4). Score card for BESS.

Errors: An error is credited to the subject when any of the following occur:

- moving the hands off the iliac crests
- opening the eyes
- step, stumble, or fall
- abduction or flexion of the hip beyond 30°
- lifting the forefoot or heel off the testing surface
- remaining out of the proper testing position for greater than 5 seconds [12, 13].

Table 1. Normal scores for each possible testing surface.

-	Firm Surface	Foam Surface
Double Leg Stance	.009 ± .12	.33 ± .90
Single Leg Stance	2.45 ± 2.33	5.06 ± 2.80
Tandem Stance	.91 ± 1.36	3.26 ± 2.62
Surface Total	3.37 ± 3.10	8.65 ± 5.13
BESS Total Score	**(12.03 ± 7.340)**	

Psychometric Properties

- Reliability: ranges from moderate (< 0.75) to good (> 0.75) [14 - 16].

THE MINI-BALANCE EVALUATION SYSTEMS TEST (MINI-BESTEST)

The Balance Evaluation Systems Test (BESTest) was developed to identify the postural control system(s) that underlie poor functional balance, enabling physiotherapists to target treatment to a person's specific balance deficit. It is a quantitative assessment tool. By identifying the disordered systems underlying balance control, therapists can direct specific types of intervention for different types of balance problems. A limitation of the BESTest is the time to administer it (30 to 45 minutes); therefore, a shorter version of the BESTest was developed *via* a Rasch analysis, the Mini-Balance Evaluation Systems Test2 (Mini-BESTest). The Mini-BESTest was developed in 2010 by Franchignoni *et al.* Therapists have found it easy to learn and feel that it provides relevant and valuable information that is consistent with the functional level. The Mini-BESTest is reliable and able to predict falls [17, 18].

Description

Intended Population: It can be used in ambulatory patients of varied ages and severity with neurological conditions, *e.g.*, Parkinson's Disease, stroke, cerebellar ataxia, neuropathies, head injury, multiple sclerosis, cerebral palsy, vestibular disorders, cognitive impairments, and the elderly [17, 18].

- The Mini BESTest is a 14-item test scored on a 3-level ordinal scale.
- Mini BESTest assesses dynamic balance, a unidimensional construct, and includes 14 items addressing 4 of the 6 sections of the original BESTest:

1) Anticipatory postural adjustments
2) Reactive postural control
3) Sensory orientation
4) Dynamic gait

Equipment Required

- 60 cm x 60 cm block of 4" medium density Tempur foam (T41)
- Incline ramp of 10-degree slope (2 x 2 feet recommended)
- Standard chair without armrests or wheels
- Firm chair with arms. Box that is 9 inches (23 cm) in height (~2 stacked shoeboxes)

- Stopwatch
- Masking tape marked on the floor at 3 meters from the front of the chair.

Administration

Time to administer: 10 to 15 minutes.
Age Ranges:
Adult: 18 - 64years
Elderly Adult: 65+years.
Required Training: Reading an Article/Manual

Scoring

1) The original BESTest 4-level (0 - 3) scoring was revised to 3 levels (0 - 2) due to redundancy.
2) Total score = 28 points per test direction.
3) Two items have right and left assessment in which the lower score is used within the total score (directions specify which to use).
4) For research, many studies specify the use of both left and right data, thus calculating data based on 32 (*vs.* 28) points.

Mini-BESTest of Dynamic Balance – Balance Evaluation System's Test

Subjects should be tested with flat-heeled shoes OR shoes and socks off. If the subject must use an assistive device for an item, score that item one category lower. If the subject requires physical assistance to perform an item, score the lowest category (0) for that item.

SIT TO STAND

(2) Normal: Stable for 3 s with maximum height.

(1) Moderate: Comes to stand with the use of hands on the first attempt.

(0) Severe: Impossible to stand up from a chair without assistance, OR several attempts with the use of hands.

RISE TO TOES

(2) Normal: Stable for 3 s with maximum height.

(1) Moderate: Heels up, but not full range (smaller than when holding hands), OR noticeable instability for 3 s.

(0) Severe: ≤3 s.

STAND ON ONE LEG

Left Time in Seconds Trial 1: _____ Trial 2: _____

(2) Normal: 20 seconds (1) Moderate: < 20 seconds (0) Severe: Unable

Right Time in Seconds. Trial 1: _____ Trial 2: _______

(2) Normal: 20 seconds (1) Moderate: < 20 seconds (0)Severe: Unable.

COMPENSATORY STEPPING CORRECTION – FORWARD

(2) Normal: Recovers independently a single, large step (second realignment step is allowed).

(1) Moderate: More than one step is used to recover equilibrium.

(0) Severe: No step, OR would fall if not caught, OR falls spontaneously.

COMPENSATORY STEPPING CORRECTION – BACKWARD

(2) Normal: Recovers a single, large step.

(1) Moderate: More than one step is used to recover equilibrium.

(0) Severe: No step, OR would fall if not caught, OR falls spontaneously.

COMPENSATORY STEPPING CORRECTION – LATERAL

Left: (2) Normal: Recovers independently with 1 step (crossover or lateral OK). (1) Moderate: Several steps to recover equilibrium. (0) Severe: Falls, or cannot step.

Right: (2) Normal: Recovers independently with 1 step (crossover or lateral OK). (1) Moderate: Several steps to recover equilibrium. (0) Severe: Falls, or cannot step.

STANCE EYES OPEN, FIRM SURFACE (FEET TOGETHER): TIME IN SECONDS: _______

(2) Normal: 30 seconds

(1) Moderate: < 30 seconds

(0) Severe: Unable.

STANCE EYES CLOSED, FOAM SURFACE (FEET TOGETHER): Time in seconds: ________

(2) Normal: 30 seconds

(1) Moderate: < 30 seconds

(0) Severe: Unable.

INCLINE – EYES CLOSED: TIME IN SECONDS: _______

(2) Normal: Stands independently for 30 seconds and aligns with gravity.

(1) Moderate: Stands independently for <30 seconds OR aligns with the surface.

(0) Severe: Unable.

CHANGE IN GAIT SPEED

(2) Normal: Significantly changes walking speed without imbalance.

(1) Moderate: Unable to change walking speed or have an imbalance.

(0) Severe: Unable to achieve significant change in speed AND signs of imbalance.

WALK WITH HEAD TURNS – HORIZONTAL

(2) Normal: performs head turns with no change in gait speed and good balance.

(1) Moderate: performs head turns with a reduction in gait speed.

(0) Severe: performs head turns with imbalance.

WALK WITH PIVOT TURNS

(2) Normal: Turns with feet close, FAST (≤3 steps) with good balance.

(1) Moderate: Turns with feet close SLOW (≥4 steps) with good balance.

(0) Severe: Cannot turn with feet close at any speed without imbalance.

STEP OVER OBSTACLES

(2) Normal: Able to step over the box with minimal change of speed and with good balance.

(1) Moderate: Steps over shoe boxes but touches the box, OR displays cautious behaviour by slowing gait.

(0) Severe: Cannot step over shoe boxes, OR hesitates, OR steps around the box.

TIMED GET UP & GO (TUG) AND COGNITIVE GET UP & GO WITH DUAL TASK

TUG: ______ seconds; Dual Task TUG: ______seconds

(2) Normal: No noticeable change between sitting and standing in backward counting, and no change in gait speed compared with TUG with a dual task.

(1) Moderate: Dual task affects either counting OR walking.

(0) Severe: Stops counting while walking OR stops walking while counting.

Psychometric Properties [18 - 21]

1. Vestibular Disorders:
   - Test-retest Reliability: Excellent test-retest reliability ICC = 0.96 (0.94-0.99).
   - Interrater/Interrater Reliability: Excellent interrater reliability ICC = 0.98 (0.97-0.99).
   - Excellent concurrent validity of Mini-BESTest*r* = 0.85 (CI 0.78-0.90);
   - Floor/Ceiling Effects: No evidence of floor or ceiling effect.
   - Responsiveness: Excellent ability to identify those subjects with clinically meaningful improvement: AUC = 0.92 (0.84-0.97), sensitivity = 94%, specificity = 81%, discriminative accuracy to detect moderate improvement in balance = 79%
   - Discriminatory accuracy excellent; area under the ROC curve 0.92, indicating a moderate to large global rating of change improvement.

2. Stroke:
   - Cut Off Scores: Scores of ≤ 17.5 identified those with a history of falling, sensitivity 64%, specificity 64%, AUC 0.64.
   - Test-Retest Reliability: Excellent for total score ICC = 0.96.kappa = 0.37 to 1.0.
   - Interrater/Interrater Reliability: Excellent for total scores ICC = 0.96, kappa = 0.36 to 1.0.
   - Internal Consistency: Excellent Cronbach's alpha = 0.89, 0.93, 0.94 for each rater.
   - Validity: Excellent correlation with the Berg Balance Scale, r = 0.83
   - Adequate correlation with the Functional Reach Test r = 0.55
   - Excellent correlation with Timed "Up & Go" r = -0.82
   - Floor/Ceiling Effects: Skewness = - 0.81
   - Floor effect: 0 participants with the lowest score
   - Ceiling effect: 0.9% participants with the highest score.
3. Parkinson's Disease:
   - Cut-Off Scores: Preferred Fall risk cut score 63% (20/32 points total) had adequate ability to identify fallers (sensitivity = 0.88, specificity = 0.78).
   - Test-Retest Reliability: Excellent test-retest reliability (ICC = 0.92).
   - Interrater/Interrater Reliability: Excellent Inter-rater reliability (ICC = 0.91)
   - Validity: Excellent concurrent validity between Mini-BESTest and Berg (*r* = 0.79);
   - Mini-BESTest has excellent correlation with BESTest (*r* = 0.955)
   - Excellent correlation with the Berg Balance Scale, r = 0.94
   - Floor/Ceiling Effects: No evidence of ceiling effect, Skewness -0.93.

THE WALKING INDEX FOR SPINAL CORD INJURY (WISCI)

The Walking Index for Spinal Cord Injury (WISCI) is a scale that measures the type and amount of assistance (in terms of assistive devices, or human helpers) required by a person with spinal cord injury (SCI) for walking. It is an ordinal scale that rates people with SCI from being unable to walk to independent walking and is designed to indicate the grades of impairment occurring after SCI and their relationship to the function of walking. A year after the release of the 19-level WISCI, it was modified to WISCI II, which included two levels. WISCI II is the current, accepted scale [22, 23].

Description

Intended Population: The WISCI/WISCI II was designed as a tool to measure improvement in walking ability specifically for spinal cord injury [22]. It is precisely useful for the following categories of patients:

1. Individuals with SCI who can stand and walk with parallel bars are suitable for assessment with the WISCI. Only patients with reciprocal gait should be considered when scoring the WISCI II.
2. Several individuals with ASIA Impairment Scale grade A below T10 and AIS B, C, D qualify for assessment with the WISCI II.
3. Individuals with tetraplegic presentation require motor strength in their triceps up to a grade of 3 or more to be able to sufficiently support their body weight.
4. Individuals presenting with tetraplegia and arm strength in the triceps that is less than grade 3 would not be easily classified by the WISCI.

Equipment Needed

1. Walkers (conventional, if rolling walkers are used, they must be identified in the descriptors). A platform walker is considered equivalent to a walker.
2. The use of an advanced reciprocating gait orthosis (ARGO) should be excluded.
3. Axillary or Lofstrand (Canadian) crutches may be used.
4. Braces, which could mean one or two braces, should be identified in the descriptors. For other braces, such as ace wraps or splints, they should be described under "other".
5. Long leg braces, whether they are locked or unlocked at the ankle, must be indicated in the descriptors.
6. Braces must not be covered by clothing to ensure that the physical therapist and other professional staff can visually determine whether the patient has a brace.

Administration

Completion Time: The WISCI II may take about 5 to 15 minutes to complete. Especially during the acute phase, the time required could be longer or shorter during follow-up assessments.

Rank orders the ability of a person to walk 10m after a spinal cord injury from most to least severe impairment.

- Considers: 1) Amount of assistance: two persons, defined as moderate to maximum assist; 1 person, defined as minimal assist; no assist; assistive device, such as parallel bars, walker, crutches (axillary or forearm), canes.
  Braces: 1 or 2; short or long. Of note, the original scale, WISCI, consisted of items 1-20; the scale was revised to WISCI II to include 0-20.
- Time to administer: The WISCI II may take about 5 to 15 minutes to complete. Especially during the acute phase, the time required could be longer or shorter during follow-up assessments.

- Age Ranges: Adolescent- 13 to 17 years, adult- 18 to 64years, early adult- 65+years.

Level Description

0: Client is unable to stand and/or participate in assisted walking.
1: Ambulates in parallel bars, with braces and physical assistance of two persons, less than 10 meters.

1. Ambulates in parallel bars, with braces and physical assistance of two persons, 10 meters.
2. Ambulates in parallel bars, with braces and physical assistance of one person, 10 meters.
3. Ambulates in parallel bars, no braces, and with the physical assistance of one person, 10 meters.
4. Ambulates in parallel bars, with braces and no physical assistance, 10 meters.
5. Ambulates with walker, with braces and physical assistance of one person, 10 meters.
6. Ambulates with two crutches, with braces and physical assistance of one person, 10 meters.
7. Ambulates with walker, no braces, and physical assistance of one person, 10 meters.
8. Ambulates with walker, with braces and no physical assistance, 10 meters.
9. Ambulates with one cane/crutch, with braces and physical assistance of one person, 10 meters.
10. Ambulates with two crutches, no braces, and the physical assistance of one person, 10 meters.
11. Ambulates with two crutches, with braces and no physical assistance, 10 meters.
12. Ambulates with walker, no braces and no physical assistance, 10 meters.
13. Ambulates with one cane/crutch, no braces, and the physical assistance of one person, 10 meters.
14. Ambulates with one cane/crutch, with braces and no physical assistance, 10 meters.
15. Ambulates with two crutches, no braces, and no physical assistance, 10 meters.
16. Ambulates with no devices, no braces, and physical assistance of one person, 10 meters.
17. Ambulates with no devices, with braces, and no physical assistance, 10 meters.
18. Ambulates with one cane/crutch, no braces, and no physical assistance, 10 meters.

19. Ambulates with no devices, no braces, and no physical assistance, 10 meters.

Scoring

- To score the WISCI/WISCI II, the descriptors that relate to the present walking performance of an individual with SCI are observed.
- Then, an appropriate level of the highest walking performance is assigned to the patient.
- The physical therapist selects the level at which the patient is safest, as observed, with the patient's comfort level also described. If other devices, beyond those stated in the standard definitions, are used during the assessment, they should be documented as descriptors.
- Also, if there is a discrepancy between two observers, the record with the higher level should be selected. The patient should be observed with the WISCI level documented on the scale, rated from 0 to 20, at baseline (called the Baseline WISCI), and the subject is then observed again at the defined interval (called the interval WISCI).
- Gains in walking can be obtained by simply subtracting the baseline WISCI from the interval WISCI, which is known as the "changed WISCI" [23].

Psychometric Properties [23 - 26]

Spinal Injuries

- Test- retest Reliability: Self-selected WISCI Excellent, ICC =0.994; Max WISCI, Excellent, ICC = 0.995.
- Interrater/ interrater Reliability: Excellent Interrater reliability (maximum) = 1.0
- Excellent Interrater reliability = 0.98.
- Validity: Concurrent Validity is Excellent WISCI and FIM score correlations (r = 0.765)
- Construct validity: overall correlation is Excellent WISCI II *vs* TUG (r= -0.76)
- Excellent WISCI II *vs* 10MWT (r= -0.68)
- Excellent WISCI II *vs* 6MWT (r= 0.60)
- Floor/ceiling effects: Acute incomplete SCI: 17% subjects, 42/249, reached the WISCI II score of 20 by the time of discharge from inpatient rehabilitation.
- 53% (131/249) had a WISCI score of 0 at discharge from inpatient rehab; however, 82 of these individuals were classified as AIS A or B.
- Acute SCI: 44.8% of subjects reached the highest score on the WISCI II, indicating a ceiling effect.
- Chronic SCI: 48% (24/50) subjects at greater than 1 year post injury have WISCI =20 at entry into the study

- Responsiveness: Acute incomplete SCI: Found the WISCI II to be a more precise and sensitive scale for documenting changes in levels of walking over the FIM, SCIM, RMI, and BI. WISCI II scores had a greater distribution at discharge (12 levels) *versus* FIM.
- Acute to chronic incomplete SCI: Looked at the change between different time intervals post SCI of WISCI II, 10m, and 6-minute walk tests, and ASIA LEMS. The WISCI II and LEMS showed change between 1 month and 3 months, but not thereafter, while the 10m and 6min continued to show change at 6 months post-injury [25, 26].
- Bottom line – The WISCI II is less responsive in assessing walking ability among those at a higher walking level [25, 26].

SPINAL CORD INJURY FUNCTIONAL AMBULATION INVENTORY

The Spinal Cord Injury Functional Ambulation Inventory (SCI-FAI) is a clinician-administered, self-report, and performance-based SCI-specific ambulation measure focusing on gait abnormalities. The areas measured by SCI-FAI consist of gait parameters, assistive device use, and walking mobility. This scale applies only to SCI individuals who can ambulate independently. The SCI-FAI assesses functional walking ability in ambulatory individuals with SCI (Fig. 5) [27].

Description

- An observational gait assessment that includes 3 key domains of walking function.
- Higher scores denote higher levels of function in each subscale.
- Not considered meaningful to combine subscales into an overall composite score, as each domain measures different types of function.
- Area of Assessment: coordination, functional mobility, gait, range of motion.
- Equipment required: video camera, optional (improved reliability).

SCI Functional Ambulation Inventory (SCI-FAI)

Name: Session: Date:

PARAMETER	CRITERION	L	R	
A. Weight shift	shifts weight to stance limb	1	1	
	weight shift absent or only onto assistive device	0	0	
B. Step width	swing foot clears stance foot on limb advancement	1	1	
	stance foot obstructs swing foot on limb advancement	0	0	
	final foot placement does not obstruct swing limb	1	1	
	final foot placement obstructs swing limb	0	0	
C. Step rhythm (relative time needed to advance swing limb)	at heel strike of stance limb, the swing limb:			
	begins to advance in < 1 second *or*	2	2	
	requires 1–3 seconds to begin advancing *or*	1	1	
	requires > 3 seconds to begin advancing	0	0	
D. Step height	toe clears floor throughout swing phase *or*	2	2	
	toe drags at initiation of swing phase only *or*	1	1	
	toe drags throughout swing phase	0	0	
E. Foot contact	heel contacts floor before forefoot *or*	1	1	
	forefoot or foot flat first contact with floor	0	0	
F. Step length	swing heel placed forward of stance toe *or*	2	2	
	swing toe placed forward of stance toe *or*	1	1	
	swing toe placed rearward of stance toe	0	0	
	Parameter total			Sum /20

ASSISTIVE DEVICES		L		R	
Upper extremity balance/weightbearing devices	None	4		4	
	Cane(s)	3		3	
	Quad cane(s), Crutch(es) (forearm/axillary)	2		2	
	Walker		2		
	Parallel bars		0		
Lower extremity assistive devices	None	3		3	
	AFO	2		2	
	KAFO	1		1	
	RGO	0		0	
	Assistive device total				Sum /14

TEMPORAL/DISTANCE MEASURES			
Walking mobility (typical walking practice as opposed to W/C use)	Walks . . .		
	regularly in community (rarely/never use W/C)	5	
	regularly in home/occasionally in community	4	
	occasionally in home/rarely in community	3	
	rarely in home/never in community	2	
	for exercise only	1	
	does not walk	0	
	Walking mobility score		Sum /5
Two-minute walk test (distance walked in 2 minutes)	Distance walked in 2 minutes = ...	feet/minute	meters/minute

AFO: ankle-foot orthosis; KAFO: knee-ankle-foot orthosis.

Fig. (5). Spinal cord injury functional ambulation inventory.

Administration

- Subscale 1) gait parameters: (each limb scored individually and assessed by evaluating the following):
  a) weight shift
  b) step width

c) step rhythm
d) step height
e) foot contact
f) step length

- Subscale 2) assistive device: (each limb scored individually):
  a) ranks assistive devices by the degree of assistance they provide; includes the use of UE weight-bearing devices and LE orthotics
- Subscale 3) temporal distance:
  a) assesses walking mobility, described as the capability and frequency with which a patient walks during a normal day
  b) includes a 2-minute walk test

Time to administer: 15-30 minutes.

Age ranges: adolescent-13 - 17years, adult-18 - 64years, elderly adult-65+years.

Number of items included: 32

Scoring

- Subscale 1) gait parameters: max score = 20 pts.
- Subscale 2) assistive device: max score = 14 pts.
- Subscale 3) temporal distance max score = 5 pts

Psychometric properties [28]

Reliability: Interrater/intrarater reliability: adequate to excellent inter-rater reliability (ICCs ranged from 0.703 to 0.840).

Excellent intra-rater reliability (ICCs ranged from 0.850 to 0.960; comparing the rater's score of the live score to the same rater's videotape 1 scores).

Criterion validity: (predictive/concurrent): excellent: videotape 1 and walking speed (r = -0.742), excellent: videotape 2 and walking speed (r = -0.700).

Floor/ceiling effects: percentage of patients tested who reach maximal scores:

Gait parameter = 68.8%
Assistive devices = 34.4%
Walking mobility = 34.4%

- Responsiveness: The change in the gait parameter scores following a walking-focused rehabilitation program was 44.7%. changes in gait speed and lems were correlated with the change in the gait parameter score. Moderate correlation was found between % change in the gait score and change in lems(r=0.58).

THE SPINAL CORD INJURY-QUALITY OF LIFE (SCI-QOL)

The Spinal Cord Injury — Quality of Life (SCI-QOL) measurement system was developed to address the shortage of relevant, psychometrically sound patient-reported outcome measures (PROMs) for clinical care and research in spinal cord injury (SCI) rehabilitation. Using a computer-adaptive testing (CAT) approach, the SCI-QOL builds on the Patient-Reported Outcomes Measurement Information System (PROMIS) and the Quality of Life in Neurological Disorders (Neuro-QOL) initiative [29].

Description

The SCI-QOL comprises 22 subdomains across four broad domains physical-medical health, emotional health, social participation, and physical functioning. The 22 final subdomains include 19 IRT-calibrated item banks and 3 fixed-length scales. Subdomains were selected and developed based on qualitative feedback and a literature review, and large pools of items were written based on comments from individuals with SCI [29].

Number of Items: 19 items

Scoring

IRT-based scores on all SCI-QOL banks/scales use a standardised T metric, with a mean of 50 and a standard deviation of 10. Higher scores on a SCI-QOL item bank represent a greater amount of the construct being measured. A T-score of 60 would represent an individual functioning at 1 standard deviation above the mean of the SCI population. For Bladder Management Difficulties, a T-score of 60 indicates an individual performing 1 standard deviation below the mean of the SCI population.

Psychometric Properties [30, 31]

Validity ranged from low to high. A high correlation was observed between the SCI-QOL depression scales and PHQ-9 scores (r = 0.76). Item–total correlations for bladder complications ranged from low to moderate (r = 0.38–0.60), while item–total correlations for bladder management difficulties ranged from low to high (r = 0.38–0.78).

Reliability ranged from moderate to high. The bladder management difficulties scale demonstrated high internal consistency (α = 0.91) and high test–retest reliability (r = 0.77; ICC = 0.76). The bladder complications scale also showed high internal consistency (α = 0.72) and moderate test–retest reliability (r = 0.70; ICC = 0.69).

Spinal Cord Injury Spasticity Evaluation Tool (SCI-SET)

The SCI-SET can be used as a tool for medical management decisions and as a measure of current treatment effects. Spasticity is known to be highly variable, fluctuating daily and even hourly. A seven-day recall of the impact of spasticity may be overshadowed by current levels of spasticity. Repeated administration may therefore be necessary to provide a more accurate picture of the impact spasticity has on daily life. The SCI-SET, as shown in Fig. (**6**) was developed specifically for the SCI population. The scale is easy to administer and score. Definitions of 'spasm' and the scale responses are clearly outlined in the instructions. It assesses the impact of spasticity on daily life in people with SCI. It requires participants to recall their past 7 days when rating spasticity on a scale ranging from -3 (extremely problematic) to +3 (extremely helpful) [32].

Description

- The SCI-SET is composed of 35 items that assess the degree to which spasticity has affected life activities over the past 7 days.
- Responses are on a 7-point scale that ranges from +3 (extremely helpful) to -3 (extremely problematic).
- Age Ranges
- Adolescent:13 - 17 years
- Adult: 18 - 64years
- Elderly Adult: 65+ years
- Time to administer: 5-9 minutes.
- Equipment Required: None

Psychometric Properties [32 - 35]

- Test/Retest Reliability- Excellent test-retest reliability (ICC = 0.91) (Table **2**).
- Internal Consistency: Excellent Internal consistency (Cronbach's alpha = 0.90).
- Construct Validity:

For each of the following, please choose the answer that best describes how your spasticity symptoms have affected that area of your life **during the past 7 days**. When I talk about "spasticity symptoms", I mean:
a) uncontrolled, involuntary muscle contraction or movement (slow or rapid; short or prolonged).
b) involuntary, repetitive, quick muscle movement (up and down; side to side), c) muscle tightness, and
d) what you might describe as "spasms". Please let me know when a question is not applicable to you.

Extremely problematic	*Moderately problematic*	*Somewhat problematic*	*No effect*	*Somewhat helpful*	*Moderately helpful*	*Extremely helpful*
- 3	**- 2**	**- 1**	**0**	**+ 1**	**+ 2**	**+ 3**

DURING THE **PAST 7 DAYS**. HOW HAVE YOUR SPASTICITY SYMPTOMS AFFECTED:

1. your showering?	-3	-2	-1	0	+1	+2	+3	N/A
2. your dressing/undressing?	-3	-2	-1	0	+1	+2	+3	N/A
3. your transfers (to and from bed, chair, vehicle, *etc.*)?	-3	-2	-1	0	+1	+2	+3	N/A
4. your sitting positioning (in your chair, *etc.*)?	-3	-2	-1	0	+1	+2	+3	N/A
5. the preparation of meals?	-3	-2	-1	0	+1	+2	+3	N/A
6. eating?	-3	-2	-1	0	+1	+2	+3	N/A
7. drinking?	-3	-2	-1	0	+1	+2	+3	N/A
8. your small hand movements (writing, use of computer, *etc.*)?	-3	-2	-1	0	+1	+2	+3	N/A
9. your ability to perform household chores?	-3	-2	-1	0	+1	+2	+3	N/A
10. your hobbies/recreational activities?	-3	-2	-1	0	+1	+2	+3	N/A
11. your enjoyment of social outings?	-3	-2	-1	0	+1	+2	+3	N/A
12. your ability to stand/weight-bear?	-3	-2	-1	0	+1	+2	+3	N/A
13. your walking ability?	-3	-2	-1	0	+1	+2	+3	N/A
14. your stability/balance?	-3	-2	-1	0	+1	+2	+3	N/A
15. your muscle fatigue?	-3	-2	-1	0	+1	+2	+3	N/A
16. the flexibility of your joints?	-3	-2	-1	0	+1	+2	+3	N/A
17. your therapy/exercise routine?	-3	-2	-1	0	+1	+2	+3	N/A
18. your manual wheelchair use?	-3	-2	-1	0	+1	+2	+3	N/A

Fig. (6). SCI-SET.

Table 2. Correlations between SCI-SET score and related instruments.

Domain	Strength	SCI-SET
Spasticity severity	Adequate	-0.48*
Spasticity impact	Excellent	-0.61*
FIM motor score	Poor	0.21
QLI health and functioning subscale	Excellent	0.68*
PSFS	Excellent	-0.66
PSFS = Penn Spasm Frequency Scale *$p < .001$		

CLINICAL CONSIDERATIONS, STRENGTHS, LIMITATIONS, AND EMERGING PERSPECTIVES

Assessment of individuals with spinal cord injury (SCI) requires a multidimensional approach that reflects the complex interaction between neurological impairment, functional capacity, participation, and quality of life. No single assessment scale is sufficient to capture the full spectrum of consequences following SCI. Instead, a combination of neurological, functional, and patient-reported outcome measures is necessary to support clinical decision-making, rehabilitation planning, and outcome evaluation across different stages of recovery [36, 37].

The International Standards for Neurological Classification of Spinal Cord Injury (ISNCSCI/ASIA Impairment Scale) remains the cornerstone for neurological assessment in SCI. Its primary strength lies in the standardised evaluation of motor and sensory function, allowing precise injury classification and prognostication. ASIA scores are indispensable in acute care and research settings; however, they provide limited information regarding functional independence or participation. Improvements in neurological scores do not always translate into meaningful gains in daily activities, highlighting the scale's restricted ability to reflect real-world function [38 - 40].

Functional assessment tools such as the Spinal Cord Independence Measure (SCIM) address this gap by focusing on activities of daily living, mobility, and sphincter management. SCIM offers greater sensitivity than generic functional measures when evaluating rehabilitation outcomes in SCI populations. Nevertheless, its emphasis on task performance may underestimate subtle neurological recovery and does not fully capture patient-perceived well-being. Additionally, administration requires familiarity with SCI-specific functional challenges, which may affect consistency across settings [41].

The Walking Index for Spinal Cord Injury (WISCI) provides a focused evaluation of ambulation by quantifying walking ability based on assistance, devices, and braces. Its hierarchical structure allows the detection of meaningful changes in walking capacity, particularly during rehabilitation. However, WISCI is applicable only to individuals with ambulatory potential and provides no insight into non-ambulatory function, upper-limb performance, or broader participation outcomes [42].

Patient-reported outcome measures, such as the Spinal Cord Injury–Quality of Life (SCI-QOL) system, capture domains that are often overlooked by clinician-rated scales, including emotional well-being, social participation, pain, fatigue, and life satisfaction. SCI-QOL instruments enhance patient-centred assessment and provide valuable information for long-term outcome evaluation. Their subjective nature, however, means that psychological adaptation, environmental factors, and cultural context may influence responses. As a result, SCI-QOL measures are best interpreted alongside objective neurological and functional assessments rather than in isolation [43].

A key limitation across SCI assessment tools is the conceptual separation between impairment, activity, and participation. While ASIA focuses on neurological impairment, SCIM and WISCI assess functional activity, and SCI-QOL addresses participation and quality of life. Overlapping content may occur if these tools are used without a clear assessment framework, potentially increasing evaluation burden without proportional clinical benefit. Strategic selection based on assessment goals—rather than routine use of all available scales—is therefore essential [44 - 46].

Emerging perspectives in SCI assessment increasingly emphasise integrated and technology-enabled approaches. Wearable sensors and instrumented gait analysis are being explored to objectively quantify mobility, balance, and activity levels in both inpatient and community settings. Digital adaptations of established scales and remote monitoring platforms are also gaining relevance, particularly for long-term follow-up and tele-rehabilitation. In parallel, there is growing interest in linking clinical scale scores with biomarkers, neuroimaging, and electrophysiological measures to enhance prognostic accuracy [45, 46].

Recent consensus initiatives have highlighted the importance of standardising outcome selection in SCI research and clinical practice. Rather than replacing existing tools, these efforts aim to clarify the complementary roles of neurological, functional, and patient-reported measures. Such harmonisation improves comparability across studies and supports a more meaningful interpretation of rehabilitation outcomes [46].

In clinical practice, the choice of SCI assessment scales should be driven by the phase of injury and the intended purpose of assessment. The ASIA classification is essential in the acute and early recovery stages; SCIM and WISCI are most informative during rehabilitation; and SCI-QOL measures provide critical insight into long-term participation and quality of life. An integrated yet selective approach ensures comprehensive assessment while minimising redundancy and administrative burden [43, 44, 47]. A comparative summary of commonly used SCI assessment scales is presented in Table 3.

Table 3. Comparative summary of SCI assessment scales.

Scale	Primary Domain	Key Strengths	Major Limitations	Optimal Use
ISNCSCI / AIS	Neurological impairment	Global standard; prognostic value; research utility	Limited functional relevance	Acute care, classification, trials
SCIM III	Functional independence	SCI-specific; sensitive to rehab change	Requires trained raters	Inpatient and outpatient rehabilitation
WISCI II	Ambulation	Sensitive to walking recovery	Only applicable to ambulatory patients	Gait-focused rehab and trials
SCI-QOL	Quality of life & participation	Patient-centred; comprehensive domains	Subjective; context-dependent	Long-term outcomes, chronic SCI
Wearable/digital metrics	Real-world function	Objective: continuous monitoring	Limited standardization	Emerging research and tele-rehab
-	**CONCLUSION**	An accurate and comprehensive assessment of spinal cord injury (SCI) is essential for effective diagnosis, rehabilitation planning, and monitoring of recovery. The use of standardised evaluation tools, such as the ASIA, SCIM, and various balance, spasticity, gait, and quality-of-life measures, enables clinicians to obtain a detailed understanding of a patient's functional status and progress over time. By integrating these assessment scales, healthcare professionals can tailor rehabilitation strategies, optimise functional outcomes, and enhance the overall quality of life for individuals living with SCI.	**Conflict of Interest:** The authors declare no conflict of interest.	**Funding:** No funding received.

AI DISCLOSURE STATEMENT

During the preparation of this chapter, the authors used ChatGPT (OpenAI) as a support tool for language refinement, structural organisation, and clarification of ideas. All content generated with AI assistance was carefully reviewed, verified, and revised by the authors to ensure factual accuracy, originality, and consistency with the scientific literature. The authors take full responsibility for the integrity, interpretation, and final content of the published chapter.

ACKNOWLEDGEMENT

We thank the authors of the scales for providing their consent to include the scales in our chapter.

REFERENCES

[1] Golestani A, Shobeiri P, Sadeghi-Naini M, *et al.* Epidemiology of traumatic spinal cord injury in developing countries from 2009 to 2020: A systematic review and meta-analysis. Neuroepidemiology 2022; 56(4): 219-39.
[http://dx.doi.org/10.1159/000524867] [PMID: 35512643]

[2] Schuld C, Wiese J, Franz S, *et al.* Effect of formal training in scaling, scoring and classification of the International Standards for Neurological Classification of Spinal Cord Injury. Spinal Cord 2013; 51(4): 282-8.
[http://dx.doi.org/10.1038/sc.2012.149] [PMID: 23184026]

[3] The 2019 revision of the International Standards for Neurological Classification of Spinal Cord Injury (ISNCSCI)—What's new? Spinal Cord 2019; 57(10): 815-7.
[http://dx.doi.org/10.1038/s41393-019-0350-9] [PMID: 31530900]

[4] Savic G, Bergström EMK, Frankel HL, Jamous MA, Jones PW. Inter-rater reliability of motor and sensory examinations performed according to American Spinal Injury Association standards. Spinal Cord 2007; 45(6): 444-51.
[http://dx.doi.org/10.1038/sj.sc.3102044] [PMID: 17387316]

[5] El Masry WS, Tsubo M, Katoh S, El Miligui YH, Khan A. Validation of the American Spinal Injury Association (ASIA) motor score and the National Acute Spinal Cord Injury Study (NASCIS) motor score. Spine (Phila Pa 1976). 1996 Mar 1; 21(5): 614-9. [https://doi.org/10.1097/00007632-199603010-00015] [PMID: 8852318]

[6] Jacobs SR, Yeaney NK, Herbison GJ, Ditunno JF Jr. Future ambulation prognosis as predicted by somatosensory evoked potentials in motor complete and incomplete quadriplegia. Arch Phys Med Rehabil 1995; 76(7): 635-41.
[http://dx.doi.org/10.1016/S0003-9993(95)80632-6] [PMID: 7605182]

[7] Kirshblum S, Waring W III. Updates for the International Standards for Neurological Classification of Spinal Cord Injury. Phys Med Rehabil Clin N Am 2014; 25(3): 505-517, vii.
[http://dx.doi.org/10.1016/j.pmr.2014.04.001] [PMID: 25064785]

[8] Marino RJ, Jones L, Kirshblum S, Tal J, Dasgupta A. Reliability and repeatability of the motor and sensory examination of the international standards for neurological classification of spinal cord injury. J Spinal Cord Med 2008; 31(2): 166-70.
[http://dx.doi.org/10.1080/10790268.2008.11760707] [PMID: 18581663]

[9] Itzkovich M, Gelernter I, Biering-Sorensen F, *et al.* The Spinal Cord Independence Measure (SCIM) version III: Reliability and validity in a multi-center international study. Disabil Rehabil 2007; 29(24):

1926-33.
[http://dx.doi.org/10.1080/09638280601046302] [PMID: 17852230]

[10] Benz EN, Hornby TG, Bode RK, Scheidt RA, Schmit BD. A physiologically based clinical measure for spastic reflexes in spinal cord injury. Arch Phys Med Rehabil 2005; 86(1): 52-9. [http://dx.doi.org/10.1016/j.apmr.2004.01.033] [PMID: 15640989]

[11] Akpinar P, Atici A, Ozkan FU, Aktas I, Kulcu DG, Kurt KN. Reliability of the Spinal Cord Assessment Tool for Spastic Reflexes. Arch Phys Med Rehabil 2017; 98(6): 1113-8. [http://dx.doi.org/10.1016/j.apmr.2016.09.119] [PMID: 27744026]

[12] Iverson GL, Koehle MS. Normative data for the balance error scoring system in adults. Rehabil Res Pract 2013; 2013: 1-5.
[http://dx.doi.org/10.1155/2013/846418] [PMID: 23577257]

[13] Bell DR, Guskiewicz KM, Clark MA, Padua DA. Systematic review of the balance error scoring system. Sports Health 2011; 3(3): 287-95.
[http://dx.doi.org/10.1177/1941738111403122] [PMID: 23016020]

[14] Azad AM, Al Juma S, Bhatti JA, Delaney JS. Modified Balance Error Scoring System (M-BESS) test scores in athletes wearing protective equipment and cleats. BMJ Open Sport Exerc Med 2016; 2(1): e000117.
[http://dx.doi.org/10.1136/bmjsem-2016-000117] [PMID: 27900181]

[15] Finnoff JT, Peterson VJ, Hollman JH, Smith J. Intrarater and Interrater Reliability of the Balance Error Scoring System (BESS). PM R 2009; 1(1): 50-4.
[http://dx.doi.org/10.1016/j.pmrj.2008.06.002] [PMID: 19627872]

[16] Manley G, Gardner AJ, Schneider KJ, Guskiewicz KM, Bailes J, Cantu RC, Castellani RJ, Turner M, Jordan BD, Randolph C, Dvořák J, Hayden KA, Tator CH, McCrory P, Iverson GL. A systematic review of potential long-term effects of sport-related concussion. Br J Sports Med. 2017 Jun; 51(12): 969-977. [https://doi.org/10.1136/bjsports-2017-097791] [PMID: 28455362]

[17] Potter K, Brandfass K. The Mini-Balance Evaluation Systems Test (Mini-BESTest). J Physiother 2015; 61(4): 225.
[http://dx.doi.org/10.1016/j.jphys.2015.04.002] [PMID: 26044345]

[18] Yingyongyudha A, Saengsirisuwan V, Panichaporn W, Boonsinsukh R. The Mini-Balance Evaluation Systems Test (Mini-BESTest) Demonstrates Higher Accuracy in Identifying Older Adult Participants With History of Falls Than Do the BESTest, Berg Balance Scale, or Timed Up and Go Test. J Geriatr Phys Ther 2016; 39(2): 64-70.
[http://dx.doi.org/10.1519/JPT.0000000000000050] [PMID: 25794308]

[19] Duncan RP, Leddy AL, Cavanaugh JT, *et al.* Comparative utility of the BESTest, mini-BESTest, and brief-BESTest for predicting falls in individuals with Parkinson disease: a cohort study. Phys Ther 2013; 93(4): 542-50.
[http://dx.doi.org/10.2522/ptj.20120302] [PMID: 23174567]

[20] Di Carlo S, Bravini E, Vercelli S, Massazza G, Ferriero G. The Mini-BESTest: a review of psychometric properties. Int J Rehabil Res 2016; 39(2): 97-105.
[http://dx.doi.org/10.1097/MRR.0000000000000153] [PMID: 26795715]

[21] Huang M, Pang MYC. Psychometric properties of Brief-Balance Evaluation Systems Test (Brief-BEST est) in evaluating balance performance in individuals with chronic stroke. Brain Behav 2017; 7(3): e00649.
[http://dx.doi.org/10.1002/brb3.649] [PMID: 28293482]

[22] Ditunno JF Jr, Ditunno PL, Scivoletto G, *et al.* The Walking Index for Spinal Cord Injury (WISCI/WISCI II): nature, metric properties, use and misuse. Spinal Cord 2013; 51(5): 346-55. [http://dx.doi.org/10.1038/sc.2013.9] [PMID: 23459122]

[23] Ditunno JF Jr, Barbeau H, Dobkin BH, *et al.* Validity of the walking scale for spinal cord injury and

other domains of function in a multicenter clinical trial. Neurorehabil Neural Repair 2007; 21(6): 539-50.
[http://dx.doi.org/10.1177/1545968307301880] [PMID: 17507642]

[24] Ditunno JF Jr, Ditunno PL, Graziani V, *et al.* Walking index for spinal cord injury (WISCI): an international multicenter validity and reliability study. Spinal Cord 2000; 38(4): 234-43.
[http://dx.doi.org/10.1038/sj.sc.3100993] [PMID: 10822394]

[25] Kim MO, Burns AS, Ditunno JF Jr, Marino RJ. The assessment of walking capacity using the walking index for spinal cord injury: self-selected *versus* maximal levels. Arch Phys Med Rehabil 2007; 88(6): 762-7.
[http://dx.doi.org/10.1016/j.apmr.2007.03.021] [PMID: 17532899]

[26] Marino RJ, Scivoletto G, Patrick M, *et al.* Walking index for spinal cord injury version 2 (WISCI-II) with repeatability of the 10-m walk time: Inter- and intrarater reliabilities. Am J Phys Med Rehabil 2010; 89(1): 7-15.
[http://dx.doi.org/10.1097/PHM.0b013e3181c560eb] [PMID: 20026943]

[27] Field-Fote EC, Fluet GG, Schafer SD, *et al.* The Spinal Cord Injury Functional Ambulation Inventory (SCI-FAI). J Rehabil Med 2001; 33(4): 177-81.
[http://dx.doi.org/10.1080/165019701750300645] [PMID: 11506216]

[28] Kusano S, Miyata K, Yoshikawa K, Mizukami M. Construct validity, responsiveness, and interpretability of the Spinal Cord Injury Functional Ambulation Inventory (SCI-FAI). J Spinal Cord Med. 2026 Jan; 49(1): 68-80. [http://dx.doi.org/ 10.1080/10790268.2024.2448039]

[29] Tulsky DS, Kisala PA, Victorson D, *et al.* Overview of the Spinal Cord Injury--Quality of Life (SCI-QOL) measurement system. J Spinal Cord Med 2015; 38(3): 257-69.
[http://dx.doi.org/10.1179/2045772315Y.0000000023] [PMID: 26010962]

[30] Kuzu D, Kallen MA, Kalpakjian CZ, Kratz AL. Psychometric properties of the spinal cord injury-quality of life (SCI-QOL) Resilience item bank in a sample with spinal cord injury and chronic pain. Qual Life Res 2022; 31(3): 927-36.
[http://dx.doi.org/10.1007/s11136-021-02981-4] [PMID: 34545477]

[31] Kuzu D, Kallen MA, Kratz AL. Psychometric Properties of the Spinal Cord Injury-Quality of Life (SCI-QOL) Resilience Short Form in a Sample With Spinal Cord Injury. Arch Phys Med Rehabil 2024; 105(1): 59-66.
[http://dx.doi.org/10.1016/j.apmr.2023.10.002] [PMID: 37865166]

[32] Adams MM, Ginis KAM, Hicks AL. The spinal cord injury spasticity evaluation tool: development and evaluation. Arch Phys Med Rehabil 2007; 88(9): 1185-92.
[http://dx.doi.org/10.1016/j.apmr.2007.06.012] [PMID: 17826466]

[33] Akpinar P, Atici A, Kurt KN, Ozkan FU, Aktas I, Kulcu DG. Reliability and cross-cultural adaptation of the Turkish version of the Spinal Cord Injury Spasticity Evaluation Tool. Int J Rehabil Res 2017; 40(2): 152-7.
[http://dx.doi.org/10.1097/MRR.0000000000000223] [PMID: 28225536]

[34] Sweatman WM, Heinemann AW, Furbish CL, Field-Fote EC. Modified PRISM and SCI-SET Spasticity Measures for Persons With Traumatic Spinal Cord Injury: Results of a Rasch Analyses. Arch Phys Med Rehabil 2020; 101(9): 1570-9.
[http://dx.doi.org/10.1016/j.apmr.2020.05.012] [PMID: 32497601]

[35] Ansari NN, Kashi M, Naghdi S. The Spinal Cord Injury Spasticity Evaluation Tool: A Persian adaptation and validation study. J Spinal Cord Med 2017; 40(4): 380-8.
[http://dx.doi.org/10.1080/10790268.2016.1195941] [PMID: 27579622]

[36] Dawson J, Shamley D, Jamous MA. A structured review of outcome measures used for the assessment of rehabilitation interventions for spinal cord injury. Spinal Cord 2008; 46(12): 768-80.
[http://dx.doi.org/10.1038/sc.2008.50] [PMID: 18521096]

[37] Lam T, Noonan VK, Eng JJ. A systematic review of functional ambulation outcome measures in spinal cord injury. Spinal Cord 2008; 46(4): 246-54. [http://dx.doi.org/10.1038/sj.sc.3102134] [PMID: 17923844]

[38] Rupp R, Biering-Sørensen F, Burns SP, *et al.* International standards for neurological classification of spinal cord injury: revised 2019. Top Spinal Cord Inj Rehabil 2021; 27(2): 1-22. [http://dx.doi.org/10.46292/sci2702-1] [PMID: 34108832]

[39] Walden K, Schuld C, Noonan VK, Rupp R. Computer International Standards for Neurological Classification of Spinal Cord Injury (ISNCSCI) algorithms: a review. Spinal Cord. 2023 Feb; 61(2): 125-132. [https://doi.org/10.1038/s41393-022-00854-2] [PMID: 36114239]

[40] Kirshblum S, Snider B, Rupp R, Read MS. Updates of the International Standards for Neurologic Classification of Spinal Cord Injury. Phys Med Rehabil Clin N Am 2020; 31(3): 319-30. [http://dx.doi.org/10.1016/j.pmr.2020.03.005] [PMID: 32624097]

[41] Harvey LA, Anderson KD. The spinal cord independence measure. J Physiother. 2015 Apr; 61(2): 99. [https://doi.org/10.1016/j.jphys.2015.02.013] [PMID: 25801929]

[42] van Hedel HJA, Wirz M, Curt A. Improving walking assessment in subjects with an incomplete spinal cord injury: responsiveness. Spinal Cord 2006; 44(6): 352-6. [http://dx.doi.org/10.1038/sj.sc.3101853] [PMID: 16304565]

[43] Aquarone RL, Faro AC. Scales on Quality of Life in patients with spinal cord injury: integrative review. Einstein (Sao Paulo). 2014 Apr; 12(2): 245-50. [https://doi.org/10.1590/s1679-45082014rw2591] [PMID: 25003935]

[44] Chen Y, Charlifue S, Noonan VK, New PW, Gururaj G, Katoh S, Leiulfsrud H, Post MW, Biering-Sørensen F. International spinal cord injury socio-demographic basic data set (version 1.0). Spinal Cord. 2023 May; 61(5): 313-316. [https://doi.org/10.1038/s41393-023-00896-0] [PMID: 37059864]

[45] Korupolu R, Stampas A, Singh M, Zhou P, Francisco G. Electrophysiological Outcome Measures in Spinal Cord Injury Clinical Trials: A Systematic Review. Top Spinal Cord Inj Rehabil. 2019 Fall; 25(4): 340-354. [https://doi.org/10.1310/sci2504-340] [PMID: 31844386]

[46] Alexander MS, Anderson KD, Biering-Sorensen F, *et al.* Outcome measures in spinal cord injury: recent assessments and recommendations for future directions. Spinal Cord 2009; 47(8): 582-91. [http://dx.doi.org/10.1038/sc.2009.18] [PMID: 19381157]

[47] Biering-Sørensen F, Charlifue S, Chen Y, *et al.* Spinal Cord Injury Core Data Set (version 3.0)-including standardisation of reporting. Spinal Cord 2023; 61(1): 65-8. [http://dx.doi.org/10.1038/s41393-022-00862-2] [PMID: 36307730]

CHAPTER 9

Scales for Traumatic Brain Injury

Preeti Kapri[1,2], **Nidhi Sharma**[2,3,*] and **Parveen Kumar**[4]

[1] *Department of Physiotherapy, School of Allied Medical Sciences, Lovely Professional University, Phagwara, Punjab, India*

[2] *Maharishi Markandeshwar Institute of Physiotherapy and Rehabilitation, Maharishi Markandeshwar (Deemed to be University), Mullana, Ambala, Haryana, India*

[3] *Department of Physiotherapy, Amity Institute of Health Allied Sciences, Amity University, Noida, Uttar Pradesh, India*

[4] *Pal Physiotherapy and Rehabilitation Centre, Pal Healthcare, Ambala City, Haryana, India*

Abstract: Traumatic brain injury (TBI) is a complicated and diverse condition that impacts millions of people around the globe, with a variety of cognitive, emotional, and behavioural problems. The severity of TBI can vary greatly, from mild concussions to severe, life-altering injuries. Various scales, such as the Glasgow-Coma Scale, Rancho_Los_Amigos Scale, and National Institutes of Health-Stroke Scale, are used to assess the severity of TBI and guide treatment decisions. TBI can result in cognitive, emotional, and behavioural changes, impacting daily life and relationships. Proper diagnosis and evaluation are essential for creating effective treatment strategies and enhancing patient outcomes. Cognitive deficits can include memory loss, attention problems, and difficulty with problem-solving, while emotional changes can include depression, anxiety, and mood swings. Behavioural changes can include impulsivity, irritability, and aggression. Early and accurate diagnosis, as well as comprehensive treatment and rehabilitation, are essential for maximising recovery and enhancing the quality of life for those with TBI.

Keywords: Behavioural deficits, Brain injuries, Cognition, Cognitive dysfunction, Coma, Consciousness, Glasgow-coma scale, Neurological deficits, Stroke, Traumatic-brain injury.

INTRODUCTION

Traumatic-Brain Injury (TBI), a complex and diverse condition that affects millions of people worldwide, is identified as a variety of brain injuries that take place when an abrupt trauma inflicts damage on the brain. Prevalence rate of TBI

* **Corresponding author Nidhi Sharma**: Department of Physiotherapy, Amity Institute of Health Allied Sciences, Amity University, Noida, Uttar Pradesh, India; E-mail: sharmanidhiphysio@gmail.com

varies widely depending on the population and the criteria used to define TBI, with approximately 1.7 million instances of traumatic brain injury occurring annually in America, culminating in 52,000 fatalities, 275,000 inpatient admissions, and 1.3 million urgent care centre visits [1]. To assess the severity and outcome of TBI, several scales are used, including the Glasgow Coma Scale (GCS), Rancho Los Amigos Scale, Functional Independence Measure (FIM), and Glasgow Outcome Scale (GOS). These scales are important because they help healthcare professionals diagnose, monitor, and treat TBI patients effectively, enabling accurate diagnosis, effective treatment, monitoring of progress, and research and development [2].

RANCHO LOS AMIGOS SCALE (RLAS)

Rancho_Los_Amigos Scale (RLAS), commonly recognised healthcare measurement utilised to characterise behavioural-cognitive outlines observed among individuals with brain injury. RLAS can be used throughout the recovery period. Rancho_Los_Amigos Scale was initially developed to evaluate patients' recovery from coma through ("The Head Injury Team" at "Rancho_Los_Amigos National Rehabilitation Centre in Downey, California") by Dr. Chris Hagen and team in 1972. Original RLAS has 8 levels, which denote the level of function. Later, 2 levels were added to develop a more detailed 10-point system known as the Rancho_Los_Amigos-Revised Scale (RLAS-R) [3].

ICF Domain: Cognition

Number of items: 1

Instructions for Administration and Scoring

Administration

- Clinician administered
- The assessor performs a qualitative evaluation of the individual's conduct [4].

Level_[I]: No-Response: Total-Assistance

- Lack of reaction to outside stimuli

Level_[II]: Generalized-Response: Total-Assistance

- Reacts unpredictably and aimlessly to external stimuli
- Reactions are frequently identical regardless of the stimulus

Level_[III]: Localized-Response: Total-Assistance

- Reacts unpredictably and specifically to external stimuli
- Reactions are directly connected to the stimulus; for instance, the patient may withdraw or vocalise in response to painful stimuli
- Shows greater responsiveness to familiar individuals (friends and family) compared to unfamiliar ones.

Level_[IV]: Confused/Agitated: Maximal-Assistance

- The person is in a state of heightened activity, exhibiting strange and aimless behaviour.
- Displays restless actions that stem more from internal disorientation than from the surrounding environment
- Lacks short-term memory

Level_[V]: Confused-Inappropriate_Non-Agitated: Maximal-Assistance

- Exhibits improved consistency in following and reacting to basic instructions.
- Reactions are aimless and erratic to more complicated commands.
- Actions and speech are frequently unsuitable, and the individual seems disoriented and often fabricates information.
- Memory is significantly compromised, making it challenging to acquire new knowledge.
- Distinct from level IV in that the individual does not display agitation in response to internal stimuli; however, they may exhibit agitation in reaction to unpleasant external stimuli.

Level_[VI]: Confused-Appropriate: Moderate-Assistance

- Consistently adheres to basic instructions.
- Capable of remembering how to perform familiar activities they did before the injury (such as brushing teeth or washing their face), but struggle to learn new tasks.
- Shows heightened awareness of themselves, their circumstances, and their surroundings, yet lacks awareness of particular deficits and safety issues
- Reactions may be inaccurate due to memory deficits, but are suitable for the context.

Level _[VII]: Automatic-Appropriate: Minimal-Assistance for Daily-Living Skills

- Still demonstrates a lack of awareness, reduced judgment, and safety consciousness;
- Oriented in known environments;
- Able to perform daily routines automatically with minimal to no confusion;
- Exhibits retention for new tasks and learning alongside familiar activities;
- Unaware of specific deficits but has a superficial understanding of their diagnosis;
- Beginning to express interest in social and recreational activities within organised settings;
- Needs at least some supervision for safety and learning reasons.

Level_[VIII]: Purposeful-Appropriate: Stand-by Assistance

- Able to utilise memory aids to remember daily activities;
- Consistently aware of person, location, and time;
- Independently carries out familiar tasks in a non-distracting setting;
- Demonstrates progress in memory and the capacity to integrate past and future events;
- Recognises specific deficits and their impact on tasks but needs nearby assistance to cope;
- Generally irritable, restless, and has a low tolerance for frustration.

Level_[IX]: Purposeful-Appropriate: Stand-by Assistance (on-request)

- Capable of switching among activities and finishing those on their own;
- Conscious of impairments and able to employ coping mechanisms when they interfere with tasks;
- Incapable of independently anticipating potential hurdles that may develop as a result of impairment.
- Continues to exhibit despair and a low threshold for frustration;
- With support, it can reflect on the consequences of actions and choices;
- Recognises the emotional requirements of others by offering nearby assistance.

Level_[X]: Purposeful-Appropriate: Modified-Independent

- Ability to independently anticipate potential obstacles resulting from impairments and take corrective action;

- The capability to handle multiple tasks in different settings with extra time or supportive tools
- The ability to develop one's own techniques and tools for memory retention;
- The ability to make decisions on their own and act appropriately, though sometimes additional time or compensatory strategies may be needed;
- The capability to act appropriately in social situations [3].

Equipment: No equipment required

Scoring and Interpretability

- Scores range from level 1 to level 10.
- Level I represents the lowest degree of functioning, while Level 10 indicates the highest degree of functioning.
- Elevated-level shows better behavioural and cognitive state and move towards increased independence [3, 4].

Languages: The scale's original language is English [3].

Training Required: Administration must be performed by a trained healthcare professional.

Clinical Considerations

- The RLAS-R is often employed together with the Glasgow Coma Scale (GCS) to deliver an initial evaluation of cognitive function in patients with brain injuries.
- In contrast to the GCS, the RLAS-R is beneficial for assessing a patient's recovery after they first wake from a coma.
- Early screening of cognitive function offers significant benefits, including predicting recovery trajectories and aiding rehabilitation planning in a clinical setting [5].

Psychometric Properties

Reliability

- Test/Retest Reliability was excellent (Spearman rho=.82) [6]
- Inter-rater Reliability was also excellent (Spearman rho=.89) [6, 7]

Validity

- Predictive validity of level of cognitive function scale scores was assessed by examining correlations with discharge evaluations on the Stover-Zeiger scale (r=.59), Glasgow-Outcome Scale (r-0.57), and the Expanded-Glasgow-Outcome

Scale (r-0.68) [6].

- Excellent concurrent validity of the level of cognitive function scale at admission with the Stover-Zeiger scale was r-0.92 [6, 7]
- Concurrent measures of the level of cognitive function scale with Stover-Zeiger_Scale at discharge were (r-0.73), Glasgow-Outcome Scale (r-0.76), and Expanded-Glasgow-Outcome Scale(r-0.79) [6, 7].

Responsiveness: No reported values for brain injury.

Floor/ceiling effect: No reported values of brain injury.

GLASGOW COMA SCALE (GCS)

The Glasgow Coma Scale (GCS) was initially introduced in 1974 at the University of Glasgow's Institute of Neurological Sciences, located at the Southern General Hospital in the city, and developed by neurosurgery professors *Graham Teasdale* and *Bryan J. Jennett*. The Glasgow Coma Scale (GCS) is used to objectively assess the level of impaired consciousness in all types of acute medical and trauma patients. By evaluating eye-opening, motor, and verbal responses, this measure assesses patients' responsiveness across three dimensions [8].

ICF Domain: Physiological function and cognition

Number of items: 15

Instructions for Administration and Scoring

Administration

- GCS is a clinician-administered outcome measure.
- GCS assessment aid has four steps: check, observe, stimulate, and rate.
- Time taken to assess the patients is 10 to 15 minutes.
- The sixth point for "withdrawal from painful stimulus" was added to the motor response subscale in the 1976 revision, bringing it up to date following its 1974 publication [8, 9].

Equipment: No specific equipment required. Basic requirements: paper and pencil

Scoring

- A useful "shorthand" assessment of overall severity can be obtained by summing the results from each scale component to obtain the Glasgow Coma Score.
- This summary is less detailed than the individual scale scores.
- The total of the scores and each part is the score expression.
- For example, GCS10 = E3V4M3 is one way to express a score of 10 [8 - 10].

GCS divides into 3 variables [8-10]:

- Best eye response (E)
- Best vocal response (V)
- Optimal motor response (M).

Eye Response (4 Being the Best)

1. Don't open their eyes at all.
2. Only open their eyes when we apply painful pressure.
3. Open their eyes when they hear a sound.
4. Eyes open on their own, spontaneously.

Verbal Response (5 Being the Best)

1. They don't make any sounds.
2. Make sounds, but they're not understandable (like moaning or groaning).
3. Say words, but they don't make sense in the context of the situation.
4. They're confused, but they can speak. They might not know where they are or what happened.
5. They're oriented and can answer questions appropriately, knowing who they are, where they are, and the current time.

Motor Response (6 Being the Best)

1. Don't move at all.
2. When we apply painful pressure, their limbs extend or straighten out abnormally.
3. When we apply painful pressure, their limbs flex or bend abnormally.
4. They pull away from painful pressure.
5. They try to move towards the source of the pain, showing they can pinpoint where it's coming from.
6. They follow simple commands, like "squeeze my hand.

GCS scores eye, verbal, and motor responses (max scores 4, 5, and 6, respectively). "1" means no response. Total score ranges from 3 (no response) to 15 (fully awake) [11].

The Pediatric Glasgow Coma Scale was created in Adelaide [12].

Eye Opening (4 is the Best)

1. No eye-opening at all.
2. Eyes open only when we apply painful pressure.
3. Eyes open when they hear a sound.
4. Eyes open on their own.

Verbal Responses (5 is the Best)

1. No sounds whatsoever.
2. Moans in response to pain.
3. Cries in response to pain.
4. Irritable or crying.
5. Coos and babbles (babies) or uses words/phrases appropriately (older children).

Movement (6 is the Best)

1. No movement at all.
2. Limbs extend abnormally in response to painful stimuli.
3. Limbs flex abnormally in response to painful stimuli.
4. Pulls away from pain.
5. Pulls away from touch.
6. Moves spontaneously and purposefully. They aren't just reacting, they're initiating movement.

Interpretability

GCS helps classify the severity of TBI:

- **Severe TBI:** A score of 3 to 8.
- **Moderate TBI:** A score of 9 to 12.
- **Mild TBI:** A score of 13 to 15 [12].

Languages: Although it was first created in English, because of its widespread use, it has been translated into many other languages to enable application in a variety of international medical and healthcare contexts [9, 10].

Training Required: No specialised training necessary

Clinical Considerations

- When a patient has a traumatic brain injury or other neurological condition, the GCS is frequently utilised as part of the initial examination [8].
- It facilitates prompt decision-making on triage and treatment by assisting medical professionals in rapidly assessing the severity of the patient's condition [8].
- Healthcare professionals can use serial GCS evaluations to monitor improvements or declines in awareness, which can assist them in making decisions about treatments and interventions [9].
- Frequently regarded as a prognostic score, the initial GCS score provides medical professionals with an approximation of the extent of brain damage and its consequences.
- A worse prognosis and more extensive brain damage are typically linked to lower GCS scores [9, 10].
- The GCS score may affect the need for imaging tests (such as CT scans), surgery, or admission to a critical care unit, among other treatment options [8 - 10].

Psychometric Properties

Reliability

- Glasgow-Coma Scale (GCS) is generally reliable, with 86% agreement between raters [13].
- Reliability varies across components: eye (76%), verbal (67%), and motor (81%) [13].
- Test-retest reliability is moderate (66-77%) [14].
- Overall GCS score is less reliable (77% agreement) than individual components: eye (89%), motor (94%), verbal (88%) [13, 14].

Validity

- Recent investigations have challenged the idea that intubation leads to substantially disparate survival outcomes, with verbal score correlation coefficient r = 0.90 and total score correlation coefficient r = 0.97 [15].

Responsiveness

- Sensitivity of GCS is low (56.1%), and specificity is high (82.2%) [15, 16].
- An accuracy rate of 71% in forecasting functional independence after injury [15].

- GCS shows a moderate correlation with the Disability-Rating Scale (-0.28) and the cognitive aspect of the Functional-Independence Measure (0.37) [16].

Floor/ceiling effect: There were no reported values regarding the existence of floor or ceiling effects in the GCS for brain injury.

GLASGOW OUTCOME SCALE (GOS)

GOS was first published by B. Jennett and M. Bond in 1975. It serves as a widely recognized metric in fields of neurotrauma and neurosurgery for determining the prognosis and functional status of individuals who have suffered traumatic brain injuries. GOS is frequently paired with the GCS, which assesses consciousness levels immediately after the injury. There are also variations of GOS, including the Glasgow Outcome Scale-Extended (GOS-E) and a pediatric adaptation, both of which build on the original scale's strengths [17].

ICF Domain: Body Structure, Function, and Cognition

Number of items: 19

Instructions for Administration and Scoring

Administration:

- GOS is a clinician-administered outcome measure (Table **1**).
- There are several ways to administer the GOS, including by mail, in inpatient settings with a modified version, and in-person or by telephone.
- Time taken to administer GOS is 10-15 minutes [17].
- Unstructured Glasgow Outcome Scale (uGOS) was a popular tool for evaluating traumatic brain injury (TBI) outcomes; its subjective nature led to the development of more structured versions.
- Modified GOS retained the uGOS's five outcome categories (death *[D]*, vegetative state *[VS]*, severe disability *[SD]*, moderate disability *[MD]*, and good recovery *[GR]*) but used a structured interview to increase objectivity.
- The Extended GOS (GOS-E) further expanded the scale by increasing the number of outcome categories to eight [18].

Equipment: No specific equipment required.

Table 1. Levels of Glasgow outcome scale.

[1]	Death	D
[2]	Vegetative state	VS
[3]	Lower severe disability	SD -

(Table 1) cont.....

[4]	Upper severe disability	SD +
[5]	Lower moderate disability	MD -
[6]	Upper moderate disability	MD +
[7]	Lower good recovery	GR -
[8]	Upper good recovery	GR +

Scoring and Interpretability

In the extended Glasgow Outcome Scale, total scores range from 0 to 8 (Table **1**).

- Scores range from 1 to 8, with a minimum score of 1 and a maximum score of 8 [19].

Post-discharge structured interview for GOS-E [20]

Consciousness

1. Can the head-injured person follow commands or speak? (Yes/No).

(If yes, they're not vegetative. Eye movements alone don't indicate responsiveness. Confirm with caregivers. Full assessment needed to diagnose vegetative state.

Independence at home

2a. Can the person manage daily activities at home *independently*? (Yes/No - "No" means they need daily assistance).

[*Independence means they could manage for 24 hours alone, even if they don't currently*.]

2b. Do they need someone present at home *most* of the time? (Yes/No - *"No" means they could be left alone for up to 8 hours during the day*).
2c. Were they independent at home *before* the injury? (Yes/No).

Independence outside home

3a. Can they shop *independently* (plan, pay, behave appropriately)? (Yes/No).
3b. Were they able to shop independently *before*? (Yes/No).
4a. Can they travel *locally* without help (driving, public transport, taxi)? (Yes/No).
4b. Were they able to travel locally alone *before*? (Yes/No).

Work

5a. Can they work/care for others at their *previous* level? (Yes/No).
5b. If no, are they working less, in a sheltered job, or unable to work? (Reduced/Sheltered/Unable).
5c. Is this a *change* from their pre-injury work status? (Yes/No).

Social and Leisure activities

6a. Can they resume regular social/leisure activities *outside* the home? (Yes/No).
6b. If no, are they participating a bit less, much less, or not at all? (Bit Less/Much Less/None).
6c. Is this a *change* in their social/leisure activities compared to before the injury? (Yes/No).

Family and friendships

7a. Has there been family/friend *disruption* due to psychological problems (*e.g.*, temper, anxiety, depression)? (Yes/No).
7b. Is the disruption occasional, frequent, or constant? (Occasional/Frequent/Constant).
7c. Is this disruption a *change* from before the injury? (Yes/No).

Return to normal life

8a. Are there *other* post-injury problems affecting daily life (*e.g.*, headaches, dizziness, memory)? (Yes/No).
8b. If similar problems existed before, have they become *markedly worse*? (Yes/No).
9. What is the *most important* factor affecting outcome: head injury, other injury/illness, or a combination? (Head Injury/Other/Combination)

MCID: For GOS-E - 0.5 [19]

Languages: GOS was first released in English.

Training Required: No specific training required.

Clinical Considerations

- GOS is an essential tool for evaluating and sharing patients' overall results after traumatic brain injury.
- It supports clinical judgment calls, rehabilitation plans, and brain injury outcome-related research projects.
- To assess subjects' status following acute-phase damage, the GOS is usually

administered at predetermined intervals, such as 6 months or 1 year after the accident.

- When performing TBI assessments, GCS and GOS are frequently combined. The GOS assesses the long-term functional result.
- Healthcare practitioners can better comprehend the correlation between the extent of an injury and its subsequent healing by combining GCS and GOS.
- Clinical decision-making, including choices regarding continued medical care, rehabilitation therapies, and discharge planning, may be influenced by the GOS outcome categories [19, 20].

Psychometric Properties

Reliability

- Test-retest reliability is high, whether comparing postal surveys (κ = .98) or phone and mail surveys (κ = .92) [21, 22].
- Mild to moderate traumatic brain injury; test-retest reliability is also excellent (ICC = 0.92) [23, 24].
- Interrater reliability is consistently good to excellent, with weighted kappa coefficients ranging from 0.70 to 0.95 across various studies [23].
- Specifically, studies comparing psychologist and nurse ratings (one in-person, one by phone) found excellent interrater reliability, with kappa values between 0.84 and 0.92 overall, and even more specifically for minor (κ = .89) and severe (κ = .92) injuries [24, 25].
- Another study reported excellent interrater reliability (κ = .85). One study on mild to moderate TBI found excellent interrater reliability (κ = 0.84), adequate internal consistency (Cronbach's alpha = 0.80), but lower person reliability (0.63) [22 - 25].

Validity

- Strong negative correlation with Disability Rating Scale (DRS) (r = -0.89) and a strong negative correlation with Beck Depression Inventory (r= -0.64) [26].
- Correlations with other measures are more moderate. A moderate negative correlation with a duration of post-traumatic amnesia (PTA) (r = -0.52), and moderate positive correlations with self-reported subscales of the Neurobehavioral Functioning Inventory (NFI) (r = 0.37-0.63) and the Barthel Index (r = 0.46) [27, 28].
- Instrument also exhibits moderate to strong positive correlations with subscales of the SF-36 Health Survey (r = 0.47-0.71) and with relative/friend-reported subscales of the NFI (r = 0.47-0.69) [28].
- Separate analysis found a strong negative Spearman's rank correlation of -0.88 at three months post-injury [27, 28].

Responsiveness

- Significant improvement from 3 to 6 months post-injury on FSE ($p < 0.001$, Wilcoxon signed-rank test), mean change = 1.97 [26].
- Significant improvement from 3 to 6 months post-injury on GOSE ($p < 0.001$, Wilcoxon signed-rank test), mean change = -0.42 [26, 27].
- Significant difference in change between FSE and GOSE for moderate to severe TBI ($p < 0.001$, Wilcoxon signed-rank test) [27].

Floor/Ceiling Effect

- High ceiling effect (69%) necessitates the use of the more detailed GOS-E [28].
- Adequate, slight ceiling effect (4.5%) for mild to moderate traumatic brain injury [29]
- No floor effect

MONTREAL-COGNITIVE ASSESSMENT (MOCA)

MoCA is a tool used to evaluate cognitive abilities. Developed in 2005 as an update to the 1975 Mini-Mental State Examination (MMSE), MoCA was designed by Dr. Ziad S. Nasreddine and his team to quickly identify mild cognitive impairment (MCI) and early dementia. It is a cognitive screening instrument specifically aimed at detecting MCI [30].

ICF Domain: Body structure, function, and cognition

Number of Items: 16

Instructions for Administration and Scoring

Administration

- MoCA, a cognitive screening tool administered by clinicians in about ten minutes, evaluates individuals aged 55 to 85 suspected of early-stage dementia [31].
- This condition is marked by a gradual decline in intellectual capabilities, notably memory and abstract reasoning [31].
- The 30-item assessment examines various cognitive domains, such as memory, language, executive functions, visuospatial abilities, calculation skills, abstract thinking, attention span, concentration, and orientation [31] (Table **2**).
- Modified versions of the trail-making, cube-copying, clock-drawing, and object-naming tasks assess visuospatial and executive functions [31].
- Digit span (forward and backward) measures attention [31, 32].

- A tapping task with the letter A and serial sevens subtraction evaluates concentration and calculation [32].
- Language proficiency is gauged through sentence repetition and letter F word fluency. Abstract thought is assessed by identifying similarities between objects. Delayed recall tests memory [32].

Table 2. Montreal Cognitive Assessment (MOCA) [32].

Cognitive Domain	Task	Points
1. Visuospatial/Executive	Trail Making (alternating numbers & letters)	1
	Cube Copying	1
	Clock Drawing (numbers, hands, contour)	3
	Total	/5
2. Naming	Identifying 3 animals (lion, rhinoceros, camel)	3
	Total	/3
3. Attention	Digit Span (forward & backward)	2
	Letter A Tapping (vigilance task)	1
	Serial 7s (count backwards from 100 by 7s)	3
	Total	/6
4. Language	Sentence Repetition	2
	Verbal Fluency (words starting with "F")	1
	Total	/3
5. Abstraction	Explaining relationships between two word pairs (*e.g.*, banana & orange → fruit)	2
	Total	/2
6. Delayed Recall/ Memory	Remembering 5 words without cues	5
	Total	/5
7. Orientation	Date, month, year, day, place, city	6
	Total	/6
Grand Total		/30

Equipment: Basic requirements are: a scorecard, timer, writing instrument, and a notepad.

Scoring: (Table **2**)- The MoCA, a 30-point cognitive screening instrument, uses 16 tasks divided into 11 categories to assess several cognitive functions [31, 32]:

- **Visuospatial/Executive Skills:** These are evaluated through alternating trail making and figure copying (like a cube).
- **Naming:** Individuals are asked to name animals.

- **Memory:** Recall of a previously presented word list is tested after a delay.
- **Attention:** This domain is assessed using forward and backward digit spans, a vigilance task, and subtracting serial sevens.
- **Language:** Sentence repetition and word fluency (starting with a specific letter) are used.
- **Abstraction:** The ability to identify similarities is measured.
- **Orientation:** Individuals are asked to recall the current place and date [31, 32].

MoCA has standardized scoring for each section and comes in three forms to reduce practice effects [32].

Interpretability

MoCA scores are interpreted as follows:

- Normal cognitive function is indicated by scores of 26-30.
- Scores of 18-25 suggest mild cognitive impairment.
- Moderate impairment associated with scores of 10-17.
- A score below 10 signifies severe cognitive impairment [31, 32].

Languages: The Montreal Cognitive Assessment is available in over 60 languages and dialects, including Hebrew and English. The translations of MoCA are linguistically and culturally adapted versions of the original MoCA full version [32].

Training Required: Proper training and a certificate are required.

Clinical Considerations

- In instances where cognitive function is not the main outcome measure in Parkinson's disease (PD), the task force led by Chou *et al.* (2010) advised the utilization of the MoCA as a preferred alternative to several other cognitive evaluation tools, including the MMSE, MMP, PANDA, and SCOPA-cog, for diagnosing MCI in patients.
- Cognitive impairment is an issue; the MoCA has been widely utilized and researched in populations of older adults and people with Parkinson's disease. The MoCA has more focus on executive function and attentiveness.
- The MoCA seems to be more sensitive for people with early stages of dementia, non-AD dementia, and high premorbid IQ in those with modest impairments.
- The MoCA comes in many simultaneous variants, which is advantageous if a patient needs to utilize it more than once [31, 32].

Psychometric Properties

Reliability

- High test-retest reliability (ICC = 0.92, $p < 0.001$) [33]
- Good internal consistency (Cronbach's alpha = 0.82) [33].

Validity

- High correlation with MMSE ($r = 0.87$, $p < 0.001$) [34, 35]
- High convergent validity with MMSE ($r = 0.66$, $p < 0.001$) [35]

***Responsiveness*: (**For mild cognitive impairment)

- Excellent sensitivity (90%) [35]
- Good specificity (87%) [35]

Floor/Ceiling Effect

- No floor effect for total MoCA score in brain injury patients.
- Floor effect in abstraction and delayed recall subdomains (20% of the sample) [36].
- Ceiling effect common in most domains (especially naming: 80.8%, and orientation: 89%), except delayed recall [36].

MINI-MENTAL STATE_EXAMINATION (MMSE)

Original "MMSE"—which was developed in 1975 by Dr. Marshall Folstein *et al.*—had poor inter-rater reliability. In an effort to lower variability and boost reliability, the Standardised MMSE (SMMSE) was created in 1997 by Dr D.W.Molloy and Timothy I.M. Standish with precise scoring instructions and unmistakable administration criteria. The features of MMSE are to increase the effectiveness of screening techniques for dementia and cognitive issues [37].

MMSE is a tool used to assess older persons' cognitive decline. Folstein and his team highlight its utility in assessing cognitive decline among older adults. This tool can identify cognitive issues, measure the extent of impairment at a specific time, track cognitive changes over time, and evaluate a person's response to therapeutic interventions. It evaluates several cognitive functions, including language, orientation, memory, attention, and visuospatial ability. It is also advised for the evaluation of cognitive function in individuals with depression. It is also useful for tracking a person's cognitive changes over time and for estimating the degree and course of cognitive impairment; these uses make it a valuable tool for recording a patient's response to therapy [38].

ICF Domain: Physiological response and cognition

Number of items: 11

Instructions for Administration and Scoring

Administration

- A 30-point questionnaire (Folstein Test) was administered to the subjects in a calm area of their house during the first phase of the trial by one of the three home nurses (Table **3**).
- At follow-up, the research psychologist administered an MMSE as a prelude to a clinical neuropsychological evaluation conducted at the participant's residence.
- The patented mini-mental state evaluation takes ten to fifteen minutes to administer [39].

Table 3. Mini-Mental State Examination (MMSE) [40].

Patient's name-		Date-
Maximum Score	**Patient's Score**	**Questions**
		Orientation
5		What is the (year) (season) (date) (day) (month)?
5		Where are we (state) (country) (town) (hospital) (floor)?
		Registration
3		Name 3 objects: 1 second to say each. Then ask the patient all 3 after you have said them. Give 1 point for each correct answer. Then repeat them until he/she learns all 3. Count trials and record trials
		Attention and Calculation
5		Serial 7's. 1 point for each correct answer. Stop after 5 answers. Alternatively, spell "world" backward.
		Recall
3		Ask for the 3 objects repeated above. Give 1 point for each correct answer.
		Language
2		Name a pencil and a watch.
1		Repeat the following: "No ifs, ands, or buts"

(Table 3) cont.....

Patient's name-		Date-
Maximum Score	**Patient's Score**	**Questions**
3		Follow a 3-stage command: "Take a paper in your hand, fold it in half, and put it on the floor."
1		Read and obey the following: CLOSE YOUR EYES.
1		Write a sentence.
1		Copy the design shown. (Overlapping Pentagons)
Total score		
30		

Equipment: Score sheet that demonstrates a figure to copy and a writing instrument [38].

Scoring: Total score is 30 points (Table **3**) [40].

Interpretability

- A cognitive assessment score of 24 or higher (out of 30) is considered normal.
- Scores between 19 and 23 suggest mild cognitive impairment, while scores between 10 and 18 indicate moderate impairment.
- A score of 9 or below suggests severe cognitive impairment [37, 38].

MCID: MCID for the MMSE, a measure not specifically designed for brain injury, varies. Using baseline standard deviations, the MCID is 1.6 points at 0.4 standard deviations and 2 points at 0.5 standard deviations. When calculated using mean change standard deviations, the MCID is slightly lower, at 1.4 points (0.4 standard deviations) and 1.8 points (0.5 standard deviations) [41].

Languages: MMSE was created in English. However, it has been translated into over 50 languages, including Spanish, Arabic, Chinese, and Nigerian [37].

Training Required: No specialised training needed

Clinical Considerations

- MMSE is adequate for screening purposes, but lacks the precision needed for confirming diagnoses of dementia, moderate cognitive impairment, or delirium.
- The MMSE's capacity to identify dementia is restricted when used alone; however, this capacity can be greatly increased by including a brief assessment of memory, executive function, and IADL [41].

- While factors such as age, education, culture, and socioeconomic status can influence MMSE scores, gender does not appear to be a contributing factor.
- It is an analysis of outcome measures associated with stroke [42].

Psychometric Properties

Reliability

- MMSE demonstrates moderate internal consistency, with Cronbach's alpha values of 0.748 at admission and 0.653 at discharge [43].

Validity

- Data on the validity of the MMSE specifically within a brain injury population is currently unavailable.

Responsiveness

- For dementia, MMSE has a reported sensitivity of 88.3% (95% CI, 81.3% to 92.9%) and specificity of 86.2% (95% CI, 81.8% to 89.7%).
- Meta-analysis of numerous studies found slightly different values: 81% sensitivity (95% CI, 78% to 84%) and 89% specificity (95% CI, 87% to 91%) [44, 45].

Floor/Ceiling Effect

- There is no current data available regarding the floor or ceiling effects of the MMSE in individuals with brain injuries.

GALVESTON ORIENTATION AND AMNESIA TEST (GOAT)

Levin, O'Donnell, and Grossman developed the GOAT in 1979. GOAT was designed to assess cognition in stages: head-injury (closed) patients recover in the subacute phase. This important assessment tool evaluates memory for events that occurred both before and after the injury, along with orientation to individuals, locations, and timeframes. Several items measuring memory, biographical recall, and temporal and spatial orientation were included in the test. Both anterograde and retrograde amnesia fall under the category of posttraumatic amnesia, which is the condition of disorientation and confusion that follows a head injury [46].

ICF Domain: Orientation

Number of items: 10

Instructions for Administration and Scoring

Administration

- GOAT is a clinician-reported outcome measure.
- Post-traumatic amnesia and orientation following TBI are evaluated using the 10-item GOAT.
- Each question is worth 1 point, and a maximum of 100 points can be earned.
- The cutoff point for emerging from post-traumatic amnesia is thought to be a score of more than 78 for three days in a row [47].

Equipment: Paper and pen

Scoring

- This test comprises a total of 16 questions. If a negative value is assigned to any question, it is referred to as an error score (Table **4**).
- The overall score is determined by subtracting the total of the error scores from 100 [46, 47].
- Should a patient achieve a total score of 75 or above for two consecutive days, they are deemed to have exited the PTA-phase and are considered to be in a NORMAL state [46].
- Scores ranging from 66 to 75 indicate a borderline status, classified as BORDERLINE [46, 47].
- Conversely, if the score falls below 66, the patient is still regarded as being in the PTA-phase, categorised as IMPAIRED [46, 47].

Table 4. Galveston Orientation & Amnesia Test (GOAT) [48].

Question	Error Score	Notes
What is your name?	/ 2	Must give both first name and surname.
When were you born?	/ 4	Must give day, month, and year.
Where do you live?	/ 4	The town is sufficient.
Where are you now?		
(a) City	/ 5	Must give actual town.
(b) Building	/ 5	Usually in hospital or a rehab centre. Actual name necessary.
When were you admitted to this hospital?	/ 5	Date.

(Table 4) cont.....

<table>
<tr><th>Question</th><th>Error Score</th><th>Notes</th></tr>
<tr><td>How did you get here?</td><td>/ 5</td><td>Mode of transport.</td></tr>
<tr><td>What is the first event you can remember after the injury?</td><td>/ 5</td><td>Any plausible event is sufficient (record answer).</td></tr>
<tr><td>Can you give some details?</td><td>/ 5</td><td>Must give relevant details.</td></tr>
<tr><td>Can you describe the last event you can recall before the accident?</td><td>/ 5</td><td>Any plausible event is sufficient (record answer).</td></tr>
<tr><td>What time is it now?</td><td>/ 5</td><td>1 for each half-hour error, etc.</td></tr>
<tr><td>What day of the week is it?</td><td>/ 3</td><td>1 for each day error, etc.</td></tr>
<tr><td>What day of the month is it? (i.e., the date)</td><td>/ 5</td><td>1 for each day error, etc.</td></tr>
<tr><td>What is the month?</td><td>/ 15</td><td>5 for each month error, etc.</td></tr>
<tr><td>What is the year?</td><td>/ 30</td><td>10 for each year error.</td></tr>
<tr><td>Total score:</td><td colspan="2"></td></tr>
<tr><td rowspan="4">Total error:
100 - Total error (Can be a negative number.)
76-100 = Normal
66-75 = Borderline
< 66 = Impaired</td><td colspan="2">Patient's last name:</td></tr>
<tr><td colspan="2">Patient first name:</td></tr>
<tr><td colspan="2">Date of birth:</td></tr>
<tr><td colspan="2">Date:</td></tr>
</table>

Interpretability: Post-traumatic amnesia (PTA) is defined as the period following a coma during which an individual's GOAT score remains below 75.

- Participant receives a score of 75 or higher on three separate administrations, PTA is deemed to have stopped [48, 49].
- At an early follow-up, hospitalisation and post-concussion syndrome are linked to a low GOAT score.
- For the GOAT, ranges:

- After two days with a score of at least 75, the person is no longer in the PTA phase.
- A score between 66 and 75 on two consecutive days is considered borderline.
- Score < 66 indicates that the patient was still in the PTA phase for two days in a row [49].

Languages: GOAT has been translated into several languages, including Farsi and Portuguese.

Training Required: No special qualifications needed

Clinical Considerations

- GOAT is a valuable assessment tool for evaluating sequential cognitive processes during the subacute phase of recovery from a closed head injury.
- The exam assesses memory for events both preceding and following the injury, along with orientation to people, places, and times.
- The GOAT is used to measure post-traumatic and retrograde amnesia in individuals with traumatic brain injury and, more broadly, to examine their overall cognitive status.
- At an early follow-up, hospitalisation and post-concussion syndrome are linked to a low GOAT score.
- Patients with closed head injuries from traumatic brain traumas are the main patients treated with the GOAT.
- The purpose of this test is to provide a credible and practical scale that can be used by medical professionals from multiple specialties at the bedside of patients or in emergency care settings [46, 47, 49].

Psychometric Properties

Reliability

- Inter-rater reliability: $r = 0.98$ (Kappa = 0.73) [49, 50]
- Individual item reliability (Kendall's coefficient): 0.99 [50].

Validity

- Positive correlation with Glasgow Coma Scale (GCS): $r = 0.456$, $p < 0.002$ [49]
- Positive correlation with Functional Independence Measure (FIM):
  - Admission: $r = 0.701$ [50, 51]
  - Discharge: $r = 0.531$ [49 - 51]

Responsiveness: No data reported for brain injury.

Floor/ceiling effect: No data reported for brain injury.

GENERAL_PRACTITIONER_ASSESSMENT_OF_COGNITION (GPCOG) SCORE

Designed for rapid assessment of cognitive decline, the GPCOG was developed by Brodaty and colleagues in 2002. GPCOG comprises an informant interview in addition to a cognitive exam for the patient [52].

ICF Domain: Cognition

Number of items: 9

Instructions for Administration and Scoring

Administration

- The test is clinician-administered and includes an informant rating
- The cognitive portion of the assessment consists of nine tasks:
  - These include drawing a clock (evaluating time orientation, proper numbering and spacing, and accurate hand placement), recalling a recent news event, and remembering a name and address (specifically, the first name, last name, number, street, and neighbourhood)
- Six historical questions are posed to an informant during an informant interview.
- Informant interview touches on several topics, such as memory loss, trouble finding words, money management issues, difficulty taking medications on one's own, and needing help getting around.
- GPCOG is a rapid and easy-to-use screening tool. The cognitive assessment takes less than 4 minutes, and the informant interview takes less than 2 minutes [52].

Equipment: Paper and pencil

Scoring [53]

A. Interview of the patient-
  - 1 point is awarded for each of the nine items.
  - When correct responses are added together, the maximum score is 9.
  - A person is deemed cognitively intact if they score 9 on the GPCOG. Additional actions are not necessary, although it is advised to retest after a year.
  - A score between five and eight denotes some impairment; however, more details are needed.
  - The informant interview is to be conducted by the user/general practitioner—someone with 4 points or less likely to have cognitive impairment.

B. Interview of the informant –
  - If more details regarding the patient's function are needed, an informant interview should be held.
  - There are VI questions. In all, the options are:
    - "Yes" (impairment)
    - "No" (with no impairment)

    - "Don't know."
    - "N/A"
  - One point is awarded for each question. Since "yes" answers indicate impairment, they receive a score of 0, while all other answers receive a score of 1.
  - Higher scores signify less impairment.
  - When a patient's score in the informant interview is between 0 and 3, and the informant interview score is between 5 and 8, it suggests cognitive impairment and calls for additional testing.
  - For the time being, the patient can be regarded as cognitively intact if they score between 4 and 6, indicating they have difficulty in fewer than 3 areas. It is nevertheless advised to retest after a year [35].

Interpretability

- If an individual receives the maximum possible nine points, no additional evaluation is required.
- If the score is between five and eight, more details are needed. Next, the test administrator will go on to the test's second component. They will enquire about the patient's symptoms from a caregiver or family member. This segment is known as the "Informant Interview."
- The exam indicates that a person may be cognitively impaired if their result is between 0 and 4. It is not necessary to conduct an informant interview, but the medical professional may wish to run additional diagnostic procedures [52].

Languages

- GPCOG was initially published in the English language in 2002 [52].
- Other versions have been validated in French and Italian [52, 53].

Training Required: No prerequisites needed

Clinical Considerations

- GPCOG is primarily used to assess older persons for cognitive impairment.
- During typical office visits, general practitioners utilise this test to swiftly assess cognitive performance.
- Frequent evaluations may help identify cognitive changes over time, enabling early intervention and appropriate management [52].

Psychometric Properties

Reliability

- The GPCOG patient section showed acceptable internal consistency, with a Cronbach's alpha of 0.68 (indicating that the items within that section measure the same underlying construct reasonably well) [54].
- The overall GPCOG-C (likely a composite score) demonstrated excellent test-retest reliability (0.98); this indicates that the test produces very consistent results over time [54].

Validity

- GPCOG has a positive predictive value of 72% (meaning that when the test indicates a patient has cognitive impairment, it is correct 72% of the time) [53].
- The test has a high negative predictive value of 99% (meaning that if the test suggests a patient does *not* have cognitive impairment, it is very likely correct (99% of the time)) [53, 54].

Responsiveness

- The English version of the GPCOG has a sensitivity ranging from 0.81 to 0.98 (meaning it's good at correctly identifying individuals who *do* have cognitive impairment (81% to 98% of the time)) [54].
- The specificity of the English GPCOG ranges from 0.72 to 0.95; this indicates its ability to correctly identify individuals without cognitive impairment (72% to 95% of the time) [54].

Floor/Ceiling Effect

- The GPCOG has no ceiling effect.
- The GPCOG may have a floor effect, meaning that it may not be sensitive enough to detect mild cognitive impairment [54].

WESTERN NEURO SENSORY STIMULATION PROFILE (WNSSP)

WNSSP was created in 1989 by Ansel and Keenan. It aims to assess cognitive function in individuals with severe head injuries, intended to monitor progress and predict future outcomes. It also aims to evaluate cognitive function in individuals with serious brain injuries (Rancho levels II–V). Individuals who are slow to recover are those who stay at RLA (level II and III) for a longer duration. These individuals may benefit from programs involving sensory stimulation [55].

ICF Domain: Body structure and function

Number of items: 33

Instructions for Administration and Scoring

Administration

- The WNSSP is a 33-item observational test that is given at the patient's bedside. Scoring is based on the type of stimulation (general or specific), the speed of response, and whether prompting is needed.
- Time duration=45 min.
- Every test section comprises multiple items, such as
    - Communication (vocalisation or mouthing words)
    - Visual Responses (tracking and responses to written commands)
    - Tactile Responses (touch perception and object use)
    - Olfactory Responses (odour perception) [55, 56]

Arousal/Attention

1. **Responsiveness:** Awakening ease (eye/face/body movement) *via* voice/touch/shaking/bed/cloth. Scores: Repeated stimuli (0), two or more stimuli (1), one stimulus (2), spontaneously awake (3).
2. **Sustained Wakefulness**: Longest unprompted awake time. Scores: <10 min (0), 11-20 min (1), >21 min/all session (2).
3. **Visual Interaction**: Eye contact. Scores: Closed (0), open/unfocused (1), focused >50% (2), unable to open (N).
4. **Concentration**: Visual/task focus. Scores: <50% time (0), >50% time (1)
   Auditory Response:
5. **Voice:** Reaction to "Hello, my name is…". Scores: No response <20s (0), undifferentiated response (1), differentiated response (2).
6. **Sound:** Best reaction to non-verbal sound (music/bell/clicker/recorder/sneeze/door). Scores: No response <20s (0), undifferentiated response (1), differentiated response (2).

Auditory Comprehension: (Single-stage commands, one repeat allowed, score coinciding responses, penalty for perseveration)

- No response <20s (0)
- Incorrect response (1)
- Cued, delayed (>5s) (2)
- Cued, prompt (3)
- Spontaneous, delayed (>5s) (4)

- Spontaneous, prompt (5)
    1. Grip my hand
    2. **Part/shut mouth** (use "part" if mouth usually shut)
    3. Extend tongue
    4. **Shut/open eyes** (use "shut" if eyes usually open)
    5. Lift brows
    6. **Shift body part** (patient can move on their own)

III. EXPRESSIVE

Communication

1. **Sound Production: Scores**: No response (0), best spontaneous non-meaningful vocalisation (1), best spontaneous inappropriate verbalisation/mouthing (2), vocalises on command/appropriate verbalisation/mouthing (3).
2. **Non-verbal Expression**: (excluding yes/no head nods). Scores: No response (random grimaces/reflexes only) (0), one gesture/facial expression (1), more than one gesture/facial expression with intent (2).
3. **Affirmative/Negative Response:** Verbal or non-verbal (finger signals, eye gaze, buzzer) to 3 questions. Scores: Neither response (0), either "yes" or "no" (1), both "yes" and "no" (2).

Visual Response Tracking

- Horizontal Tracking: (Repeated trials) Scores: No response <20s (0), follows to one side (1), follows to both sides (2), follows across midline (3). Using: **Mirror (16), person (17), picture (18), object (19), mirror (20).**
- Vertical Tracking: Scores: No response <20s (0), follows up or down (1), follows up and down (2). Using: **Picture (21), object (22).**

Visual Comprehension: (Written commands, "Read & do," one repeat, no reading aloud) Scores: No response <20s (0), incorrect (1), cued, delayed (>5s) (2), cued, prompt (3), spontaneous, delayed (>5s) (4), spontaneous, prompt (5). Commands: **Open mouth (23), stick out tongue (24), close eyes (25), raise eyebrows (26), move body part (27).**

Tactile Response

1. **Touch**: (Non-painful tap/brush/towel/comb). Scores: No response <20s (0), undifferentiated response (1), differentiated response (2).
2. **Oral Stimulation:** (Q-tip on lips). Scores: Withdrawal/abnormal reflexes (0), primitive reflexes (1), tolerates stimulation (2).

Object Manipulation: ("Show me how you use it.") Scores: No response <20s (0), holds/releases (1), moves inappropriately (2), reaches/pushes (3), cued use (4), spontaneous use (5), both arms casted/splinted (N). Objects: **Spoon (30), comb (31), pencil (32).**

Olfactory Response: (Pleasant/unpleasant scents). Scores: No response <20s (0), undifferentiated response (1), differentiated response (2), not applicable (tracheostomy) (N)

Interpretation

Total score=0-113, *(Higher scores -better cognitive function).*

TIME OF ADMINISTRATION

The administration of the WNSSP typically takes **30-60 minutes,** depending on the individual's responsiveness and the specific sensory modalities being assessed. The evaluation can be conducted in a single session or spread over multiple sessions to ensure a thorough assessment without overwhelming the individual.

Equipment: Moist fabric, Non-spoken audio (melody/gong/clicker, *etc.*), a portable reflector, an image, Bristled implement, Coarse terrycloth, Hair arranger, Cotton swab, Eating utensil, Writing tool, Scent, Acidic liquid, Spice, Pungent bulb, Brew

Scoring:

- WNSSP is made up of nine sections: Arousal/Attention (4 questions), Hearing Response (2 questions), Hearing Understanding (6 questions), Speaking (3 questions), Sight Tracking (7 questions), Sight Understanding (5 questions), Touch Response (2 questions), Object Handling (3 questions), and Smell Response (1 question) [57].
- The score is determined by the type of stimulation used (basic or targeted), how long it takes to elicit a response, and whether any prompts are necessary. The final score ranges from 0-113 (the lower the score, the poorer the *ability*) [57, 58] (Table **5**).

Interpretability

- Multipoint systems, which differ from item to item and range from 0-1 to 0-5, are used to assess each item.
- Better cognitive performance is linked to higher scores.
- A score of zero is the smallest, and 110 is the maximum.

- Subscale scores provide a way to assess a patient's response pattern [57, 58].

Table 5. Six categories of points at Western Neuro Sensory Stimulation Profile (WNSSP).

Subscales Category	Maximum Score
Comprehending sounds	30
Perception of visual information	25
Visual Guidance	18
Manipulating objects	15
Attention/Arousal	8
Tactile/Olfactory	6

Language: English [57]

Training Required: No specific prior training

Clinical Considerations

- Applied to the assessment and planning of sensory stimulation interventions in therapeutic or rehabilitation settings.
- A person's tolerance levels, preferred sensory experiences, and any particular neurological problems would all be taken into account [56, 57].

Psychometric Properties

Reliability

- WNSSP demonstrated high internal consistency ($\alpha = 0.933$ for total score, 0.73-0.95 for subscales, though Tactile/Olfactory was low at 0.59) [59, 60].
- Interrater reliability was excellent for the total score ($r = 0.94$-0.99) and ranged from adequate to excellent for the Arousal/Attention subscale ($r = 0.78$-0.90), but was poor to adequate for the Tactile/Olfactory subscale ($r = 0.64$-0.86) [59, 60].

Validity

- Concurrent validity with the FIM was weak but significant at admission for the total score (rs = -0.146, $p = 0.0424$), and modest at discharge for Motor (rs = 0.374, $p = 0.045$) and Cognition (rs = 0.412, $p = 0.026$) subscales. Concurrent validity with the RLAS was strong at both admission (rs = 0.693, $p = 0.01$) and discharge (rs = 0.788, $p = 0.01$) [59, 60].

- Convergent validity with a communication score was excellent (k = 0.99, $p < 0.0001$), but more limited with arousal (k = 0.93) and awareness (k = 0.77) scores [59].

Floor/Ceiling Effect

- WNSSP had a poor ceiling effect, with 50% of participants at follow-up at the ceiling and 33% scoring between 110 and 112 [60].

CLINICAL CONSIDERATIONS, STRENGTHS, LIMITATIONS, AND EMERGING PERSPECTIVES

Traumatic brain injury (TBI) is a heterogeneous condition characterised by varying degrees of altered consciousness, cognitive impairment, physical disability, emotional disturbances, and long-term participation restrictions. Consequently, assessment in TBI must be phase-specific and purpose-driven, as no single scale adequately captures the evolving clinical profile across the continuum from acute injury to chronic recovery [61, 62].

In the acute and critical care setting, scales of consciousness such as the Glasgow Coma Scale (GCS) and the Full Outline of UnResponsiveness (FOUR) score remain essential for rapid neurological assessment, severity stratification, and prognostication. The FOUR score offers advantages in intubated patients by incorporating brainstem reflexes and respiratory patterns, addressing some limitations of the GCS. However, both scales provide limited information regarding higher cognitive function, behavioural sequelae, or long-term disability [63].

As patients transition to subacute and rehabilitation phases, functional outcome measures become increasingly relevant. Instruments such as the Disability Rating Scale (DRS) and the Functional Independence Measure (FIM) are widely used to track recovery across domains of arousal, cognition, self-care, and mobility. While these scales are valuable for monitoring broad functional trends, they may lack sensitivity to subtle cognitive deficits, executive dysfunction, and psychosocial limitations commonly observed after moderate to severe TBI [64, 65].

Cognitive and participation-focused measures, including neuropsychological test batteries and patient-reported outcome measures, address aspects of recovery that are often underrepresented in clinician-rated scales. Patient-reported tools capture symptoms such as fatigue, emotional dysregulation, and perceived cognitive difficulty, which may persist despite favourable functional scores. However, self-report measures may be influenced by reduced insight, mood disorders, and contextual factors, necessitating cautious interpretation [66].

A key limitation across TBI assessment tools is the fragmentation of outcome domains. Measures of consciousness, function, cognition, and quality of life are frequently applied independently, which can result in overlapping assessments or incomplete representation of patient recovery. Strategic selection of complementary tools, aligned with the International Classification of Functioning, Disability and Health (ICF) framework, is therefore essential to balance comprehensiveness with feasibility [62, 67].

Emerging perspectives in TBI assessment emphasize standardization, digitalisation, and ecological validity. Recent initiatives advocate for common data elements (CDEs) to improve comparability across studies and clinical settings. In parallel, wearable sensors, mobile cognitive assessments, and remote monitoring platforms are being explored to capture real-world function, activity levels, and symptom fluctuations outside clinical environments. Advances in neuroimaging and fluid biomarkers are also increasingly integrated with clinical scales to refine prognostication and treatment stratification [68, 69].

In clinical practice, scale selection should reflect the stage of recovery and clinical objective. Acute assessment prioritises consciousness and neurological stability, rehabilitation focuses on functional independence and cognitive recovery, and long-term follow-up emphasises participation, quality of life, and community reintegration. An integrated yet selective assessment strategy improves clinical relevance while minimising redundancy and patient burden [61, 65, 67] (Table **6**).

Table 6. Comparative summary of commonly used TBI assessment scales.

Scale	Primary Domain	Key Strengths	Major Limitations	Optimal Clinical Use
Glasgow Coma Scale (GCS)	Level of consciousness	Rapid, widely accepted, prognostic	Limited use in intubated patients; no cognition	Acute and emergency assessment
FOUR Score	Consciousness & brainstem function	Applicable in intubation; brainstem assessment	Less familiar; training required	Neurocritical care
Disability Rating Scale (DRS)	Global disability	Tracks recovery from coma to the community	Limited sensitivity to subtle deficits	Longitudinal outcome tracking
Functional Independence Measure (FIM)	Functional ability	Standardised rehab utility	Ceiling effects; limited cognition detail	Inpatient rehabilitation

(Table 6) cont.....

Scale	Primary Domain	Key Strengths	Major Limitations	Optimal Clinical Use
Rancho Los Amigos Scale	Cognitive recovery	Simple staging of cognitive function	Descriptive; limited responsiveness	Cognitive recovery monitoring
Neuropsychological batteries	Cognition & executive function	Detailed cognitive profiling	Time-consuming; resource-intensive	Post-acute & chronic TBI
Patient-reported outcome measures	Symptoms & participation	Patient-centred; captures hidden deficits	Insight and mood dependent	Long-term follow-up

CONCLUSION

In conclusion, this chapter thoroughly examines various assessment tools used to evaluate brain injury, commonly employed in clinical practice and research to identify cognitive, emotional, and behavioural deficits. These scales include their ability to provide a standardised and objective assessment of TBI severity, guide treatment decisions, and monitor progress over time. They also have good reliability and validity, making them useful tools for clinicians and researchers.

However, there are some limitations and areas for improvement. For instance, the MMSE can struggle to identify minor cognitive improvements due to its upper limit, while the GPCOG might miss subtle cognitive decline because of its lower limit. The WNSSP has a poor ceiling effect, with 50% of participants reaching the maximum score at follow-up. Additionally, the GOAT has limited responsiveness, with no values reported for its responsiveness in brain injury. The GCS has been found to have limited sensitivity and specificity, particularly in patients with intubation.

Thus, future research recommendations include developing more sensitive and specific scales to detect mild cognitive impairment, such as revising the GPCOG to improve its sensitivity, investigating the cultural and linguistic adaptations of existing scales, developing more comprehensive and multidimensional scales to assess TBI, and investigating the use of technology-based assessments to improve efficiency and accuracy.

AI DISCLOSURE STATEMENT

During the preparation of this chapter, the authors used ChatGPT (OpenAI) as a support tool for language refinement, structural organisation, and clarification of ideas. All content generated with AI assistance was carefully reviewed, verified, and revised by the authors to ensure factual accuracy, originality, and consistency with the scientific literature. The authors take full responsibility for the integrity, interpretation, and final content of the published chapter.

ACKNOWLEDGEMENT

The authors wish to express their gratitude to neurologists, neuropsychologists, rehabilitation physicians, and researchers whose dedicated work in the field of traumatic brain injury assessment and recovery has significantly shaped current clinical practices. Their ongoing contributions to developing and validating standardised scales have enhanced the precision of diagnosis, recovery monitoring, and rehabilitation outcomes for individuals living with TBI.

REFERENCES

[1] Faul M, Coronado V. Epidemiology of traumatic brain injury. In: Grafman J, Salazar AM, Eds. Handbook of Clinical Neurology. New York: Elsevier 2015; Vol. 127: pp. 3-13.

[2] Dams-O'Connor K, Cantor JB, Brown M, Dijkers MP, Spielman LA, Gordon WA. Screening for traumatic brain injury: findings and public health implications. J Head Trauma Rehabil 2014; 29(6): 479-89.
[http://dx.doi.org/10.1097/HTR.0000000000000099] [PMID: 25370440]

[3] Lin K, Wroten M. Ranchos Los Amigos. StatPearls Publishing 2022.

[4] Hagen C, Malkmus D, Durham P. Levels of cognitive functioning. Rehabilitation of the head-injured adult: comprehensive physical management. Downey, CA: Professional Staff Association of Rancho Los Amigos Hospital 1979; pp. 87-8.

[5] Boake C, High WM Jr, Levin HS, *et al.* Comparison of the Rancho Los Amigos and the Functional Independence Measure in traumatic brain injury. Arch Phys Med Rehabil 1995; 76(12): 1153-9.

[6] Gouvier WD, Blanton PD, LaPorte KK, Nepomuceno C. Reliability and validity of the Disability Rating Scale and the Levels of Cognitive Functioning Scale in monitoring recovery from severe head injury. Arch Phys Med Rehabil 1987; 68(2): 94-7.
[PMID: 3813863]

[7] Gouvier WD, Blanton PD, LaPorta NK, Nepomuceno C. Reliability and validity of the Rancho Los Amigos Scale in traumatic brain injury. Int J Rehabil Res 1987; 10(3): 231-6.

[8] Teasdale G, Knill-Jones R, van der Sande J. Observer variability in assessing impaired consciousness and coma. J Neurol Neurosurg Psychiatry 1978; 41(7): 603-10.
[http://dx.doi.org/10.1136/jnnp.41.7.603] [PMID: 690637]

[9] Matis G, Birbilis T. The Glasgow Coma Scale--a brief review. Past, present, future. Acta Neurol Belg 2008; 108(3): 75-89.
[PMID: 19115670]

[10] Teasdale G, Murray G, Parker L, Jennett B. Adding up the Glasgow Coma Score. Acta Neurochir Suppl (Wien) 1979; 28(1): 13-6.
[PMID: 290137]

[11] Crossman J, Bankes M, Bhananker S, *et al.* The Glasgow Coma Scale: reliable evidence-informed guidance for everyday clinical practice. J Clin Nurs 2012; 21(11-12): 1726-34.
[PMID: 22225909]

[12] Reilly PL, Simpson DA, Sprod R, Thomas L. Assessing the conscious level in infants and young children: a paediatric version of the Glasgow Coma Scale. Childs Nerv Syst 1988; 4(1): 30-3.
[http://dx.doi.org/10.1007/BF00274080] [PMID: 3135935]

[13] Gill MR, Reiley DG, Green SM. Interrater reliability of Glasgow Coma Scale scores in the emergency department. Ann Emerg Med 2004; 43(2): 215-23. [http://dx.doi.org/10.1016/S0196-0644(03)00814-X] [PMID: 14747811]

[14] Reith FCM, Van den Brande R, Synnot A, Gruen R, Maas AIR. The reliability of the Glasgow Coma Scale: a systematic review. Intensive Care Med 2016; 42(1): 3-15. [http://dx.doi.org/10.1007/s00134-015-4124-3] [PMID: 26564211]

[15] Meredith W, Rutledge R, Fakhry SM, Emery S, Kromhout-Schiro S. The conundrum of the Glasgow Coma Scale in intubated patients: a linear regression prediction of the Glasgow verbal score from the Glasgow eye and motor scores. J Trauma Inj Infect Crit Care 1998; 44(5): 839-45. [http://dx.doi.org/10.1097/00005373-199805000-00016] [PMID: 9603086]

[16] McNett M. A review of the predictive ability of Glasgow Coma Scale scores in head-injured patients. J Neurosci Nurs 2007; 39(2): 68-75. [http://dx.doi.org/10.1097/01376517-200704000-00002] [PMID: 17477220]

[17] McMillan T, Wilson L, Ponsford J, Levin H, Teasdale G, Bond M. The Glasgow Outcome Scale — 40 years of application and refinement. Nat Rev Neurol 2016; 12(8): 477-85. [http://dx.doi.org/10.1038/nrneurol.2016.89] [PMID: 27418377]

[18] Lindsay KW, Bone I, Fuller G. Neurology and Neurosurgery Illustrated. 5th ed., Edinburgh: Churchill Livingstone 2010.

[19] Jennett B, Snoek J, Bond MR, Brooks N. Disability after severe head injury: observations on the use of the Glasgow Outcome Scale. J Neurol Neurosurg Psychiatry 1981; 44(4): 285-93. [http://dx.doi.org/10.1136/jnnp.44.4.285] [PMID: 6453957]

[20] Wilson JTL, Pettigrew LL, Teasdale GM. Structured interviews for the Glasgow Outcome Scale and the extended Glasgow Outcome Scale: guidelines for their use. J Neurotrauma 1998; 15(8): 573-85. [http://dx.doi.org/10.1089/neu.1998.15.573] [PMID: 9726257]

[21] Wilson JT, Pettigrew LE, Teasdale GM. Reliability of ratings on the Glasgow Outcome Scales from in-person and telephone structured interviews. J Head Trauma Rehabil 2000; 15(5): 589-95.

[22] Wilson JTL, Edwards P, Fiddes H, Stewart E, Teasdale GM. Reliability of postal questionnaires for the Glasgow Outcome Scale. J Neurotrauma 2002; 19(9): 999-1005. [http://dx.doi.org/10.1089/089771502760341910] [PMID: 12482113]

[23] Hong I, Li CY, Velozo CA. Item-Level Psychometrics of the Glasgow Outcome Scale. OTJR (Thorofare, NJ) 2016; 36(2): 65-73. [http://dx.doi.org/10.1177/1539449216632449] [PMID: 27504879]

[24] Lu J, Marmarou A, Lapane K, Turf E, Wilson L. A method for reducing misclassification in the extended Glasgow Outcome Score. J Neurotrauma 2010; 27(5): 843-52. [http://dx.doi.org/10.1089/neu.2010.1293] [PMID: 20334503]

[25] Pettigrew LEL, Wilson JTL, Teasdale GM. Reliability of ratings on the Glasgow Outcome Scales from in-person and telephone structured interviews. J Head Trauma Rehabil 2003; 18(3): 252-8. [http://dx.doi.org/10.1097/00001199-200305000-00003] [PMID: 12802167]

[26] Wilson JTL, Pettigrew LE, Teasdale GM. Emotional and cognitive consequences of head injury in relation to the Glasgow outcome scale. J Neurol Neurosurg Psychiatry 2000; 69(2): 204-9. [http://dx.doi.org/10.1136/jnnp.69.2.204] [PMID: 10896694]

[27] Dikmen S, Machamer J, Manley GT, *et al.* Functional Status Examination *versus* Glasgow Outcome Scale Extended as Outcome Measures in Traumatic Brain Injuries: How Do They Compare? J Neurotrauma 2019; 36(16): 2423-9. [http://dx.doi.org/10.1089/neu.2018.6198] [PMID: 30827167]

[28] Hall KM, Bushnik T, Lakisic-Kazazic B, Wright J, Cantagallo A. Assessing traumatic brain injury outcome measures for long-term follow-up of community-based individuals. Arch Phys Med Rehabil

2001; 82(3): 367-74.
[http://dx.doi.org/10.1053/apmr.2001.21525] [PMID: 11245760]

[29] Jennett B, Bond M. Assessment of outcome after severe brain damage. damage Lancet 1975; 1(7905): 480-.
[http://dx.doi.org/10.1016/S0140-6736(75)92830-5]

[30] Julayanont P, Phillips N, Chertkow H, Nasreddine ZS. Montreal cognitive assessment (MoCA): Concept and clinical review. In: Larner AJ, Ed. Cognitive Screening Instruments. New York: Springer-Verlag 2013; pp. 111-52.
[http://dx.doi.org/10.1007/978-1-4471-2452-8_6]

[31] Gluhm S, Goldstein J, Loc K, Colt A, Liew CV, Corey-Bloom J. Cognitive performance on the mini-mental state examination and the montreal cognitive assessment across the healthy adult lifespan. Cogn Behav Neurol 2013; 26(1): 1-5.
[http://dx.doi.org/10.1097/WNN.0b013e31828b7d26] [PMID: 23538566]

[32] Nasreddine ZS, Phillips NA, Bédirian V, *et al.* The Montreal Cognitive Assessment, MoCA: a brief screening tool for mild cognitive impairment. J Am Geriatr Soc 2005; 53(4): 695-9.
[http://dx.doi.org/10.1111/j.1532-5415.2005.53221.x] [PMID: 15817019]

[33] Luis CA, Keegan AP, Mullan M. Cross validation of the Montreal Cognitive Assessment in community dwelling older adults residing in the Southeastern US. Int J Geriatr Psychiatry 2009; 24(2): 197-201.
[http://dx.doi.org/10.1002/gps.2101] [PMID: 18850670]

[34] Yin Z, Zhao Y, Lu X, Duan H. A hybrid intelligent diagnosis approach for quick screening of Alzheimer's disease based on multiple neuropsychological rating scales. Comput Math Methods Med 2015; 2015: 1-13.
[http://dx.doi.org/10.1155/2015/258761] [PMID: 25815043]

[35] Lam B, Middleton LE, Masellis M, *et al.* Criterion and convergent validity of the Montreal cognitive assessment with screening and standardized neuropsychological testing. J Am Geriatr Soc 2013; 61(12): 2181-5.
[http://dx.doi.org/10.1111/jgs.12541] [PMID: 24320735]

[36] Tsai CF, Lee WJ, Wang SJ, Shia BC, Nasreddine Z, Fuh JL. Psychometrics of the Montreal Cognitive Assessment (MoCA) and its subscales: validation of the Taiwanese version of the MoCA and an item response theory analysis. Int Psychogeriatr 2012; 24(4): 651-8.
[http://dx.doi.org/10.1017/S1041610211002298] [PMID: 22152127]

[37] William Molloy D, Standish TIM. A Guide to the Standardized Mini-Mental State Examination. Int Psychogeriatr 1997; 9(S1) (Suppl. 1): 87-94.
[http://dx.doi.org/10.1017/S1041610297004754] [PMID: 9447431]

[38] Arevalo-Rodriguez I, Smailagic N, Roqué-Figuls M, *et al.* Mini-Mental State Examination (MMSE) for the early detection of dementia in people with mild cognitive impairment (MCI). Cochrane Database Syst Rev 2021; 7(7): CD010783.
[PMID: 34313331]

[39] Schultz-Larsen K, Lomholt RK, Kreiner S. Mini-Mental Status Examination: A short form of MMSE was as accurate as the original MMSE in predicting dementia. J Clin Epidemiol 2007; 60(3): 260-7.
[http://dx.doi.org/10.1016/j.jclinepi.2006.06.008] [PMID: 17292020]

[40] Folstein MF, Folstein SE, McHugh PR. "Mini-mental state". J Psychiatr Res 1975; 12(3): 189-98.
[http://dx.doi.org/10.1016/0022-3956(75)90026-6] [PMID: 1202204]

[41] Dujardin JP, *et al.* The Role of the Subthalamic Nucleus in the Control of Movement. In: Lindsay KW, Ed. Neurology and Neurosurgery Illustrated. 5th ed., Edinburgh: Churchill Livingstone 2010.

[42] Salter D, *et al.* Maintaining Rank in Dominance Hierarchy: Subordinate Behavioural Tactics. In: Larner AJ, Ed. Cognitive Screening Instruments: A Practical Approach. New York: Springer-Verlag

2021.

[43] Tombaugh TN, McIntyre NJ. The mini-mental state examination: a comprehensive review. J Am Geriatr Soc 1992; 40(9): 922-35.
[http://dx.doi.org/10.1111/j.1532-5415.1992.tb01992.x] [PMID: 1512391]

[44] Tsoi KKF, Chan JYC, Hirai HW, Wong SYS, Kwok TCY. Cognitive Tests to Detect Dementia. JAMA Intern Med 2015; 175(9): 1450-8.
[http://dx.doi.org/10.1001/jamainternmed.2015.2152] [PMID: 26052687]

[45] Sleutjes DKL, Harmsen IJ, van Bergen FS, Oosterman JM, Dautzenberg PLJ, Kessels RPC. Validity of the Mini-Mental State Examination-2 in Diagnosing Mild Cognitive Impairment and Dementia in Patients Visiting an Outpatient Clinic in the Netherlands. Alzheimer Dis Assoc Disord 2020; 34(3): 278-81.
[http://dx.doi.org/10.1097/WAD.0000000000000403] [PMID: 32826418]

[46] Levin HS, O'DONNELL VM, Grossman RG. The Galveston Orientation and Amnesia Test. A practical scale to assess cognition after head injury. J Nerv Ment Dis 1979; 167(11): 675-84.
[http://dx.doi.org/10.1097/00005053-197911000-00004] [PMID: 501342]

[47] Zasler ND, Katz DI, Zafonte RD. Brain Injury Medicine: Principles and Practice. New York: Demos Medical Publishing 2007.

[48] Fürbringer e Silva SC, de Sousa RM. Galveston orientation and amnesia test: applicability and relation with the Glasgow coma scale. Rev Lat Am Enfermagem 2007; 15(4): 651-7.
[http://dx.doi.org/10.1590/s0104-11692007000400020]

[49] Levin HS, High WM, Goethe KE, *et al.* The Galveston Orientation and Amnesia Test: a study of its reliability and validity. Arch Phys Med Rehabil 1987; 68(10): 771-5.

[50] Moin P, Khalighinejad N, Yusefi A, Farajzadegan Z, Barekatain M. Converting three general-cognitive function scales into persian and assessment of their validity and reliability. Int J Prev Med 2011; 2(2): 82-7.
[PMID: 21603013]

[51] Novack TA, Bergquist TF, Bennett G, Gouvier WD.. Primary caregiver distress following severe head injury. J Head Trauma Rehabil 1991; 6(3): 1-9.

[52] Brodaty H, Pond D, Kemp NM, *et al.* The GPCOG: a new screening test for dementia designed for general practice. J Am Geriatr Soc 2002; 50(3): 530-4.
[http://dx.doi.org/10.1046/j.1532-5415.2002.50122.x] [PMID: 11943052]

[53] Seeher K M, Brodaty H. The General Practitioner Assessment of Cognition (GPCOG). In: Larner, A.J. (eds) Cognitive Screening Instruments. New York: Springer-Verlag 2017.
[http://dx.doi.org/10.1007/978-3-319-44775-9_10]

[54] Brodaty H, Kemp NM, Pond D, *et al.* Diagnostic accuracy of the General Practitioner Assessment of Cognition (GPCOG). Alzheimers Dement 2006; 2(3): 238-42.

[55] Ansell BJ, Keenan JE. The western neuro sensory stimulation profile: A tool for assessing slow-to-recover head-injured patients. Arch Phys Med Rehabil 1989; 70(2): 104-8.
[PMID: 2916926]

[56] Cusick A, Lannin NA, Hanssen R, Allaous J. Validating the Western Neuro Sensory Stimulation Profile for patients with severe traumatic brain injury who are slow-to-recover. Aust Occup Ther J 2014; 61(4): 276-83.
[http://dx.doi.org/10.1111/1440-1630.12128] [PMID: 24809954]

[57] Cusick A, Lannin NA, Hanssen R, Allaous J. Validating the Western Neuro Sensory Stimulation Profile for patients with severe traumatic brain injury who are slow-to-recover. Aust Occup Ther J 2014; 61(4): 276-83.
[http://dx.doi.org/10.1111/1440-1630.12128] [PMID: 24809954]

[58] Rappaport M, Dougherty AM, Kelting DL. Evaluation of coma and vegetative states. Arch Phys Med Rehabil 1992; 73(7): 628-34.
[PMID: 1622317]

[59] Patrick PD, Wamstad JB, Mabry JL, *et al.* Assessing the relationship between the WNSSP and therapeutic participation in adolescents in low response states following severe traumatic brain injury. Brain Inj 2009; 23(6): 528-34.
[http://dx.doi.org/10.1080/02699050902926325] [PMID: 19484626]

[60] Lammi MH, Smith VH, Tate RL, Taylor CM. The minimally conscious state and recovery potential: A follow-up study 2 to 5 years after traumatic brain injury. Arch Phys Med Rehabil 2005; 86(4): 746-54.
[http://dx.doi.org/10.1016/j.apmr.2004.11.004] [PMID: 15827927]

[61] Maas AIR, Menon DK, Adelson PD, *et al.* Traumatic brain injury: integrated approaches to improve prevention, clinical care, and research. Lancet Neurol 2017; 16(12): 987-1048.
[http://dx.doi.org/10.1016/S1474-4422(17)30371-X] [PMID: 29122524]

[62] Menon DK, Schwab K, Wright DW, Maas AI. Position statement: definition of traumatic brain injury. Arch Phys Med Rehabil 2010; 91(11): 1637-40.
[http://dx.doi.org/10.1016/j.apmr.2010.05.017] [PMID: 21044706]

[63] Wijdicks EFM, Bamlet WR, Maramattom BV, Manno EM, McClelland RL. Validation of a new coma scale: The FOUR score. Ann Neurol 2005; 58(4): 585-93.
[http://dx.doi.org/10.1002/ana.20611] [PMID: 16178024]

[64] van Baalen B, Odding E, Stam HJ. Cognitive status at discharge from the hospital determines discharge destination in traumatic brain injury patients. Brain Inj 2008; 22(1): 25-32.
[http://dx.doi.org/10.1080/02699050701810662]

[65] Cicerone KD, Goldin Y, Ganci K, *et al.* Evidence-based cognitive rehabilitation: systematic review of the literature from 2009 through 2014. Arch Phys Med Rehabil 2019; 100(8): 1515-33.
[http://dx.doi.org/10.1016/j.apmr.2019.02.011] [PMID: 30926291]

[66] Silverberg ND, Panenka WJ. Mild traumatic brain injury and concussion: consensus, controversies, and challenges. Lancet Neurol 2019; 18(8): 760-72.
[http://dx.doi.org/10.1016/S1474-4422(19)30115-2] [PMID: 31160204]

[67] Laxe S, Zasler N, Selb M, Tate R, Tormos JM, Bernabeu M. Development of the International Classification of Functioning, Disability and Health core sets for traumatic brain injury: An International consensus process. Brain Inj 2013; 27(4): 379-87.
[http://dx.doi.org/10.3109/02699052.2012.750757] [PMID: 23472615]

[68] McCrea M, Broglio SP, McAllister TW, *et al.* Association of blood biomarkers with acute sport-related concussion in collegiate athletes. JAMA Netw Open 2020; 3(1): e1919771.
[http://dx.doi.org/10.1001/jamanetworkopen.2019.19771] [PMID: 31977061]

[69] Rabinowitz AR, Levin HS. Cognitive sequelae of traumatic brain injury. Psychiatr Clin North Am 2014; 37(1): 1-11.
[http://dx.doi.org/10.1016/j.psc.2013.11.004] [PMID: 24529420]

CHAPTER 10

Scales for Multiple Sclerosis

Priyanka Negi[1], **Saumya Kothiyal**[2] and **Gurjant Singh**[1,2,*]

[1] *Maharishi Markandeshwar Institute of Physiotherapy and Rehabilitation, Maharishi Markandeshwar (Deemed to be University), Mullana, Ambala, Haryana, India*

[2] *Department of Physiotherapy, University Institute of Allied Health Sciences, Chandigarh University, Mohali, Punjab, India*

Abstract: Multiple sclerosis (MS) is a chronic, autoimmune disease that affects the central nervous system, leading to demyelination and neurodegeneration. Depending on the extent and location of the demyelination, these symptoms might range from minor sensory disturbances to severe physical and cognitive impairments. Symptoms of MS include motor and sensory impairments, fatigue, cognitive dysfunction, and visual disturbances. The progression of MS differs significantly between individuals; some may undergo relapsing-remitting phases, while others might develop a more steadily advancing form of the disease. MS is usually diagnosed through a combination of clinical assessments, imaging methods such as MRI, and analysis of cerebrospinal fluid *via* lumbar puncture. Multiple Sclerosis (MS) is evaluated using various scales that assess disease progression, symptom intensity, and its impact on the patient's quality of life. The most widely used instruments, the Expanded Disability Status Scale (EDSS) and the Hauser Ambulation Index (HAI), focus on mobility, physical disability, and Ambulation. While the Scripps scale assesses more general neurological deficits, the Multiple Sclerosis Spasticity Scale (MSSS-88) is intended to measure the degree and impact of spasticity on daily activities in MS patients. Another useful instrument for assessing illness progression is the Troiano Scale, which focuses on motor and sensory deficiencies. These scales work together to support clinicians in tracking the course of diseases, customising treatment regimens, and assessing treatments.

Keywords: Autoimmune diseases, Central nervous system, Cognitive dysfunction, Comprehensive clinical tool, Humans, Magnetic resonance imaging, Multiple sclerosis, Neurological scale, Quality of life, Spasticity.

INTRODUCTION

Multiple sclerosis (MS) is a complicated autoimmune disease of the central nervous system [1]. It affects around 2.8 million people worldwide, with a preva-

* **Corresponding author Gurjant Singh:** Department of Physiotherapy, University Institute of Allied Health Sciences, Chandigarh University, Mohali, Punjab, India; E-mail: singh.guri547@gmail.com

Nidhi Sharma, Simranjeet Kaur & Parveen Kumar (Eds.)

lence of 35.9 per 100,000. It is more frequent in North America and Europe, where rates can reach 200 per 100,000 people, and less common in Asia and Africa. In India, the prevalence is lower, estimated at 8-20 per 100,000 people. Women are more affected than men, with a ratio of about 3:1 [2]. To effectively manage and track the progression of this condition, healthcare professionals and researchers rely on various assessment scales. These scales provide objective measurements of the disease's numerous components, including physical disability, cognitive impairment, and overall quality of life [3]. Using these standardised methods, clinicians and therapists may evaluate therapy efficacy, track changes over time, and make educated decisions about patients' care. MS scales are critical for identifying the various ways the disease affects patients, enabling more individualised treatment and better clinical outcomes.

Expanded Disability Status Scale (EDSS)

The Expanded Disability Status Scale (EDSS) is a neurological scale widely employed to quantify disability in individuals with multiple sclerosis (MS) [4]. Originally developed by John Kurtzke in 1983, the EDSS has become a standard tool for assessing the extent of neurological impairment in MS patients. It assesses coordination, gait, mental health, vision, and perception. EDSS was later converted into the FSS [5].

It evaluates various functional systems, including ambulation, pyramidal, cerebellar, brainstem, sensory, bowel and bladder, visual, and mental functions, as shown in Table **1**. The composite score provides a comprehensive overview of MS's impact on an individual's daily life [4].

IFC Domain

Physical functioning and disability

Number of Items: 8

Instructions for Administration and Scoring

Administration

- Administered by a neurologist, the EDSS involves a detailed examination of different functional domains.
- The EDSS includes a single grading scale, while the FSS evaluates eight items.
- It takes 15 to 30 minutes to administer.

Table 1. Expanded Disability Status Scale (EDSS).

Expanded Disability Status Scale (EDSS)
0.0: No neurological evaluation (all FS scores are 0).
1.0: No disability; slight signs in 1 FS (1 grade).
1.5: No disability; mild signs in multiple FS (more than one grade 1).
2.0: Mild disability in 1 FS (one grade 2, others 0 or 1).
2.5 Mild disability in 2 FS (two grade 2, others 0 or 1).
3.0: Fully ambulatory with moderate disability in 1 functional system (grade 3) or mild disability in three or four FS (grade 2), with others at grade 0 or 1.
3.5: Able to walk independently but has moderate disability in 1 FS (grade 3) along with one or 2 FS at grade 2, or 2 FS at grade 3, or 5 FS at grade 2, while the rest remain at grade 0 or 1.
4.0: Fully ambulatory, independent, and active for about 12 hours daily despite severe disability (1 FS at grade 4 or a combination exceeding previous levels); can walk 500 meters without aid or rest.
4.5: Fully ambulatory, and active most of the day, and able to work but may have some limitations (1 FS at grade 4 or a combination exceeding previous levels); can walk 300 meters without aid.
5.0: Able to walk 200 meters unassisted but has severe disability limiting full daily activities, such as working a full day without accommodations; typically 1 FS at grade 5 or a combination exceeding step 4.0.
5.5: Able to walk 100 meters unassisted but has severe disability and impair full daily activities; typically 1 FS at grade 5 or a combination exceeding step 4.0.
6.0: Requires intermittent or one-sided assistive support (cane, crutch, or brace) to walk about 100 meters, with or without rest; typically involves more than 2 FS at grade 3 or higher.
6.5: Requires constant bilateral support (canes, crutches, or braces) to walk about 20 meters without rest; typically involves more than 2 FS at grade 3 or higher.
7.0: Mostly wheelchair-dependent, unable to walk beyond 5 meters even with aid; can self-propel and transfer independently, staying active in a wheelchair for about 12 hours daily; typically involves multiple FS at grade 4 or higher.
7.5: Limited to a wheelchair, able to take only a few steps; needs help to transfer; can self-propel but not for a full day; requires a motorised wheelchair; typically involves multiple FS at grade 4 or higher.
8.0: Primarily confined to bed or wheelchair but may be up for much of the day; retains many self-care abilities and generally has functional arm use; typically involves multiple FS at grade 4 or higher.
8.5: Mostly confined to bed but can use arms and perform some self-care. Typically involves multiple FS at grade 4 or higher.
9.0: Completely bedridden but able to communicate and eat. Most functional systems are severely affected (mostly grades 4+).
9.5: Fully dependent and bedridden, with severe communication difficulties and inability to eat or swallow. Nearly all functional systems are profoundly impaired (all grades +4).
10.0: Mortality due to multiple sclerosis [4].

EDSS levels ranging from 1.0 to 4.5 relate to individuals with MS who can walk independently. These levels are determined by assessing disability across eight distinct functional systems [5]. These systems include:

- Pyramidal, which indicates muscle weakness or mobility issues.
- Cerebellar, characterised by ataxia, balance difficulties, coordination problems, or tremors.
- Brainstem, which involves challenges with speech, nystagmus, and swallowing.

- Sensory, indicating numbness or sensory loss.
- Bowel and bladder functions.
- Visual function, which addresses issues with sight.
- Cerebral functions, which relate to cognitive impairments affecting thinking and memory.
- Others

Equipment

EDSS and FSS assessment and pen/pencil

Scoring

EDSS is structured on a scale that spans from 0 to 10, with 0 representing normal health and 10 denoting death attributable to the MS disease, with higher scores indicating greater disability. The term functional system (FSS) denotes a network of neurons in the brain that governs particular functions. The assessment of each of the eight items is conducted on an ordinal scale from 0 to 5 or 6, with 0 representing the absence of disability and 5 or 6 indicating a more pronounced disability [5].

When a patient requires assistance for walking and uses aids such as a cane, crutches, or a walking frame, the score is 0 to 6.5. If the patient is predominantly reliant on a wheelchair, except for a few steps, the score is classified between 7.0 and 8.5. A score of 9 is assigned to patients who are confined to bed, while a score of 10 reflects mortality due to MS [4].

Interpretability

MCID: Not established

SEM: EDSS intra-rater reproducibility with 40 patients, 72.5% females diagnosed with 10% relapse-remitting MS and 90% progressive [6].

SEM for rater 1 - 0.24 and rater 2 - 0.62

FSS inter-rater reproducibility was assessed with 125 participants, mean age 43.8 years; comprised 64% females diagnosed with 7.2% relapse-remitting MS and 92.8% progressive MS [6].

- Each functional system has the following SEM values: Pyramidal - 0.52, Cerebellar - 0.99, Brainstem - 0.56, Visual - 1.02, Bladder and Bowels - 0.78, Sensory - 1.29, Mental - 0.76 [6]

MDC: Francis indicated that 95% of raters scored within 1.5 points of the accurate value on the EDSS; however, he observed greater variability in scores for EDSS levels below 6.0 than for those with higher EDSS levels [7].

Language: English

Training Required: No training required

Clinical Considerations

Lower EDSS scores are determined by neurological abnormalities observed during the physician's examination, while the higher scores reflect the disease's effect on disability [8].

FSS and EDSS are the most widely used assessment tools for assessing how MS impacts individuals, and it is expected that these instruments will continue to be extensively utilised in clinical assessment and research. However, because of their suboptimal psychometric properties, the tests are acknowledged to contain numerous flaws [4].

Comorbidities have an impact on disability and should be addressed in the entire clinical assessment. Some symptoms may be caused by comorbid disorders rather than the core MS diagnosis [8].

Psychometric Properties

Reliability

Inter-rater Reliability - EDSS inter-rater reliability is adequate (kappa coefficient is 0.65), for FSS (kappa coefficient ranging from 0.41 to 0.67).

EDSS has excellent inter-rater reliability scores (ICC = 0.99) for FSS (ICC ranging from 0.81 to 0.95) [9].

Intra-rater Reliability - Intra-rater reliability is adequate for EDSS (Kappa = 0.67), for FSS (kappa range 0.42 to 0.66).

Excellent (ICC = 0.99) intra-rater reliability on EDSS; for FSS, intra-rater reliability scores are adequate to excellent (ICC = 0.67-0.92) [9].

Validity

Construct validity – Correlation of EDSS scores with Barthel Index (r = -0.74), London Handicap Scale (r = -0.69), and the physical functioning component of the SF-36 (r = -0.82) demonstrates strong validity [9].

The correlation between EDSS scores and the physical role limitation item of SF-36 demonstrates adequate, statistically significant validity (r = -0.50). Conversely, the correlation between EDSS and the social functioning item of SF-36 shows poor, yet statistically significant, validity, indicated by a correlation coefficient of (r = -0.47) [9].

Floor/ceiling effects

Floor and ceiling effect is excellent, *i.e.*, 0% [6].

Responsiveness

EDSS demonstrates a lack of sensitivity to clinical changes, as indicated by an effect size of 0.11 and a P-value of 0.051 [9].

MULTIPLE SCLEROSIS SPASTICITY SCALE (MSSS-88)

MSSS-88 was developed by Hobart, Riazi, Thompson, *et al.*, in 2006. This tool relies on patients' own descriptions to measure how muscle stiffness and tension affect their everyday activities [10].

It examines how spasticity affects many elements of bodily function/structure, ADLs, and participation. It assesses the frequency, intensity, and impact of spasticity on these activities, providing a comprehensive evaluation of its impact on an individual's life [10].

IFC Domain

Body function and structure; Spasticity

Number of Items: 88

Instructions for Administration and Scoring

It is administered by a clinician or performed independently; the MSSS-88 involves a thorough evaluation of spasticity symptoms across multiple muscle groups. Scoring is based on the observed severity and impact of spasticity, contributing to a comprehensive assessment.

It consists of 88 items subdivided into 8 domains:

12 items related to muscle tightness, 9 items addressing pain/discomfort, 14 items focused on muscle cramps, 11 items concerning activities of daily living, 10 items for walking, 11 items for physical movements, 13 items about emotional health, and 8 items related to social functioning.

Three address spasticity-specific symptoms, including muscular stiffness, discomfort, and spasms.

Three address the individual's physical functioning, including everyday activities, walking, and bodily movements.

Two address the psychological impact, namely mental health and social functioning [10].

Equipment

- MSSS-88 questionnaire
- Pencil/pen

Scoring

Total score: 0 –352. A higher score reflects a greater impact of spasticity.

Every item has a four-point Likert scale rating.

1- not worried
2- a bit disturbed
3- moderately disturbed
4- severely disturbed

Three techniques of scoring

1- To obtain an ordinal-level total score, aggregate the responses from the entire questionnaire. The mean score can be utilised to estimate missing responses when at least 50% of the items have been answered.
2- To calculate subscale values independently.
3- Employ Rasch software for evaluation [10]

Interpretability

MCID: 18% or more

MDC: not established

SEM: not established

Language

Available in German [11], Italian [12], Serbian [13], and Persian [14], *etc.*

Training Required: No training required

Clinical Considerations

Essential for tailoring interventions to the specific spasticity-related needs of MS patients, the MSSS-88 assists in monitoring symptom progression, adjusting treatment plans, and enhancing overall functional outcomes.

It should be able to generate quality reports and support quality improvement initiatives by tracking and analysing clinical outcomes, adherence to clinical guidelines, and patient safety measures.

Psychometric Properties

Reliability

The subscales of MSSS-88 are characterised by good reliability, with person separation indices for all subscales equal to or greater than 0.92. Moreover, these subscales show varying levels of correlation with the FAMS, GHQ-12, MSIS-29, SF-36, and Barthel Index [15].

Validity

Convergent validity - A strong correlation was observed between the 12-item Multiple Sclerosis Walking Scale, the EDSS, and the "Walking," "ADL," and "Movement" subscales, but none with the Barthel Index. Each subscale had a comparable, moderately significant correlation (r = 0.41–0.53, P = .05–.01) with the MS, except for pain [15].

Floor/Ceiling Effect

MSSS-88 did not yield any reported values concerning the existence of floor or ceiling effects within the MS population.

Responsiveness

Responsiveness of MSSS-88 and the laboratory assessment of spasticity in individuals diagnosed with multiple sclerosis (n = 20).

MSSS-88 Stiffness – (0.07), Pain – (0.2), Spasms – (0.1); Total – (0.1), for ankle spasticity – (0.3) [12]

WASHINGTON CONFERENCE (POSER) CRITERIA

The Washington Conference (Poser) Criteria are diagnostic standards designed for the categorisation of multiple sclerosis (MS) [16]. These criteria, developed during the 1983 Washington Conference on Multiple Sclerosis, have helped to standardise the diagnosis of MS and guide clinicians in separating it from other neurological diseases [17].

The criteria fall into four categories: clinically definite, laboratory-supported definite, clinically probable, and laboratory-supported probable multiple sclerosis, as given in Table **2** [17].

Table 2. Washington conference (Poser) criteria.

A. Clinically defined MS
• **CDMS A1** - Diagnosis requires **two clinical attacks** and **clinical evidence of MS in two locations**. No paraclinical evidence or confirmation through CSF oligoclonal bands/increased IgG levels is necessary.
• **CDMS A2** - Diagnosis requires **two clinical attacks, clinical evidence of MS in one location**, and **one paraclinical evidence of MS**. CSF oligoclonal bands or increased IgG levels are not required.
B. Laboratory-supported defined MS
• **LSDMS B1** - Requires two clinical attacks along with either one clinical or one paraclinical sign of MS, plus positive laboratory findings are CSF oligoclonal bands/increased IgG.
• **LSDMS B2** - Requires one clinical attack with evidence of MS in two clinical locations, and positive laboratory results are CSF oligoclonal bands or increased IgG.
• **LSDMS B3** - Requires one clinical attack, one clinical sign of MS, one paraclinical sign, and positive laboratory findings, such as CSF oligoclonal bands/increased IgG.
C. Clinically Probable MS
• **CPMS C1** – Requires two clinical attacks and clinical evidence of MS in one location. No paraclinical evidence or CSF oligoclonal bands/increased IgG is needed.
• **CPMS C2** – Requires one clinical attack with clinical evidence of MS in two locations. Paraclinical evidence or CSF oligoclonal bands/increased IgG is not required.
• **CPMS C3** – Requires one clinical attack, clinical evidence in one location, and one paraclinical sign of MS. CSF oligoclonal bands/increased IgG is not necessary.
D. Laboratory-Supported Probable MS
• **LSPMS** – Diagnosis requires two clinical attacks along with the presence of CSF oligoclonal bands or increased IgG. Diagnosis of MS does not necessitate the presence of clinical or paraclinical evidence [17].

The classification of patients according to the Poser criteria involves four categories, which are established by evaluating the number of clinical attacks that endure for more than 24 hours, the number of distinct lesions that elicit clinical signs, the results from supportive imaging studies or physician evaluations (known as paraclinical evidence), and the presence of oligoclonal bands in the cerebrospinal fluid, while excluding serum, along with a rise in immunoglobulin G levels in the CSF [16, 18].

Diagnosis of clinically definite MS requires the occurrence of two distinct episodes, each supported by clinical or paraclinical evidence of separate lesions.

IFC Domain

Diagnostic criteria for multiple sclerosis

Instructions for Administration and Scoring

Administration

Neurologists and other healthcare experts administer the criteria, which include a thorough examination of clinical, laboratory, and imaging data.

It may take 5–10 minutes to identify which diagnostic level the individual fulfills. For new patients, 40 to 60 minutes of history, neurologic examination, and record review [17].

There are four categories depending on the clinical attacks: clinical evidence, paraclinical evidence, and CSF OB/IG.

Definite MS

- Two or more distinct clinical assaults affecting various regions of the CNS system.
- Objective clinical evidence of 2 or more lesions that are characteristic of MS.
- Positive findings on CSF examination (oligoclonal bands or elevated IgG index.

Probable MS

- Either normal CSF findings or only one positive CSF finding (elevated IgG index and oligoclonal bands).

Possible MS

- Only one clinical attack and objective clinical evidence of one lesion.
- Normal CSF findings.

Equipment

Standard diagnostic tools, including neuroimaging equipment and facilities for cerebrospinal fluid analysis

Scoring: not applicable

Interpretability

MCID: not established

SEM: not established

MDC: not established

Language: English

Training Required

To ensure the correct and consistent implementation of the Washington Conference (Poser) Criteria, healthcare personnel must be trained in neurology and the specific diagnostic guidelines [17].

Clinical Considerations

Essential for establishing a consistent and standardised diagnosis of MS, the criteria aid clinicians in making accurate diagnostic decisions, facilitating appropriate treatment plans and interventions. It can be utilised in both research and clinical settings [16].

Sensitivity and Specificity

The sensitivity and specificity of the Poser Criteria can affect their ability to detect real cases of MS while eliminating people who do not have the illness. Clinicians should understand the criteria's performance features, as well as any potential false positives or negatives [18].

Psychometric Properties

Reliability/Validity

No values were available.

Responsiveness & Floor/Ceiling Effect

No values were available.

SCRIPPS NEUROLOGICAL RATING SCALE (NRS)

The Scripps Neurological Rating Scale was developed to evaluate neurologic function in individuals with multiple sclerosis under a physician's supervision. It serves as a quantifiable assessment of neurologic status for MS patients [19, 20].

The Scripps Neurological Rating Scale (SNRS) is a comprehensive clinical tool designed to assess and quantify neurological function in patients with various neurological disorders. The findings are derived from a planned neurological assessment, which includes subjective evaluations of sexual, bowel, and bladder issues [20].

The SNRS covers a broad range of neurological domains, including motor function, sensory function, reflexes, coordination, and cranial nerve function. It utilises a systematic approach to evaluate the functioning of different neurological systems, providing a holistic perspective on the patient's neurological health [19].

IFC Domain

- Body Functions and Structure
- Neurological examination of multiple domains

Number of Items: 22

Instructions for Administration and Scoring

Administered by healthcare professionals, the SNRS involves a thorough neurological examination.

It is a performance-based measure; the time required for examination and scoring is 30 to 40 minutes.

This scale is made up of 10 components, with each component rated between 0 and 5, resulting in a total potential score of 50 [19].

- Mood/Mentation – 10
- Cranial nerves associated with the eyes - 21
- Lower cranial nerves - 5
- Motor or Strength of limb – 20
- Deep tendon reflexes - 8
- Babinski sign – 4
- Sensory function - 12
- Cerebellar function - 10
- Gait and balance - 10
- Special category (bowel/bladder/sexual dysfunction)

Total neurological rating = sum of all points for all components

Equipment

Standard neurological examination tools, reflex hammers, tuning forks, and other sensory assessment instruments.

Scoring

Scores range from 10 to 100, with a maximum of 100 for a normal subject. Up to 10 points may be deducted for bladder, bowel, or sexual function issues (Table **3**). Higher scores indicate better function.

Table 3. Scripps Neurologic Rating Scale (NRS).

Scripps Neurologic Rating Scale (NRS)			**Degree of Impairment**		
System Examined	**Maximum Point**	**Normal**	**Mild**	**Moderate**	**Severe**
Mentation & Mood	10	10	7	4	0
Cranial Nerves Visual acuity Fields, Discs, pupils Eye Movements Nystagmus	21	5 6 5 5	3 4 3 3	1 2 1 1	0 0 0 0
Lower Cranial Nerves	5	5	3	1	0
Motor RU LU RL LL	20	5 5 5 5	3 3 3 3	1 1 1 1	0 0 0 0
DTRS UE LE	8	4 4	3 3	1 1	0 0
Babinski R/L	4	4	0	0	0
Sensory RU LU RL LL	12	3 3 3 3	2 2 2 2	1 1 1 1	0 0 0 0
Cerebellar UE LE	10	5 5	3 3		0 0
Gait, Trunk, Balance	10	10	7	4	0
Special Category					
Bladder/Bowel/Sexual					
Dysfunction	0	0	-3	-7	-10
Totals	100				

The scoring weights are arbitrary, and the scale is characterised by imprecise terms such as mild, moderate, and severe. This is problematic because a change from mild to moderate deficiencies in motor and cerebellar scores on this scale could result in a 12-point change in overall scoring [21].

Interpretability

MCID: not established

MDC: not established

SEM: not established

Language: English

Training Required

Healthcare professionals administering the SNRS require training in neurological examination techniques to ensure accurate and consistent assessments [22].

Clinical Considerations

Essential for comprehensive neurological assessments, the SNRS aids in identifying specific deficits, tracking changes over time, and informing targeted interventions for patients with neurological conditions.

Ensure that the scale has been validated and is reliable for the intended purpose. It has certain drawbacks, including low sensitivity to change, poor correlation with scales, and low reliability.

Also, ensure that individuals administering the scale are properly trained and certified.

Psychometric Properties

Reliability

According to reports, this scale has a moderate level of sensitivity to clinical change, a nearly normal distribution, and high Intra-rater reliability (weighted kappa coefficient is 0.98 & ICC range between 0.52- 0.92) and Inter-rater reliability (weighted kappa coefficient is 0.83) [9].

Validity

Concurrent Validity – Moderate correlation with the London Handicap Scale (r-0.71 and the Barthel Index (r-0.69).

The SF-36 physical functioning items show a strong correlation (r = 0.82) [9].

Responsiveness and Floor/Ceiling Effect

No values were reported.

HAUSER AMBULATION INDEX

The Hauser Ambulation Index (HAI) is a specialised scale developed to evaluate how well individuals with multiple sclerosis (MS) can walk and move. Hauser and his team introduced it in 1983 [23].

The HAI focuses specifically on ambulation, considering factors such as walking distance, walking speed, and the use of assistive devices. It provides a nuanced evaluation of walking ability, taking into account both quantitative aspects of walking performance and qualitative aspects of gait, as outlined in Table **4** [23].

Table 4. Hauser ambulation index assessment.

Hauser Ambulation Index
0 - Asymptomatic, fully active
1 - Walks normally but experiences fatigue that hinders athletic or other strenuous activities
2 - Exhibits an abnormal gait or occasional imbalance, noticeable to family and friends; able to walk 25 feet (8 meters) within 10 seconds
3 - Walks independently and can cover 25 feet in 20 seconds or less
4 - Requires one-sided support (like a cane or single crutch) to walk; able to cover 25 feet in 20 seconds or less.
5 - Use bilateral aid (like a cane, crutches, or walker) to walk 25 feet within 25 seconds, or takes longer than 20 seconds with unilateral support.
6 - Uses bilateral support and requires more than 20 seconds walking 25 feet; may sometimes use a wheelchair.
7 - Able to take only a few steps with bilateral support; cannot walk 25 feet and primarily relies on a wheelchair for most activities.
8 - Wheelchair-dependent but capable of transferring independently.
9 - Wheelchair-dependent and unable to transfer independently.
10 – Bedridden [23]

IFC Domain

Mobility and ambulation activity.

Number of Items

N/A

Instructions for Administration and Scoring

Administration

- Clinician administered.
- The time required for administration may vary based on the patient's abilities; it should take 1-5 minutes.
- It is a mobility rating tool that measures the time required to walk 25 feet.
- The scoring system ranges from 0, indicating an asymptomatic and fully active state, to 10, which signifies a bedridden condition. The patient is instructed to walk a 25-foot defined course as swiftly and securely as possible, and the examiner records the time and needed assistance (*e.g.*, cane, walker, crutches) [23].

While the patient's walking is measured by time, that time is not used by itself. It works with other factors to evaluate the patient on a 10-point scale.

Equipment

- Stopwatch and the patient's self-selected assistive device

Scoring

- Motivation and lifestyle might have an impact on wheelchair use. Patients in Grade 7 are anticipated to use wheelchairs more often than those in Grades 5 and 6. Instead of considering how much a patient uses a wheelchair, a grade in the range of 5 to 7 is determined by the person's ability to walk a specific distance [23].
- Score range: 0 for no symptoms and 9 for confined to a wheelchair and unable to move independently.

Interpretability

MCID: not established

SEM: not established

MDC: not established

Language: English

Training Required: No training required

Clinical Considerations

Assess whether the information provided by the index is clinically relevant and useful for treatment planning or monitoring progress. A clinical tool should have practical implications for patient care [23].

It considers the ease of use and feasibility of incorporating the Hauser Ambulation Index into clinical practice. If a tool is cumbersome or time-consuming, it may be less practical for routine use.

Population-specific Considerations: aware of any limitations or specific considerations related to the population for which the index is intended. Different indices may be more appropriate for certain age groups, disease states, or types of impairment [25].

Psychometric Properties

Reliability

Test-retest reliability (ICC-0.91), inter-rater reliability (ICC = 0.96; K = 0.73; repeatability coefficient = 1 point), intra-rater reliability (ICC = 0.93; K = 0.59; repeatability coefficient = 1.5 points), and [9, 24] are all excellent.

Validity

<u>Criterion Validity</u>

EDSS and AI had a significant correlation of 0.68; all $p < 0.001–0.008$ [9]. There is an excellent correlation between AI and the London Handicap, Barthel Index (r = 0.72), Scripps Neurological Rating Scale (r =0.67), and Functional Independence Measure (r = 0.73).

Adequate correlation was observed with patients' capacity to work (r = 0.59), perform household (r = 0.55), impairment (r = 0.54), and handicap (r = 0.55) as measured by the Cambridge MS Basic Score [9].

Construct Validity

EDSS levels between 1 and 2.5 (mean = 0.8 (0.7)), 3.0 and 6.0 (mean = 3.1 (1.3)), and above 6.0 (mean = 7.0 (1.5)) all showed excellent correlation [25].

Floor/Ceiling effects

28% of individuals had a poor ceiling effect, achieving a maximum score of 9 on the AI.

0% of individuals achieved a minimum score, indicating an excellent floor effect [26].

Responsiveness

According to reports, the Ambulation Index is less responsive than the Rivermead Mobility Index but more capable of detecting changes than the 10-meter walk test and EDSS. The AI was able to identify changes in 18.5% of MS patients, compared to 39% for the Rivermead Mobility Index, 16.5% for the 10-meter walk test, and 7.5% for the EDSS [26].

CLINICAL CONSIDERATIONS, STRENGTHS, LIMITATIONS, AND EMERGING TRENDS

Multiple sclerosis (MS) is a chronic, immune-mediated neurological disorder characterised by heterogeneous patterns of disability progression, symptom fluctuation, and functional impact. The variability in disease course necessitates a structured yet flexible assessment approach that captures neurological impairment, mobility, symptom burden, and functional consequences over time. No single scale adequately reflects all dimensions of MS-related disability; therefore, a combination of clinician-rated and patient-reported measures is essential for comprehensive assessment [27, 28].

The Expanded Disability Status Scale (EDSS) remains the most widely used disability scale in MS, particularly in clinical trials and longitudinal disease monitoring. Its principal strength lies in its standardised neurological examination and ability to quantify disease progression across functional systems. However, EDSS is heavily weighted toward ambulation and lower-limb function, resulting in reduced sensitivity to upper-limb impairment, cognition, fatigue, and quality-of-life changes. This reliance on walking ability limits its responsiveness in early disease and in patients with predominantly non-motor symptoms [27, 29].

Symptom-specific instruments, such as the Multiple Sclerosis Spasticity Scale (MSSS-88), address domains insufficiently captured by global disability measures. MSSS-88 provides a patient-centred evaluation of spasticity-related symptoms and their functional impact, offering valuable insight into treatment response from the patient perspective. Nevertheless, its subjective nature and focus on a single symptom domain necessitate complementary use with objective neurological or functional assessments [30].

Historical diagnostic frameworks, including the Poser (Washington Conference) criteria, played an important role in standardising MS diagnosis. While largely superseded by revised McDonald criteria, understanding these earlier systems remains relevant for interpreting legacy data and older clinical studies. Their principal limitation lies in reduced sensitivity to early disease and limited incorporation of modern imaging biomarkers [31].

Clinician-rated neurological scales, such as the Scripps Neurological Rating Scale (NRS), and mobility-focused tools, such as the Hauser Ambulation Index, provide additional perspectives on neurological impairment and walking ability. These instruments are relatively quick to administer and useful for monitoring functional change. However, they demonstrate ceiling and floor effects and offer limited insight into cognitive, emotional, and participation-level outcomes, which are increasingly recognised as critical determinants of quality of life in MS [28, 32].

A recurring limitation across MS assessment tools is the partial separation between impairment, activity, and participation domains. While EDSS and NRS emphasise neurological impairment, mobility indices focus on activity, and symptom-specific scales reflect patient experience. Without a clear assessment framework, overlapping or incomplete measurements may occur, increasing the burden without proportionate clinical value. Purpose-driven scale selection aligned with the stage of disease and therapeutic goals is therefore essential [29, 33].

Emerging trends in MS assessment increasingly emphasise multidimensional and technology-enabled approaches. Digital gait analysis, wearable activity monitors, and smartphone-based assessments are being explored to detect subtle functional changes and capture real-world mobility patterns. In parallel, patient-reported outcome measures and cognitive screening tools are gaining prominence as endpoints in both clinical practice and research. Integration of clinical scale data with imaging markers and fluid biomarkers is also being investigated to improve disease monitoring and prognostication [34, 35].

In routine practice, assessment strategies should be tailored to the disease phase and clinical intent. EDSS remains central for longitudinal disability tracking,

MSSS-88 is valuable for symptom-specific evaluation, and mobility indices support functional monitoring. Combining these tools with emerging digital and patient-reported measures provides a more holistic and clinically meaningful representation of disease impact while minimising redundancy (Table **5**).

Table 5. Comparative summary of commonly used multiple sclerosis assessment scales.

Scale	Primary Domain Assessed	Key Strengths	Major Limitations	Optimal Clinical Use
Expanded Disability Status Scale (EDSS)	Global neurological disability	Widely accepted; prognostic value; trial standard	Overemphasis on ambulation; limited cognitive sensitivity	Longitudinal disease monitoring, trials
Multiple Sclerosis Spasticity Scale (MSSS-88)	Spasticity and symptom impact	Patient-centred; symptom-specific sensitivity	Subjective; narrow scope	Spasticity assessment and treatment response
Poser (Washington Conference) Criteria	Diagnostic classification	Historical relevance; standardised early framework	Superseded; limited sensitivity	Interpretation of legacy studies
Scripps Neurological Rating Scale (NRS)	Neurological impairment	Structured neurological assessment	Ceiling/floor effects	Clinical monitoring
Hauser Ambulation Index	Walking ability	Simple, rapid administration	Mobility-only focus	Functional ambulation tracking
Digital/wearable measures	Real-world function	Objective: continuous monitoring	Limited standardization	Emerging research and follow-up

CONCLUSION

This chapter has delineated an overview of several pivotal assessment instruments used for evaluating patients who have Multiple Sclerosis (MS), encompassing the Expanded Disability Status Scale (EDSS), Multiple Sclerosis Spasticity Scale (MSSS-88), Washington Conference (Poser) Criteria, Scripps Neurological Rating Scale (NRS), and Hauser Ambulation Index (HAI). These instruments create an integrated framework for assessing the multifaceted nature of multiple sclerosis, covering everything from overall disability to specific symptoms, including spasticity and walking ability.

The scales effectively quantify and monitor MS symptom progression, which is essential for use in research and clinical settings. In MS, the EDSS is a standardised disability measure, while the MSSS-88 evaluates the impact of spasticity on daily life. The Poser Criteria have standardised MS diagnosis, and scales such as the Scripps NRS and HAI assess neurological function and mobility. However, these scales possess notable limitations. A significant issue is their insensitivity to minor clinical changes, especially in mid-range scores. Moreover, a clinician's interpretation of subjectivity can lead to inter-rater variability, while some scales' comprehensiveness may reduce specificity.

These limitations highlight substantial research gaps. Future work should focus on developing more sensitive, objective, and comprehensive scales that incorporate patient-reported outcomes, cognitive evaluations, and modern psychometric and digital technologies. Furthermore, validating these instruments across other groups would increase their global usefulness in clinical treatment and research.

AI DISCLOSURE STATEMENT

During the preparation of this chapter, the authors used ChatGPT (OpenAI) as a support tool for language refinement, structural organisation, and clarification of ideas. All content generated with AI assistance was carefully reviewed, verified, and revised by the authors to ensure factual accuracy, originality, and consistency with the scientific literature. The authors take full responsibility for the integrity, interpretation, and final content of the published chapter.

ACKNOWLEDGEMENT

The authors express their sincere gratitude to neurologists, rehabilitation specialists, and researchers whose work has advanced the understanding and assessment of multiple sclerosis. Their continued efforts in developing and validating disease-specific scales such as the EDSS, HAI, and MSSS-88 have significantly enhanced clinical evaluation, treatment planning, and long-term monitoring of patients with multiple sclerosis.

REFERENCES

[1] Houtchens MK, Lublin FD, Miller AE, Khoury SJ. Multiple sclerosis and other inflammatory demyelinating diseases of the central nervous system. Neurol Clin Pract 2012; vol: 1283-313. [http://dx.doi.org/10.1016/b978-1-4377-0434-1.00079-7]

[2] Vos T, Allen C, Arora M, *et al.* Global, regional, and national incidence, prevalence, and years lived with disability for 310 diseases and injuries, 1990–2015: a systematic analysis for the Global Burden of Disease Study 2015. Lancet 2016; 388(10053): 1545-602. [http://dx.doi.org/10.1016/S0140-6736(16)31678-6] [PMID: 27733282]

[3] Johnston RB Jr, Joy JE, Eds. Multiple sclerosis: current status and strategies for the future. Washington (DC): National Academies Press; 2001. [http://dx.doi.org/10.3109/9780203212974]

[4] Kapposl, *et al.* Neurostatus-EDSS; Standardized training and scoring of the Expanded Disability Status Scale. Basel, Switerzerland: Neurostatus-UBH; 2024. Available at: https://www.neurostatus.net

[5] National Multiple Sclerosis Society. Functional Systems Scores (FSS) and Expanded Disability Status Scale EDSS. New York: National Multiple Sclerosis Society; 2018.

[6] Hobart J, Freeman J, Thompson A. Kurtzke scales revisited: the application of psychometric methods to clinical intuition. Brain 2000; 123(5): 1027-40. [http://dx.doi.org/10.1093/brain/123.5.1027] [PMID: 10775547]

[7] Francis DA, Bain P, Swan AV, Hughes RAC. An assessment of disability rating scales used in multiple sclerosis. Arch Neurol 1991; 48(3): 299-301. [http://dx.doi.org/10.1001/archneur.1991.00530150067020] [PMID: 2001188]

[8] Meyer-Moock S, Feng YS, Maeurer M, Dippel FW, Kohlmann T. Systematic literature review and validity evaluation of the Expanded Disability Status Scale (EDSS) and the Multiple Sclerosis Functional Composite (MSFC) in patients with multiple sclerosis. BMC Neurol 2014; 14(1): 58. [http://dx.doi.org/10.1186/1471-2377-14-58] [PMID: 24666846]

[9] Sharrack B, Hughes RAC, Soudain S, Dunn G. The psychometric properties of clinical rating scales used in multiple sclerosis. Brain 1999; 122(1): 141-59. [http://dx.doi.org/10.1093/brain/122.1.141] [PMID: 10050902]

[10] Hobart JC, Riazi A, Thompson AJ, *et al.* Getting the measure of spasticity in multiple sclerosis: the Multiple Sclerosis Spasticity Scale (MSSS-88). Brain 2006; 129(1): 224-34. [http://dx.doi.org/10.1093/brain/awh675] [PMID: 16280352]

[11] Henze T, von Mackensen S, Lehrieder G, Zettl UK, Pfiffner C, Flachenecker P. Linguistic and psychometric validation of the MSSS-88 questionnaire for patients with multiple sclerosis and spasticity in Germany. Health Qual Life Outcomes 2014; 12(1): 119. [http://dx.doi.org/10.1186/s12955-014-0119-y] [PMID: 25080934]

[12] Pellicciari L, Ottonello M, Giordano A, Albensi C, Franchignoni F. The 88-item Multiple Sclerosis Spasticity Scale: a Rasch validation of the Italian version and suggestions for refinement of the original scale. Qual Life Res 2019; 28(1): 221-31. [http://dx.doi.org/10.1007/s11136-018-2005-2] [PMID: 30238266]

[13] Rodic SZ, Knezevic TI, Kisic-Tepavcevic DB, *et al.* Validation of the Serbian Version of Multiple Sclerosis Spasticity Scale 88 (MSSS-88). PLoS One 2016; 11(1): e0147042. [http://dx.doi.org/10.1371/journal.pone.0147042] [PMID: 26771661]

[14] Kiani I, Pouretezad M, Goharpey S, Salehi R, Negahban Siuki H, Majdi Nasab N. Reliability and Validity of the Persian Version of Multiple Sclerosis Spasticity Scale in Iranian Patients with Multiple Sclerosis. Majallah-i Ilmi-i Pizishki-i Jundi/Shapur 2017; 16(2): 197-208. [http://dx.doi.org/10.18869/acadpub.ajps.16.2.197]

[15] Freeman J, Gorst T, Ofori J, Marsden J. Evaluation of the multiple sclerosis spasticity scale 88: a short report. Rehabil Process Outcome 2019; 8: 1179572718823510. [http://dx.doi.org/10.1177/1179572718823510] [PMID: 34497457] [PMCID: PMC8276976]

[16] Herndon RM, Demos DG. Multiple sclerosis and demyelinating diseases.Handbook of Neurologic Rating Scales. New York, NY: Demos Vermande 1997; pp. 109-10.

[17] Poser CM, Paty DW, Scheinberg L, *et al.* New diagnostic criteria for multiple sclerosis: Guidelines for research protocols. Ann Neurol 1983; 13(3): 227-31. [http://dx.doi.org/10.1002/ana.410130302] [PMID: 6847134]

[18] Fangerau T, Schimrigk S, Haupts M, *et al.* Diagnosis of multiple sclerosis: comparison of the Poser criteria and the new McDonald criteria. Acta Neurol Scand 2004; 109(6): 385-9. [http://dx.doi.org/10.1111/j.1600-0404.2004.00246.x] [PMID: 15147460]

[19] Sipe JC, Knobler RL, Braheny SL, Rice GPA, Panitch HS, Oldstone MBA. A neurologic rating scale (NRS) for use in multiple sclerosis. Neurology 1984; 34(10): 1368-72. [http://dx.doi.org/10.1212/WNL.34.10.1368] [PMID: 6541311]

[20] Amato MP, Portaccio E. Clinical outcome measures in multiple sclerosis. J Neurol Sci 2007; 259(1-2): 118-22. [http://dx.doi.org/10.1016/j.jns.2006.06.031] [PMID: 17376487]

[21] Sipe J, Romine JS, Koziol JA, McMillan R, Zyroff J, Beutler E. Cladribine in treatment of chronic progressive multiple sclerosis. Lancet 1994; 344(8914): 9-13. [http://dx.doi.org/10.1016/S0140-6736(94)91046-4] [PMID: 7912347]

[22] Herndon RM, Demos DG. Multiple sclerosis and demyelinating diseases.Handbook of Neurologic Rating Scales. New York, NY: Demos Vermande 1997; pp. 113-8.

[23] Hauser SL, Dawson DM, Lehrich JR, *et al.* Intensive immunosuppression in progressive multiple sclerosis. A randomized, three-arm study of high-dose intravenous cyclophosphamide, plasma exchange, and ACTH. N Engl J Med 1983; 308(4): 173-80. [http://dx.doi.org/10.1056/NEJM198301273080401] [PMID: 6294517]

[24] Syndulko K, Ke D, Ellison GW, Baumhefner RW, Myers LW, Tourtellotte WW. Comparative evaluations of neuroperformance and clinical outcome assessments in chronic progressive multiple sclerosis: I. reliability, validity and sensitivity to disease progression. Mult Scler 1996; 2(3): 142-56. [http://dx.doi.org/10.1177/135245859600200305] [PMID: 9345379]

[25] Schwartz CE, Vollmer T, Lee H. Reliability and validity of two self-report measures of impairment and disability for MS. Neurology 1999; 52(1): 63-70. [http://dx.doi.org/10.1212/WNL.52.1.63] [PMID: 9921850]

[26] Vaney C, Blaurock H, Gattlen B, Meisels C. Assessing mobility in multiple sclerosis using the Rivermead Mobility Index and gait speed. Clin Rehabil 1996; 10(3): 216-26. [http://dx.doi.org/10.1177/026921559601000306]

[27] Goldman MD, LaRocca NG, Rudick RA, *et al.* Evaluation of multiple sclerosis disability outcome measures using pooled clinical trial data. Neurology 2019; 93(21): e1921-31. [http://dx.doi.org/10.1212/WNL.0000000000008519]

[28] Kalb R, Brown TR, Coote S, *et al.* Exercise and lifestyle physical activity recommendations for people with multiple sclerosis throughout the disease course. Mult Scler 2020; 26(12): 1459-69. [http://dx.doi.org/10.1177/1352458520915629]

[29] Sormani MP, De Stefano N. Defining and scoring response to IFN-β in multiple sclerosis. Nat Rev Neurol. 2013 Sep; 9(9): 504-12. doi: 10.1038/nrneurol.2013.146. Epub 2013 Jul 30. PMID: 23897407.

[30] Hobart J C, Riazi A, Thompson A J, *et al.* Getting the measure of spasticity in multiple sclerosis: The multiple sclerosis spasticity scale (MSSS-88). Brain 2006; 129(1): 224-34. [http://dx.doi.org/10.1093/brain/awh675]

[31] Thompson AJ, Banwell BL, Barkhof F, *et al.* Diagnosis of multiple sclerosis: 2017 revisions of the McDonald criteria. Lancet Neurol 2018; 17(2): 162-73. doi: 10.1016/S1474-4422(17)30470-2. PMID: 29275977

[32] Bethoux F, Bennett S. Evaluating walking in patients with multiple sclerosis: which assessment tools are useful in clinical practice? Int J MS Care 2020; 22(1): 20-6. doi: 10.7224/1537-2073-13.1.4. [PMID: 24453700 PMCID: PMC3882949]

[33] Kuspinar A, Rodriguez AM, Mayo NE. The effects of clinical interventions on health-related quality of life in multiple sclerosis: a meta-analysis. Mult Scler 2020; 26(9): 1096-110. doi: 10.1177/1352458512445201 [PMID: 23235779]

[34] Motl RW, Pilutti LA. The benefits of exercise training in multiple sclerosis. Nat Rev Neurol 2022; 18(6): 325-37. doi: 10.1007/s11910-015-0585-6 [PMID: 26223831]

[35] Bove R, White CC, Giovannoni G, *et al.* Evaluating real-world mobility and disability in multiple sclerosis using digital health technologies. Mult Scler 2023; 29(6): 789-99. doi: 10.1177/13524585221140925.

CHAPTER 11

Scales for Guillain-Barré Syndrome

Sukhpreet Kaur[1,2], **Poornima Maurya**[2,3], **Sukhpal Singh**[2] and **Simranjeet Kaur**[2,4,*]

[1] *Sri Guru Granth Sahib World University, Fatehgarh Sahib, Punjab, India*

[2] *Maharishi Markandeshwar Institute of Physiotherapy and Rehabilitation, Maharishi Markandeshwar (Deemed to be University), Mullana, Ambala, Haryana, India*

[3] *Department of Physiotherapy, School of Allied and Healthcare Sciences, Lovely Professional University, Phagwara, Punjab, India*

[4] *Pal Physiotherapy and Rehabilitation Centre, Pal Healthcare, Ambala City, Haryana, India*

Abstract: Guillain-Barré syndrome (GBS) is a life-threatening autoimmune disorder that requires immediate care. Proper assessment is necessary to give the best possible treatment. The most commonly and widely used tools for the assessment of GBS patients are the GBS Disability Score, the Erasmus Guillain-Barré Syndrome Respiratory Insufficiency Score, and the Modified Erasmus Guillain-Barré Syndrome Outcome Score. The domains covered by these scales are severity of symptoms, respiratory function, motor function, and the ability of the patient to walk independently. Each scale has its own scoring criteria, which give us insight into the severity and progression of the disease, as well as into treatment.

Keywords: Autoimmune neuropathy, Disability score, Functional recovery, Guillain-Barré syndrome, Motor assessment, Respiratory function.

INTRODUCTION

Guillain-Barré syndrome (GBS) is an autoimmune condition that causes inflammation and destruction of the peripheral nerves. It is characterised by symmetrical motor weakness of limbs, sensory involvement (may or may not be present), cranial nerve involvement, and respiratory paralysis, which may eventually result in death. Assessment of this condition is important for understanding the progression and severity of the disease, which will help provide the most appropriate treatment [1].

* **Corresponding Author Simranjeet Kaur:** Pal Physiotherapy and Rehabilitation Centre, Pal Healthcare, Jandli, Ambala City, Haryana-134005, India; E-mail: Simranjeetkaursaini825@gmail.com

In this chapter, we have included the most used outcome measures for GBS patients, focusing on the severity of the disease, respiratory function, and the ability to walk independently.

ERASMUS GBS RESPIRATORY INSUFFICIENCY SCORE (EGRIS)

The Erasmus Guillain-Barré Syndrome Respiratory Insufficiency Score (EGRIS) is a predictive measure for predicting respiratory failure in patients with Guillain-Barré Syndrome. It specifically anticipates the likelihood of requiring mechanical ventilation within the first week of hospital admission. The assessment is based on facial/bulbar weakness, period from onset to admission, and Medical Research Council (MRC) sum score at admission [1].

Number of Items

There are three predictors for assessing the Erasmus GBS Insufficiency Score (Table **1**):

Table 1. Erasmus GBS respiratory insufficiency score [2].

Predictor	Categories	Score
Time from onset of weakness to hospital admission, days	>7	0
	4-7	1
	<3	2
Facial and or bulbar weakness at hospital admission	Absent	0
	Present	1
MRC sum score at hospital admission	51-60	0
	41-50	1
	31-40	2
	21-30	3
	<20	4
EGRIS total score		0-7

- Time from onset of weakness to hospital admission
- Facial and/or bulbar weakness at hospital admission
- MRC sum score at hospital admission

Scoring and Interpretation

- The EGRIS total score ranges from 0 to 7.
- A higher score indicates a greater risk of respiratory failure within the first week of hospitalisation.
- The score corresponds to an estimated risk of respiratory failure ranging from 1% to 90% [1].

THE MODIFIED ERASMUS GBS RESPIRATORY INSUFFICIENCY SCORE (MEGRIS)

The mEGRIS assesses four clinical aspects at admission (Table **2**):

Table 2. The modified EGRIS score [3].

The modified EGRIS score		
Predictor	**Categories**	**Score**
Bulbar weakness	Yes	5
	No	0
Time from weakness- admission (days)	0	7
	1	6
	2	5
MRC sum score at hospital admission	3	4
	4	3
	5	2
	6	1
	>7	0
Neck flexion MRC score (0-5)	0	10
	1	8
	2	6
	3	4
	4	2
	5	0

(Table 2) cont.....

The modified EGRIS score		
Predictor	**Categories**	**Score**
Bilateral hip flexion MRC score (0-10)	0	10
	1	9
	2	8
	3	7
	4	6
	5	5
	6	4
	7	3
	8	2
	9	1
	10	0
Total (The modified ERGIS Score)		**0-32**

- Time from weakness beginning to admission
- Bulbar palsy
- Neck flexion weakness
- Bilateral hip flexion weakness.

Advantages of mEGRIS as compared to Original EGRIS are –

- It requires testing of only three muscle groups, yet model accuracy is comparable
- It accurately forecasts the risk of MV at various time intervals. (For example, <1 day, <3 days, <1 week)
- It is equally relevant in GBS variations and minimally affected people [3].

MODIFIED ERASMUS GBS OUTCOME SCORE (MEGOS)

The Modified Erasmus Guillain-Barré Syndrome Outcome Score (mEGOS) was first created in 2011 using three clinical predictors: age, Medical Research Council (MRC) total score, and previous diarrhea [4, 5]. The mEGOS can be utilised at hospital admission and on day 7. The model predicts the risk of being unable to walk independently at 4 weeks, 3 months, and 6 months post-onset weakness (Table **3**).

Table 3. Modified Erasmus GBS Outcome Score (mEGOS) [4].

Prognostic Factor	Score at Hospital Admission	Score at Week 1
Age at onset (year)		
≤40	0	0
41–60	1	1
>60	2	2
Preceding diarrhea		
Absent	0	0
Present	1	1
MRC sum score		
51–60	0	0
41–50	2	3
31–40	4	6
00–30	6	9
mEGOS	0–9	0–12

GUILLAIN-BARRÉ SYNDROME DISABILITY SCORING TEST

A commonly used scoring system to evaluate the functional state of patients with Guillain-Barré syndrome (GBS) is the GBS disability score given in Table **4**. Hughes *et al.* first described it in 1978 [6].

Table 4. GBS disability score [6].

Score	Description
0	A healthy state
1	Minor symptoms and capable of running
2	Able to walk 10m or more without assistance, but unable to run
3	Able to walk 10m across an open space with help
4	Bedridden or chairbound
5	Requiring assisted ventilation for at least part of the day
6	Dead

CLINICAL CONSIDERATIONS, STRENGTHS, LIMITATIONS, AND EMERGING TRENDS

Guillain–Barré syndrome (GBS) is an acute immune-mediated polyradiculoneuropathy characterised by rapidly progressive weakness, variable sensory involvement, and potential life-threatening complications such as respiratory failure and autonomic dysfunction. Given its dynamic and often unpredictable course, assessment in GBS must prioritise early risk stratification, monitoring of disease progression, and prediction of short- and long-term outcomes. No single scale adequately captures all clinically relevant dimensions, making the selective use of complementary assessment tools essential [7, 8].

Prognostic tools such as the Erasmus GBS Respiratory Insufficiency Score (EGRIS) and its modified version (mEGRIS) play a critical role in the early identification of patients at risk for respiratory failure. These scales are particularly valuable in the acute phase, as they rely on readily available clinical variables and allow timely decision-making regarding intensive monitoring and ventilatory support. Their strength lies in simplicity and early applicability; however, they do not account for treatment effects or evolving clinical changes beyond the initial presentation, limiting their utility later in the disease course [9, 10].

The Modified Erasmus GBS Outcome Score (MEGOS) is widely used to predict functional outcomes at defined time points following disease onset. By incorporating age, preceding diarrhoea, and early disability status, MEGOS provides clinically meaningful prognostic information that can assist in counselling patients and planning rehabilitation. Nevertheless, its predictive accuracy may vary across populations, and it offers limited insight into residual symptoms such as fatigue, pain, and psychosocial impact, which are increasingly recognised as important determinants of long-term recovery [11].

The Guillain–Barré Syndrome Disability Score (GBS-DS) remains the most commonly used functional scale for grading disease severity and monitoring recovery. Its ordinal structure allows straightforward classification of walking ability and dependence, making it suitable for both clinical practice and research. However, the scale's focus on ambulation results in reduced sensitivity to upper-limb dysfunction, cranial nerve involvement, and non-motor symptoms. Ceiling and floor effects may also limit its responsiveness, particularly in mild cases or during early recovery [8, 12].

A key limitation across GBS assessment tools is their emphasis on either early prognosis or gross functional outcome, with limited integration of patient-reported symptoms and quality-of-life measures. While prognostic scores guide acute management, they do not reflect patient experience, participation, or long-term disability. Similarly, functional scales may fail to capture fatigue, neuropathic pain, and psychological sequelae that persist after apparent motor recovery. A structured, goal-oriented approach to scale selection is therefore necessary to balance feasibility with clinical relevance [11, 13].

Emerging trends in GBS assessment highlight the need for longitudinal and multidimensional outcome evaluation. Recent research emphasises extended follow-up beyond the acute phase, recognising that a substantial proportion of patients experience incomplete recovery or long-term disability. Digital health tools, remote functional monitoring, and patient-reported outcome measures are increasingly being explored to complement traditional clinician-rated scales. In parallel, efforts to harmonise outcome measures across clinical trials aim to improve comparability and facilitate evidence synthesis in this relatively rare condition [14, 15].

In clinical practice, assessment strategies should be aligned with disease phase and clinical objectives. EGRIS and mEGRIS are most relevant during early hospitalisation, MEGOS supports prognostic counselling and rehabilitation planning, and GBS-DS is useful for tracking functional recovery. An integrated yet selective use of these tools enhances clinical decision-making while minimising redundancy and assessment burden (Table **5**).

Table 5. Comparative summary of commonly used Guillain–Barré syndrome assessment scales.

Scale	Primary Domain Assessed	Key Strengths	Major Limitations	Optimal Clinical Use
EGRIS	Risk of respiratory failure	Early prediction; simple variables	Acute-phase only; no treatment effect	ICU triage and monitoring
Modified EGRIS (mEGRIS)	Respiratory insufficiency risk	Improved sensitivity	Limited longitudinal value	Early clinical decision-making
MEGOS	Functional outcome prediction	Prognostic counselling; rehab planning	Population variability	Outcome prediction
GBS Disability Score (GBS-DS)	Functional mobility	Simple; widely used	Ambulation-focused; ceiling effects	Severity grading and recovery tracking
Patient-reported measures	Symptoms and participation	Captures patient perspective	Not standardised in GBS	Emerging adjunct outcomes

CONCLUSION

GBS is a debilitating neurological disorder and requires a proper assessment to monitor the prognosis of the disease and the effect of the treatment. The scales described in the chapter are the most commonly used and well-established assessment scales for GBS patients with good psychometric properties and feasibility.

AI DISCLOSURE STATEMENT

During the preparation of this chapter, the authors used ChatGPT (OpenAI) as a support tool for language refinement, structural organisation, and clarification of ideas. All content generated with AI assistance was carefully reviewed, verified, and revised by the authors to ensure factual accuracy, originality, and consistency with the scientific literature. The authors take full responsibility for the integrity, interpretation, and final content of the published chapter.

ACKNOWLEDGEMENT

The authors extend their appreciation to neurologists, critical care specialists, and rehabilitation professionals who have contributed to the assessment and management of Guillain-Barré syndrome. Their continued efforts in refining clinical and functional outcome scales have enhanced early diagnosis, guided therapeutic decision-making, and improved the overall quality of care for individuals affected by this autoimmune neuropathy.

REFERENCES

[1] Doets AY, Walgaard C, Lingsma HF, *et al.* International Validation of the Erasmus Guillain–Barré Syndrome Respiratory Insufficiency Score. Ann Neurol 2022; 91(4): 521-31. [http://dx.doi.org/10.1002/ana.26312] [PMID: 35106830]

[2] Walgaard C, Lingsma HF, Ruts L, *et al.* Prediction of respiratory insufficiency in Guillain-Barré syndrome. Ann Neurol 2010; 67(6): 781-7. [http://dx.doi.org/10.1002/ana.21976] [PMID: 20517939]

[3] Luijten LWG, Doets AY, Arends S, *et al.* Modified Erasmus GBS Respiratory Insufficiency Score: a simplified clinical tool to predict the risk of mechanical ventilation in Guillain-Barré syndrome. J Neurol Neurosurg Psychiatry 2023; 94(4): 300-8. [http://dx.doi.org/10.1136/jnnp-2022-329937] [PMID: 36428088]

[4] Papri N, Doets AY, Mohammad QD, *et al.* Validation and adjustment of modified Erasmus GBS outcome score in Bangladesh. Ann Clin Transl Neurol 2022; 9(8): 1264-75. [http://dx.doi.org/10.1002/acn3.51627] [PMID: 35908170]

[5] Doets AY, Lingsma HF, Walgaard C, *et al.* Predicting outcome in Guillain-Barré syndrome: International validation of the modified Erasmus GBS Outcome Score. Neurology 2022; 98(5): e518-32. [http://dx.doi.org/10.1212/WNL.0000000000013139] [PMID: 34937789]

[6] Hughes RAC, Newsom-Davis JM, Perkin GD, Pierce JM. Controlled trial prednisolone in acute

polyneuropathy. Lancet 1978; 312(8093): 750-3.
[http://dx.doi.org/10.1016/S0140-6736(78)92644-2] [PMID: 80682]

[7] Leonhard SE, Papri N, Querol L, *et al.* Guillain–Barré syndrome. Nat Rev Dis Primers 2024; 10(1): 97.
[http://dx.doi.org/10.1038/s41572-024-00580-4] [PMID: 39702645]

[8] Walgaard C, Lingsma HF, Ruts L, *et al.* Prediction of respiratory insufficiency in Guillain-Barré syndrome. Ann Neurol. 2010 ; 67(6): 781-7. doi: 10.1002/ana.21976. PMID: 20517939.

[9] Walgaard C, Lingsma HF, Ruts L, van Doorn PA, Steyerberg EW, Jacobs BC. Early recognition of poor prognosis in Guillain-Barre syndrome. Neurology. 2011; 76(11): 968-75. [http://dx:doi.org/10.1212/WNL.0b013e3182104407] [PMID: 21403108]

[10] van Koningsveld R, Steyerberg EW, Hughes RAC, Swan AV, van Doorn PA, Jacobs BC. A clinical prognostic scoring system for Guillain-Barré syndrome. Lancet Neurol 2007; 6(7): 589-94.
[http://dx.doi.org/10.1016/S1474-4422(07)70130-8] [PMID: 17537676]

[11] van Doorn PA, Van den Bergh PYK, Hadden RDM, *et al.* European Academy of Neurology/Peripheral Nerve Society Guideline on diagnosis and treatment of GUILLAIN–BARRé syndrome. J Peripher Nerv Syst 2023; 28(4): 535-63.
[http://dx.doi.org/10.1111/jns.12594] [PMID: 37814551]

[12] Hughes RAC, Cornblath DR, Jacobs BC, van Doorn PA. Guillain-Barré Syndrome Disability Scale: Recommended version and benchmark for new scales. J Peripher Nerv Syst 2025; 30(4): e70064. Advance online publication
[http://dx.doi.org/10.1111/jns.70064]

[13] Willison HJ, Jacobs BC, van Doorn PA. Guillain-Barré syndrome. Lancet 2016; 388(10045): 717-27.
[http://dx.doi.org/10.1016/S0140-6736(16)00339-1] [PMID: 26948435]

[14] Bellanti R, Rinaldi S. Guillain-Barré syndrome: a comprehensive review. Eur J Neurol 2024; 31(8): e16365.
[http://dx.doi.org/10.1111/ene.16365] [PMID: 38813755]

[15] Ariatti A, Mazzoli M, Bastia E, *et al.* Predictors of poor prognosis in Guillain-Barre' syndrome: a study of 22 years from a single Italian Center. J Neurol Sci 2025; 475: 123588.
[http://dx.doi.org/10.1016/j.jns.2025.123588] [PMID: 40633182]

Neurological Assessment Scales, **2026, 269-287**

CHAPTER 12

Scales for Balance and Coordination

Sudhamoy Maity[1] and **Mandeep Jangra**[1,*]

[1] *Maharishi Markandeshwar Institute of Physiotherapy and Rehabilitation, Maharishi Markandeshwar (Deemed to be University), Mullana, Ambala, Haryana, India*

Abstract: Balance and coordination are critical components of functional mobility, particularly in populations with neurological and musculoskeletal impairments. This chapter provides a comprehensive overview of widely used clinical scales designed to assess these parameters, including the Forward Reach Test, Timed Up and Go (TUG) Test, Berg Balance Scale, and the Modified Clinical Test of Sensory Interaction in Balance (MCTSIB). Each scale is explored in terms of its methodology, clinical utility, and the specific aspects of balance and coordination it measures. The Forward Reach Test assesses an individual's stability and limits of forward reach. The TUG Test evaluates functional mobility and fall risk, requiring participants to rise from a chair, walk, and return within a timed window. The Berg Balance Scale provides a multidimensional assessment of static and dynamic balance through 14 tasks, each targeting everyday activities. Lastly, the MCTSIB examines postural control under varying sensory conditions, highlighting the individual's ability to maintain balance with visual, proprioceptive, and vestibular input. This chapter emphasises the importance of these scales in clinical practice and research, outlining their relevance for diagnosing balance deficits, guiding rehabilitation, and tracking progress in patients with various disorders.

Keywords: Balance, Berg balance scale, Coordination, Forward reach test, Modified clinical test of sensory interaction in balance, Timed up and go test.

INTRODUCTION

Balance and coordination are essential components of motor control that allow individuals to maintain postural stability and perform everyday activities. Deficits in these areas can result from a wide range of neurological or musculoskeletal conditions, including stroke, Parkinson's disease, essential tremor, and balance disorders. Assessing balance and coordination through standardised scales is crucial for identifying impairments, tracking progress, and guiding rehabilitation strategies.

* **Corresponding author Mandeep Jangra:** Maharishi Markandeshwar Institute of Physiotherapy and Rehabilitation, Maharishi Markandeshwar (Deemed to be University), Mullana, Ambala, Haryana, India; E-mail: mandeep.jangra@mmumullana.org

Nidhi Sharma, Simranjeet Kaur & Parveen Kumar (Eds.)

Several clinical scales and tests have been developed to evaluate balance and coordination. These scales provide objective measures that can help healthcare professionals assess the severity of impairments, evaluate the effectiveness of interventions, and make informed clinical decisions. Commonly used scales include the Forward Reach Test (FRT), which measures dynamic stability; the Timed Up and Go (TUG) Test, which assesses mobility and fall risk; the Berg Balance Scale (BBS), which evaluates static and dynamic balance in older adults; and the Modified Clinical Test of Sensory Interaction in Balance (MCTSIB), which assesses the integration of sensory inputs for balance control.

Each of these tools provides valuable insights into different aspects of balance and coordination, helping to create individualised rehabilitation plans that address specific deficits. By using these scales, clinicians can monitor patient progress over time and adapt interventions to optimise functional outcomes.

FUNCTIONAL REACH TEST

The Functional Reach Test is a test developed as a quick screen for balance problems in older adults to determine a person's ability to reache forward [1]. In 1990, Pamela Duncan and colleagues first developed the Functional Reach test [2 - 4].

ICF Domain

Body Function
Activity

Target Population

- Older adults
- Individuals at risk of falls
- Parkinson's disease patients
- Frail or low-mobility individuals

Clinical Setting

- Community screening programs
- Outpatient physiotherapy clinics
- Geriatric assessment centres

Instructions for Administration and Scoring

Administration

- The patient is instructed to stand next to, but not touching, a wall and to position the arm closest to the wall at 90 degrees of shoulder flexion with a closed fist.
- The assessor records the starting position at the 3rd metacarpal head on the yardstick.
- Instruct the patient to "Reach as far as you can forward without taking a step."
- The location of the 3rd metacarpal is recorded.
- Scores are determined by assessing the difference between the start and end position, which is the reach distance, usually measured in inches.
- Three trials are done, and the average of the last two is noted.

MODIFIED FUNCTIONAL REACH TEST (MFRT)

The FRT was originally designed as a simple reach test to assess standing balance. This modified version is designed to assess sitting balance in individuals with SCI (*i.e.*, modified FRT). The MFRT mimics a highly functional activity required in daily living. It can distinguish between individuals who have abdominal and back extensors (*i.e.*, high tetraplegia/high paraplegia *versus* low paraplegia), but not between individuals with high lesions. Its psychometric properties are mentioned in Table **1**.

Table 1. Psychometric property summary of mFRT [2].

Property	Metric	Value
Reliability	Agreement (ordinal level tests)	100% agreement
	Intra-class Correlation Coefficient (ICC)	0.93 – 0.99
	Correlation with comparator tests	r = 0.32 – 0.74 ($p \leq 0.05$)
	Test–retest reliability	r = 0.89
	Inter-rater agreement	0.98
Validity	Sensitivity	76%
	Accuracy	46%
	Specificity	34%
	Positive Predictive Value (PPV)	33%

Target Population

- Individuals with spinal cord injury (SCI)
- Patients with impaired trunk control
- People unable to perform standing balance tests
- High tetraplegia, high paraplegia *vs.* low paraplegia differentiation

Clinical Setting

- Inpatient neurorehabilitation units
- Spinal cord injury rehabilitation centres
- Outpatient neuro-physiotherapy clinics
- Research settings evaluating seated balance

Description

Hips, knees, and ankles are positioned at 90 degrees of flexion, with feet positioned flat on the floor.

The initial reach is measured with the patient sitting against the back of the chair with the upper extremity flexed to 90 degrees. The measurement was taken from the distal end of the third metacarpal along the yardstick.

Consists of three conditions over three trials:

- Sitting with the unaffected side near the wall and leaning forward
- Sitting with the back to the wall and leaning right
- Sitting with the back to the wall leaning left.
- Instructions should include leaning as far as possible in each direction without rotation
- and without touching the wall
- Record the distance in centimetres covered in each direction
- If the patient is unable to raise the affected arm, the distance covered by the acromion during learning is recorded
- The first trial in each direction is a practice trial and should not be included in the final result
- A 15-second rest break should be allowed between trials.

MODIFIED CLINICAL TEST FOR SENSORY INTERACTION ON BALANCE

In 1986, physiotherapists Shumway-Cook and Horak developed this test to assess fall risk in older adults and to establish rehabilitation guidelines for balance deficits and lower limb injuries [5]. Over time, the test has evolved to incorporate four distinct conditions, measuring both static and dynamic stability using foam pads. It is used for balance analysis and to determine the dependence of the individual on all sensory systems (vision, vestibular, and somatosensory) that maintain balance [6].

ICF Domain

Body Function
Activity

Target Population

- Older adults with balance impairments
- Individuals with vestibular disorders
- Patients with sensory integration deficits
- People at risk of falls due to multisensory dysfunction
- Neurological conditions affecting postural control

Clinical Setting

- Vestibular and balance rehabilitation clinics
- Community fall-risk screening programs
- Outpatient physiotherapy settings
- Research evaluating sensory contributions to balance

Instructions for Administration and Scoring

Administration

This test is designed to assess how well an older adult is using sensory inputs when one or more sensory systems are compromised. In condition one, all sensory systems (*i.e.*, vision, somatosensory, and vestibular) are available for maintaining balance. In condition two, vision has been removed, and the older adult must rely on the somatosensory and vestibular systems to balance. In condition three, the somatosensory system has been compromised, and the older adults must use vision and the vestibular system to balance. In condition four, vision has been removed, and the somatosensory system has been compromised. The older adults must not rely primarily on the vestibular inputs to balance.

Condition One: Eyes Open, Firm Surface Trial One Total Time: _______ / 30 sec Trial Two Total Time: _______ / 30 sec Trial Three Total Time: _______ / 30 sec

Condition Two: Eyes Closed, Firm Surface Trial One Total Time: _______ / 30 sec Trial Two Total Time: _______ / 30 sec Trial Three Total Time: _______ / 30 sec

Condition Three: Eyes Open, Foam Surface Trial One Total Time: _______ / 30 sec Trial Two Total Time: _______ / 30 sec Trial Three Total Time: _______ / 30 sec

Condition Four: Eyes Closed, Foam Surface Trial One Total Time: _______ / 30 sec Trial Two Total Time: _______ / 30 sec Trial Three Total Time: _______ / 30 sec

TOTAL: _______ / 120

Measurement Property Summary

Validity

The validity of the m-CTSIB test was significantly and positively correlated with the mini-BESTest-GR, with r= -0.652 and p<0.001 [7].

TIMED UP AND GO (TUG) TEST

This test is used to assess fall risk and track improvements in balance, including movements like sitting to standing and walking [8]. It is a straightforward screening tool that provides a sensitive and accurate assessment of the likelihood of falls in older adults [9].

ICF Domain

Body Function
Activity

Target Population

- Older adults and geriatric populations
- Individuals with Parkinson's disease
- Stroke survivors
- Patients with orthopaedic conditions affecting mobility
- People with general mobility or gait impairments

Clinical Setting

- Community-based fall-risk screening
- Outpatient physiotherapy and rehabilitation clinics

- Acute, subacute, and inpatient rehabilitation units
- Research assessing functional mobility outcomes

Instructions for Administration and Scoring

Administration

It is a clinician-administered test, and age-matched norms are shown in Table **2**.

Table 2. Age-matched norms.

	Age in Years	Mean in Seconds
Time's up, and go	60-69	7.9 +/- 0.9
	70-79	7.7+/-2.3
	80-89	No device: 11.0+/-2.2 With device:19.9+/-6.4
	90-101	No device: 14.7+/-7.9 With device:19.9+/-2.5

Equipment: Stopwatch, Standard Chair, Measured distance of 3 meters (10 feet)

Patient Instructions: "My commands for this test are going to be 'ready, set, go'. When I say go, I want. You have to stand up from the chair. You may use the arms of the chair to stand up or sit down. Once you are up, you may take any path you like, but I want you to move as QUICKLY as you feel safe and comfortable.

Until you pass this piece of tape (or the end of the marked course) with both feet, turn around and walk back to the chair. I will stop the clock when your back touches the back of the chair. You will complete one practice run and two that are counted."

Therapist Instructions: Start timing on the word "GO" and stop timing when the subject is seated again correctly in the chair with their back resting against the back of the chair. The subject wears their regular footwear and may use any gait aid they normally use during ambulation, but may not be assisted by another person. There is no time limit. They may stop and rest (but not sit down) if they need to [10].

Scoring

≤10 seconds=normal

≤20seconds = good mobility, can go out alone, mobile without gait aid

≤ 30 seconds = problems, cannot go outside alone, requires gait aid

A score of ≥ 14 seconds has been shown to indicate high risk of falls [9, 10]

Psychometric Properties

Reliability

The TUG test performed by clocking time manually, but the use of technologies and software (mobile application, inertial sensors, video recording system, iTUG device) developed to perform this test has now improved its reliability. Test-retest, intrarater, and interrater reliability are "good" at ranges of 0.90–0.97, 0.80–0.99, and 0.95–0.99, respectively [11].

Intra-rater and inter-rater reliability (ICC) have been reported as high, in elderly populations, from (0.92-0.99) [12].

BERG BALANCE SCALE (BBS)

The Berg Balance Scale (BBS) is used to objectively determine a patient's ability (or inability) to safely balance during a series of predetermined tasks. It does not include the assessment of gait [13].

ICF Domain:
Activity

Number of Items

14 items

Target Population

- Older adults with balance impairments
- Stroke survivors
- Individuals with Parkinson's disease
- Patients with multiple sclerosis or other neurological conditions
- People at risk of falls require a comprehensive balance assessment

Clinical Setting

- Inpatient rehabilitation units
- Outpatient physiotherapy clinics
- Geriatric assessment centres
- Neurological rehabilitation programs
- Research studies requiring detailed balance outcome measures

Instructions for Administration and Scoring

Administration

It is a clinician-administered

- The Berg Balance Scale is a 14-item scale designed to measure static and dynamic balance.
- It includes 6 static balance items and 8 dynamic balance items.
- It mainly focuses on the maintenance of body position and postural adjustment to voluntary movement.

Scoring

It is a 14-item list, with each item consisting of a five-point ordinal scale ranging from 0 to 4, with 0 indicating the lowest level of function and 4 indicating the highest level; it takes approximately 20 minutes to complete.

- A score of 56 indicates functional balance.
- A score of<45 indicates that individuals may be at greater risk of falling.
- A score of ≤49 indicates a risk of falls in individuals with stroke. Its psychometric properties are mentioned in Table **3**.

Table 3. Psychometric Properties of Berg Balance Scale (BBS) [23-25].

Property	Metric	Value
Reliability	Test–retest reliability	ICC=0.94
	Inter-rater reliability	ICC=0.95
	Internal consistency (Day 1)	Cronbach's alpha = 0.86
	Internal consistency (Day 2)	Cronbach's alpha = 0.87
Validity	Sensitivity	0.64
	Specificity	0.67
	Convergent validity with 2MWT	r=0.78

Equipment Required

- Stopwatch
- Standard height chair (18-20 inches) with armrests
- Standard height chair (18-20 inches) without armrests
- Step or stool of average height (7.75 - 9 inch step stool)
- Ruler

- Slipper or a shoe
- Ruler

Language

- Hindi [14]
- Urdu [15]
- Greek [16]
- Persian [17]
- Italian [18]
- Brazilian [19]
- Taiwan [20]
- Norwegian [21]
- Turkish [22]

Scale

SITTING TO STANDING

INSTRUCTIONS: Please stand up. Try not to use your hands for support.

( ) 4 able to stand without using hands and stabilise independently
( ) 3 able to stand independently using hands
( ) 2 able to stand using hands after several tries
( ) 1 needs minimal aid to stand or to stabilise
( ) 0 needs moderate or maximal assist to stand

STANDING UNSUPPORTED

INSTRUCTIONS: Please stand for two minutes without holding.

( ) 4 able to stand safely 2 minutes
( ) 3 able to stand 2 minutes with supervision
( ) 2 able to stand 30 seconds unsupported
( ) 1 needs several tries to stand 30 seconds unsupported
( ) 0 unable to stand 30 seconds unassisted

SITTING WITH BACK UNSUPPORTED BUT FEET SUPPORTED ON FLOOR OR ON A STOOL

INSTRUCTIONS: Please sit with arms folded for 2 minutes.

( ) 4 able to sit safely and securely for 2 minutes
( ) 3 able to sit for 2 minutes under supervision
( ) 2 able to sit for 30 seconds
( ) 1 able to sit for 10 seconds
( ) 0 unable to sit without support for 10 seconds

STANDING TO SITTING

INSTRUCTIONS: Please sit down.

( ) 4 sits safely with minimal use of hands
( ) 3 controls descent by using hands
( ) 2 uses the back of the legs against the chair to control descent
( ) 1 sits independently but has uncontrolled descent
( ) 0 needs assistance to sit

TRANSFERS

INSTRUCTIONS: Arrange chairs(s) for a pivot transfer. Ask the subject to transfer one way toward a seat with armrests and one way toward a seat without armrests. You may use two chairs (one with and one without armrests) or a bed and a chair.

( ) 4 able to transfer safely with minor use of hands
( ) 3 able to transfer safely, definite need of hands
( ) 2 able to transfer with verbal cueing and/or supervision
( ) 1 needs one person to assist
( ) 0 needs two people to assist or supervise to be safe

STANDING UNSUPPORTED WITH EYES CLOSED

INSTRUCTIONS: Please close your eyes and stand still for 10 seconds. () 4 able to stand 10 seconds safely

( ) 3 able to stand 10 seconds with supervision
( ) 2 able to stand 3 seconds
( ) 1 unable to keep eyes closed for 3 seconds, but stays steady
( ) 0 needs help to keep from falling

STANDING UNSUPPORTED WITH FEET TOGETHER

INSTRUCTIONS: Place your feet together and stand without holding.

( ) 4 able to place feet together independently and stand for 1 minute safely () 3 able to place feet together independently and stand for 1 minute with supervision
( ) 2 able to place feet together independently, but unable to hold for 30 seconds
( ) 1 needs help to attain a position, but is able to stand for 15 seconds with feet together
( ) 0 needs help to attain a position and is unable to hold for 15 seconds

REACHING FORWARD WITH OUTSTRETCHED ARM WHILE STANDING

INSTRUCTIONS: Lift arm to 90 degrees. Stretch out your fingers and reach forward as far as you can. (Examiner places a ruler at the end of fingertips when the arm is at 90 degrees. Fingers should not touch the ruler while reaching forward. The recorded measure is the distance forward the finger reaches while the subject is in the most forward-lean position. When possible, ask the subject to use both arms when reaching to avoid rotation of the trunk.)

( ) 4 can reach forward confidently >25 cm (10 inches)
( ) 3 can reach forward >12 cm safely (5 inches)
( ) 2 can reach forward >5 cm safely (2 inches)
( ) 1 reaches forward but needs supervision
( ) 0 loses balance while trying/requires external support

PICK UP OBJECT FROM THE FLOOR FROM A STANDING POSITION

INSTRUCTIONS: Pick up the shoe/slipper that is placed in front of your feet.

( ) 4 able to pick up a slipper safely and easily
( ) 3 able to pick up a slipper but needs supervision
( ) 2 unable to pick up but reaches 2-5cm (1-2 inches) from the slipper and keeps balance independently
( ) 1 is unable to pick up and needs supervision while trying
( ) 0 unable to try/needs assist to keep from losing balance or falling

TURNING TO LOOK BEHIND OVER LEFT AND RIGHT SHOULDERS WHILE STANDING

INSTRUCTIONS: Turn to look directly behind you over toward your left shoulder. Repeat to the right. The examiner may pick an object to look at directly behind the subject to encourage a better twist and turn.

( ) 4 looks behind from both sides, and weight shifts well
( ) 3 looks behind one side, only the other side shows less weight shift
( ) 2 turns sideways, but maintains balance
( ) 1 needs supervision when turning
( ) 0 needs assistance to keep from losing balance or falling

TURN 360 DEGREES

INSTRUCTIONS: Turn completely around in a full circle. Pause. Then turn a full circle in the other direction.

( ) 4 able to turn 360 degrees safely in 4 seconds or less
( ) 3 able to turn 360 degrees safely, one side only, in 4 seconds or less
( ) 2 able to turn 360 degrees safely but slowly
( ) 1 needs close supervision or verbal cueing
( ) 0 needs assistance while turning

PLACING ALTERNATE FOOT ON STEP OR STOOL WHILE STANDING UNSUPPORTED

INSTRUCTIONS: Place each foot alternately on the step/stool. Continue until each foot has touched the step/stool four times.

( ) 4 able to stand independently and safely, and complete 8 steps in 20 seconds
( ) 3 able to stand independently and complete 8 steps in >20 seconds
( ) 2 able to complete 4 steps without aid with supervision
( ) 1 able to complete >2 steps needs minimal assistance
( ) 0 needs assistance to keep from falling/unable to try

STANDING UNSUPPORTED ONE FOOT IN FRONT

INSTRUCTIONS: (DEMONSTRATE TO SUBJECT) Place one foot directly in front of the other. If you feel that you cannot place your foot directly in front, try to step far enough ahead that the heel of your forward foot is ahead of the toes of the other foot. (To score 3 points, the length of the step should exceed the length of the other foot, and the width of the stance should approximate the subject's normal stride width.)

( ) 4 able to place foot tandem independently and hold for 30 seconds
( ) 3 able to place foot ahead of the other independently and hold for 30 seconds
( ) 2 able to take a small step independently and hold for 30 seconds
( ) 1 needs help to step, but can hold for 15 seconds
( ) 0 loses balance while stepping or standing

STANDING ON ONE LEG

INSTRUCTIONS: Stand on one leg as long as you can without holding. () 4 able to lift leg independently and hold for>10 seconds

( ) 3 able to lift leg independently and hold for 5-10 seconds
( ) 2 able to lift leg independently and hold = or >3 seconds
( ) 1 tries to lift the leg, unable to hold for 3 seconds, but remains standing independently
( ) 0 unable to try or needs assistance to prevent a fall

CLINICAL CONSIDERATIONS, STRENGTHS, LIMITATIONS, AND EMERGING TRENDS

Balance and coordination impairments are common across a wide range of neurological, musculoskeletal, and geriatric populations and are major contributors to functional limitation and fall risk. Accurate assessment of balance requires consideration of static stability, dynamic control, sensory integration, and functional mobility. No single balance scale captures all these components; therefore, the selection of assessment tools should be guided by patient characteristics, the clinical setting, and the specific purpose of the evaluation [26, 27].

Simple performance-based measures such as the Functional Reach Test (FRT) and Modified Functional Reach Test (MFRT) provide quick screening of dynamic balance and limits of stability. Their strengths lie in ease of administration, minimal equipment requirements, and applicability in outpatient and community settings. However, these tests assess balance in a single plane and do not account for gait, turning, or sensory contributions to postural control. As a result, they may lack sensitivity for detecting complex balance deficits or subtle changes following intervention [28].

The Modified Clinical Test for Sensory Interaction on Balance (mCTSIB) addresses sensory integration by systematically altering visual and surface conditions. This makes it particularly useful for identifying sensory dependence and balance strategies in individuals with vestibular, neurological, or age-related impairments. Despite its conceptual strength, mCTSIB performance can be influenced by testing environment and examiner consistency, and it provides limited information regarding functional mobility or fall risk during daily activities [29].

Functional mobility assessments such as the Timed Up and Go (TUG) test evaluate the integrated performance of balance, gait, and transitional movements. TUG is widely used due to its simplicity, strong predictive value for falls, and applicability across diverse populations. However, its global nature limits diagnostic specificity, as prolonged times may reflect deficits in strength, cognition, or mobility rather than balance alone [30].

The Berg Balance Scale (BBS) remains one of the most extensively validated balance measures in clinical practice and research. It offers a comprehensive assessment of static and dynamic balance tasks and demonstrates good reliability and validity across neurological populations. Nevertheless, ceiling effects in higher-functioning individuals and limited sensitivity to reactive balance and gait adaptability reduce its usefulness in detecting subtle deficits or changes in mildly impaired patients [31, 32].

A key limitation across commonly used balance scales is the emphasis on controlled, clinic-based tasks that may not fully reflect real-world balance demands. Many tools inadequately capture reactive postural responses, dual-task performance, and environmental variability, which are critical contributors to fall risk. Overlapping content among balance scales can also increase assessment burden if tools are selected without a clear evaluative framework [27, 33].

Emerging trends in balance assessment emphasise the integration of technology to enhance objectivity and ecological validity. Wearable sensors, inertial measurement units, and force platforms are increasingly used to quantify postural sway, gait variability, and dynamic stability in real-world environments. Digital adaptations of traditional balance tests and remote assessment platforms are also gaining relevance, particularly for fall-risk monitoring and tele-rehabilitation. These innovations aim to complement, not replace, established clinical scales by providing continuous and context-sensitive balance metrics [34, 35].

In clinical practice, balance assessment should follow a tiered approach. Screening tools such as FRT or TUG are suitable for rapid evaluation, while comprehensive scales like BBS and mCTSIB support detailed assessment and treatment planning. Combining traditional clinical measures with emerging technology-enabled tools offers a more complete understanding of balance performance while minimising redundancy and optimising clinical efficiency (Table **4**).

Table 4. Comparative summary of commonly used balance and coordination assessment scales.

Scale	Primary Domain Assessed	Key Strengths	Major Limitations	Optimal Clinical Use
Functional Reach Test	Dynamic balance	Quick, minimal equipment	Single-plane assessment	Community and outpatient screening
Modified Functional Reach Test	Sitting balance and reach	Suitable for frail or seated patients	Limited functional scope	Elderly and wheelchair users
mCTSIB	Sensory integration	Identifies sensory dependence	Limited functional relevance	Vestibular and neurological assessment
Timed Up and Go	Functional mobility	Simple; fall-risk prediction	Non-specific to balance	Geriatric and neurological screening
Berg Balance Scale	Static and dynamic balance	Well validated; comprehensive	Ceiling effects; limited gait	Rehabilitation assessment
Wearable sensor metrics	Real-world balance	Objective: continuous monitoring	Limited standardization	Emerging clinical and research use

CONCLUSION

FRT, mFRT, MCTSIB, TUG, and BBS are valuable, cost-effective tools for assessing balance and mobility in clinical and research settings. They provide objective measures and are useful in predicting falls and guiding rehabilitation. However, limitations include a focus on anterior or static balance (FRT, mFRT, and MCTSIB), as well as issues like ceiling effects (BBS) and a lack of sensitivity to subtle deficits (TUG).

Future developments should explore integrating technology, such as sensors and mobile apps, to improve precision. Additionally, more research is needed to validate these tests in real-world settings and across diverse populations.

AI DISCLOSURE STATEMENT

During the preparation of this chapter, the authors used ChatGPT (OpenAI) as a support tool for language refinement, structural organisation, and clarification of ideas. All content generated with AI assistance was carefully reviewed, verified, and revised by the authors to ensure factual accuracy, originality, and consistency with the scientific literature. The authors take full responsibility for the integrity, interpretation, and final content of the published chapter.

ACKNOWLEDGEMENT

The authors acknowledge the contributions of the academic and clinical literature that informed the development of this chapter. The chapter has been prepared through careful review and synthesis of existing research, clinical guidelines, and validated assessment frameworks related to balance and coordination. The authors also acknowledge the broader scientific community whose foundational work has advanced the understanding and clinical application of balance assessment tools. Any limitations remain the responsibility of the authors.

REFERENCES

[1] Scena S, Steindler R, Ceci M, Zuccaro SM, Carmeli E. Computerised functional reach test to measure balance stability in elderly patients with neurological disorders. J Clin Med Res 2016; 8(10): 715-20. [http://dx.doi.org/10.14740/jocmr2652w] [PMID: 27635176]

[2] Duncan PW, Weiner DK, Chandler J, Studenski S. Functional reach: A new clinical measure of balance. J Gerontol 1990; 45(6): M192-197. [http://dx.doi.org/10.1093/geronj/45.6.M192] [PMID: 2229941]

[3] de Waroquier-Leroy L, Bleuse S, Serafi R, *et al.* The functional reach test: Strategies, performance and the influence of age. Ann Phys Rehabil Med 2014; 57(6-7): 452-64. [http://dx.doi.org/10.1016/j.rehab.2014.03.003] [PMID: 24928146]

[4] Weiner DK, Duncan PW, Chandler J, Studenski SA. Functional reach: A marker of physical frailty. J Am Geriatr Soc 1992; 40(3): 203-7. [http://dx.doi.org/10.1111/j.1532-5415.1992.tb02068.x] [PMID: 1538035]

[5] Shumway-Cook A, Horak FB. Assessing the influence of sensory interaction of balance. Suggestion from the field. Phys Ther 1986; 66(10): 1548-50. [http://dx.doi.org/10.1093/ptj/66.10.1548] [PMID: 3763708]

[6] Antoniadou E, Kalivioti X, Stolakis K, Koloniari A, *et al.* Reliability and validity of the mctsib dynamic platform test to assess balance in a population of older women living in the community. J Musculoskelet Neuronal Interact 2020; 20(2): 185-93. [PMID: 32481234]

[7] Antoniadou E, Kalivioti X, Stolakis K, *et al.* Reliability and validity of the mctsib dynamic platform test to assess balance in a population of older women living in the community. J Musculoskelet Neuronal Interact 2020; 20(2): 185-93. [PMID: 32481234]

[8] Podsiadlo D, Richardson S. The timed “up & go”: A test of basic functional mobility for frail elderly persons. J Am Geriatr Soc 1991; 39(2): 142-8. [http://dx.doi.org/10.1111/j.1532-5415.1991.tb01616.x] [PMID: 1991946]

[9] Bohannon RW. Reference values for the timed up and go test: A descriptive meta-analysis. J Geriatr Phys Ther 2006; 29(2): 64-8. [http://dx.doi.org/10.1519/00139143-200608000-00004] [PMID: 16914068]

[10] Shumway-Cook A, Brauer S, Woollacott M. Predicting the probability for falls in communitydwelling older adults using the timed up & go test. Phys Ther 2000; 80(9): 896-903.

[http://dx.doi.org/10.1093/ptj/80.9.896] [PMID: 10960937]

[11] Mollinedo I, Ma Cancela J. Evaluation of the psychometric properties and clinical applications of the timed up and go test in parkinson disease: A systematic review. J Exerc Rehabil 2020; 16(4): 302-12. [http://dx.doi.org/10.12965/jer.2040532.266] [PMID: 32913835]

[12] Steffen TM, Hacker TA, Mollinger L. Age- and gender-related test performance in communitydwelling elderly people: Six-minute walk test, berg balance scale, timed up & go test, and gait speeds. Phys Ther 2002; 82(2): 128-37. [http://dx.doi.org/10.1093/ptj/82.2.128] [PMID: 11856064]

[13] Berg KO, Wood-Dauphinee SL, Williams JI, Maki B. Measuring balance in the elderly: Validation of an instrument. Can J Public Health 1992; 83(Suppl. 2): S7-S11. [PMID: 1468055]

[14] Shah SR, Joshi V1, Snowdon NJ2. Cross-cultural adaptation and reliability of the berg balance scale in hindi. Ind J Phys Ther Res 2022; 4(1): 22-9. [http://dx.doi.org/10.4103/ijptr.ijptr_60_21]

[15] Kashif M, Ahmad A, Bandpei MAM, Gilani SA, Iram H, Farooq M. Psychometric properties of the urdu translation of berg balance scale in people with parkinson's disease. Int J Environ Res Public Health 2022; 19(4): 2346. [http://dx.doi.org/10.3390/ijerph19042346] [PMID: 35206533]

[16] Lampropoulou S, Gizeli A, Kalivioti C, *et al.* Cross cultural adaptation of berg balance scale in greek for various balance impairments. J Phys Med Rehabil Disabil 2016; 2: 011. [http://dx.doi.org/10.24966/PMRD-8670/100011]

[17] Salavati M, Negahban H, Mazaheri M, *et al.* The persian version of the berg balance scale: Inter and intra-rater reliability and construct validity in elderly adults. Disabil Rehabil 2012; 34(20): 1695-8. [http://dx.doi.org/10.3109/09638288.2012.660604] [PMID: 22380626]

[18] Ottonello M, Ferriero G, Benevolo E, *et al.* Psychometric evaluation of the italian version of the berg balance scale in rehabilitation inpatients. EUR MED PHYS 2003; 39(4): 181-9.

[19] Miyamoto ST, Lombardi Junior I, Berg KO, *et al.* Brazilian version of the berg balance scale. Braz J Med Biol Res 2004; 37(9): 1411-21. Available form: https://doi.org/10.1590/S0100-879X2004000900017

[20] Wang CY, Hsieh CL, Olson SL, *et al.* Psychometric properties of the berg balance scale in a community-dwelling elderly resident population in taiwan. J Formos Med Assoc 2006; 105(12): 992-1000. [http://dx.doi.org/10.1016/S0929-6646(09)60283-7] [PMID: 17185241]

[21] Halsaa KE, Brovold T, Graver V, *et al.* Assessments of interrater reliability and internal consistency of the norwegian version of the berg balance scale. Arch Phys Med Rehabil 2007; 88(1): 94-8. Available form: https://doi.org/10.1016/j.apmr.2006.10.016

[22] Sahin F, Yilmaz F, Ozmaden A, *et al.* Reliability and validity of the turkish version of the berg balance scale. J Geriatr Phys Ther 2008; 31(1): 32-7.

[23] Taghizadeh G, Martinez-Martin P, Fereshtehnejad SM, *et al.* Psychometric properties of the berg balance scale in idiopathic parkinson' disease in the drug off-phase. Neurol Sci 2018; 39(12): 2175-81. [http://dx.doi.org/10.1007/s10072-018-3570-4] [PMID: 30244299]

[24] Wang CY, Hsieh CL, Olson SL, *et al.* Psychometric properties of the berg balance scale in a community-dwelling elderly resident population in taiwan. J Formos Med Assoc 2006; 105(12): 992-1000. [http://dx.doi.org/10.1016/S0929-6646(09)60283-7] [PMID: 17185241]

[25] La Porta F, Caselli S, Susassi S, *et al.* Is the berg balance scale an internally valid and reliable measure of balance across different etiologies in neurorehabilitation? A revisited rasch analysis study. Arch Phys Med Rehabil 2012; 93(7): 1209-6.

[http://dx.doi.org/10.1016/j.apmr.2012.02.020] [PMID: 22521926]

[26] Cohen H, Blatchly CA, Gombash LL. A study of the clinical test of sensory interaction and balance. Phys Ther 1993; 73(6): 346-51.
[http://dx.doi.org/10.1093/ptj/73.6.346] [PMID: 8497509]

[27] Blum L, Korner-Bitensky N. Usefulness of the berg balance scale in stroke rehabilitation: A systematic review. Phys Ther 2008; 88(5): 559-66.
[http://dx.doi.org/10.2522/ptj.20070205] [PMID: 18292215]

[28] Moriyama Y, Yamada T, Shimamura R, *et al.* Movement patterns of the functional reach test do not reflect physical function in healthy young and older participants. PLoS One 2022; 17(3): e0266195.
[http://dx.doi.org/10.1371/journal.pone.0266195] [PMID: 35358272]

[29] Whitney SL, Wrisley DM, Marchetti GF, Gee MA, Reding MJ, Furman JM. Clinical measurement of sit-to-stand performance in people with balance disorders: Validity of data for the five-times-st-stand test. Phys Ther 2005; 85(10): 1034-45.
[http://dx.doi.org/10.1093/ptj/85.10.1034]

[30] Herman T, Giladi N, Hausdorff JM. Properties of the 'timed up and go' test: More than meets the eye. Gerontology 2011; 57(3): 203-10.
[http://dx.doi.org/10.1159/000314963] [PMID: 20484884]

[31] Downs S. The berg balance scale. J Physiother 2015; 61(1): 46.
[http://dx.doi.org/10.1016/j.jphys.2014.10.002] [PMID: 25476663]

[32] Cho J, Ha S, Lee J, *et al.* Standing balance test predicts the berg balance scale score in patients with stroke using principal component analysis. Sci Rep 2025; 15(1): 17653.
[http://dx.doi.org/10.1038/s41598-02--99710-5] [PMID: 40399582]

[33] Mancini M, Horak FB. The relevance of clinical balance assessment tools to differentiate balance deficits. Eur J Phys Rehabil Med 2010; 46(2): 239-48.
[PMID: 20485226]

[34] Ghislieri M, Gastaldi L, Pastorelli S, *et al.* Wearable inertial sensors to assess standing balance: A systematic review. Sensors (Basel) 2019; 19(19): 4075.
[http://dx.doi.org/10.3390/s19194075] [PMID: 31547181]

[35] Nairn B, Tsakanikas V, Gordon B, *et al.* Smart wearable technologies for balance rehabilitation in older adults at risk of falls: Scoping review and comparative analysis. JMIR Rehabil Assist Technol 2025; 12: e69589.
[http://dx.doi.org/10.2196/69589] [PMID: 40435383]

CHAPTER 13

Scales to Assess Myasthenia Gravis

Yukta Sharma[1,2], **Sukhpal Singh**[2] and **Simranjeet Kaur**[2,3,*]

[1] *Department of Physiotherapy, University Institute of Allied Health Sciences, Chandigarh University, Mohali, Punjab, India*

[2] *Maharishi Markandeshwar Institute of Physiotherapy and Rehabilitation, Maharishi Markandeshwar (Deemed to be University), Mullana, Ambala, Haryana, India*

[3] *Pal Physiotherapy and Rehabilitation Centre, Pal Healthcare, Ambala City, Haryana, India*

Abstract: Myasthenia gravis (MG) is the most common uncommon neuromuscular condition. The hallmark clinical characteristic of MG is marked, variable weakness that is limited to voluntary muscles. Interestingly, this myasthenic weakness is made worse by physical exercise. Despite being a widespread illness, localised weakness is frequently how it first manifests. Most patients have ocular muscule weakness at the beginning, which results in symptoms like ptosis (drooping of the eyelids) and diplopia (double vision). "Ocular myasthenia" is the word used to describe weakness that is limited to the ocular muscles. Patients who suffer from oropharyngeal weakness may find it difficult to masticate, deglutinate, and articulate. The proximal muscle groups of the limb girdle often exhibit greater weakness than the distal muscle units in patients with generalised myasthenia gravis. The inability to breathe and difficulties swallowing can lead to a myasthenic crisis, a severe and potentially fatal worsening of myasthenia gravis. Patients with myasthenia gravis are generally affected by this in terms of quality of life. Four general assessment scales are provided in this chapter to gauge patients' quality of life. Scales like Myasthenia Gravis Quality of Life (MG-QOL), Myasthenia Gravis Impairment Index, Myasthenia Gravis Composite Score (MGC Score), and Myasthenia Gravis Quality of Life 15-Items Revised (MG-QOL15r) are included in this chapter.

Keywords: Disease severity assessment, Neuromuscular disorders, Patient-reported outcome measures, Psychometric validation, Quality of life.

INTRODUCTION

Myasthenia gravis (MG) is an autoimmune neuromuscular disorder characterized by fluctuating muscle weakness that worsens with exertion and improves with

* **Corresponding author Simranjeet Kaur:** Pal Physiotherapy and Rehabilitation Centre, Pal Healthcare, Ambala City, Haryana, India; E-mail: Simranjeetkaursaini825@gmail.com

rest. The condition primarily affects voluntary muscles, including those in the eyes, face, throat, and limbs [1]. In approximately two-thirds of patients, initial symptoms manifest as weakness of the extrinsic ocular muscles, leading to issues such as drooping eyelids (ptosis) and double vision (diplopia).

As the disease progresses, it can extend to other bulbar muscles and limb musculature, resulting in generalised myasthenia gravis (gMG), which may involve significant fatigue and difficulties with swallowing and breathing. Symptoms typically fluctuate in intensity, often being more pronounced later in the day or after physical activity. While there is no cure for MG, various treatments are available to manage symptoms effectively [1, 2]. A thorough assessment is needed to evaluate Myasthenia Gravis.

MYASTHENIA GRAVIS IMPAIRMENT INDEX

Introduction

The Myasthenia Gravis Impairment Index (MGII) is a novel tool for measuring MG-related impairments. It focuses on the impairments that matter to individual patients and has a patient-centered approach [1, 2].

ICF Domain

Body Functions: Muscle strength, respiratory function, ocular and facial muscle weakness, swallowing, and speech issues

Activities and Participation: Ability to perform daily activities like eating, dressing, and mobility. Impact on social participation, work, and communication.

Environmental factors: Support systems, availability of assistive devices, and healthcare services. Barriers in the physical environment.

Number of Items

The MGII consists of 12 items, carefully designed to capture a broad spectrum of impairments associated with Myasthenia Gravis [2].

Instructions for Administration

Administration

Clinicians administer the MGII during routine clinical examinations, focusing on specific impairments associated with Myasthenia Gravis. The assessment involves a combination of physician observations and patient self-reports [2].

Equipment

No specific equipment is required for the MGII, making it a practical tool that can be utilized in various healthcare settings. A well-equipped examination room facilitates a comprehensive evaluation.

Scoring

Each item in the MGII is scored on a scale from 0 to 4, with 0 indicating no impairment and 4 indicating severe impairment. The total score ranges from 0 to 48, with higher scores indicating greater impairment due to Myasthenia Gravis [1].

Interpretability

MCID (Minimal Clinically Important Difference)

The MCID for the MGII is considered to be a change of 3 points.

This represents a clinically meaningful alteration in a patient's Myasthenia Gravis-related impairments [1].

SEM (Standard Error of Measurement)

The SEM for the MGII is ±2 points, indicating the expected range within which an individual's true score lies with 68% confidence [1]. Table **1** details the other measuring properties.

Table 1. Psychometric properties [1 - 3].

Category	Measure	Value	Confidence Interval
Reliability	Internal consistency (Cronbach's alpha)	0.87	-
Reliability	Test-retest reliability (intraclass correlation coefficient)	0.92	95% CI: 0.79–0.94
Reliability	Interrater reliability (intraclass correlation coefficient)	0.81	95% CI: 0.79–0.94
Correlations	MGII with MG–activities of daily living	R=0.91	-
Correlations	MGII with MG-specific quality of life (15-item scale)	R=0.78	-

MDC (Minimal Detectable Change)

The MDC for the MGII is 5 points, suggesting that a change of 5 points or more is required to confidently infer a real change in a patient's impairment status [1].

Languages

Italian Cronbach's alpha=0.98 [3]

Training Required

Healthcare professionals administering the MGII should have training in neurological assessments and familiarity with Myasthenia Gravis-related impairments. Training includes understanding the scoring criteria and interpretation guidelines.

Availability

The MGII is widely available in neurology clinics and hospitals. It serves as a valuable tool for assessing the impairment profile of Myasthenia Gravis patients.

Clinical Considerations

The MGII, with its focus on impairments, provides a detailed snapshot of the physical impact of Myasthenia Gravis. Clinicians should consider the combination of physician observations and patient self-reports when interpreting results [1].

Responsiveness

The MGII exhibits excellent responsiveness to changes in Myasthenia Gravis-related impairments over time, making it a valuable tool for tracking disease progression or treatment efficacy [1].

Floor/Ceiling Effect

The MGII shows no significant floor or ceiling effects, indicating its ability to capture a broad range of impairment levels associated with Myasthenia Gravis [2].

Myasthenia Gravis Impairment Index [1]

PROBLEMS WITH YOUR EYES: Please answer regarding the past 2 weeks.

1. Double vision throughout the day

Have you experienced episodes of double vision?

[ ] No Double Vision

[ ] Episodes only in the evenings

[ ] Episodes starting in the afternoons

[ ] Constant or present most of the day

2. Double vision with activities

Have you experienced double vision while reading, driving, watching TV, or using a computer?

[ ] No Double Vision

[ ] After more than 1 hour

[ ] After less than 1 hour, but not immediately

[ ] Constant double vision or it starts immediately

3. Severity of double vision

Have you experienced double vision?

[ ] No Double Vision

[ ] Mild: it doesn't affect my daily activities

[ ] It affects my activities, but no need to cover one eye

[ ] I need to cover one eye to be able to function

4. Eyelid drooping throughout the day

Have you experienced drooping of your eyelid(s)? If yes, when does it occur (on average)?

[ ] No eyelid drooping

[ ] Only in the evenings

[ ] Drooping starts in the afternoons

[ ] Constant drooping or present most of the day

5. Eyelid drooping with activities

Have you experienced drooping of your eyelid(s) with activities such as reading, driving, watching TV, or using a computer?

[ ] No eyelid drooping

[ ] After more than 1 hour

[ ] After less than 1 hour, but not immediately

[ ] Constant drooping or it starts immediately

6. Severity of eyelid drooping

Have you experienced drooping of your eyelids? If yes, how severe has it been (at your worst)?

[] No eyelid drooping

[ ] Mild: it doesn't affect my vision

[ ] It affects my vision, but no need to lift my eyelid

[ ] I need to lift my eyelid or tilt my head to be able to see

PROBLEMS EATING: Please answer regarding the past 2 weeks

7. Difficulty swallowing

Have you experienced difficulty swallowing? How severe has it been (at your worst)?

[ ] No swallowing problems

[ ] Occasional episodes of choking/coughing with food

[ ] Liquids return through my nose, but no problems with solid food

[ ] Difficulty swallowing hard food, requiring a change in diet

[ ] Unable to swallow or using a feeding tube

8. Chewing different types of food

Have you experienced difficulty chewing? How severe has it been (at your worst)?

[] No difficulty chewing

[ ] Difficulty chewing hard foods (*e.g.*, steak, raw carrots)

[ ] Difficulty chewing soft foods (*e.g.*, hard-boiled egg)

[ ] Unable to chew (eating only liquids or feeding tube)

9. Chewing tiredness/fatigue

At your worst, how long does it take to develop fatigue or tiredness in your jaw? [ ] No difficulty chewing

[ ] Difficulty chewing at the end of the meal

[ ] Difficulty chewing from the beginning of the meal

[ ] Unable to chew (eating only liquids or feeding tube)

PROBLEMS SPEAKING AND BREATHING: Please answer regarding the past 2 weeks

10. Voice changes through the day

Have you experienced episodes of a nasal, hoarse, or weak voice? When do they occur on average?

[] No voice changes

[ ] Voice changes only in the evenings

[ ] Voice changes starting in the afternoons

[ ] Constant voice changes or present most of the day

11. Voice changes with prolonged conversation

How long can you talk (on average) before developing voice changes, such as a nasal, hoarse, or weak voice? (Normal conversation, with pauses for other speakers)

[ ] No voice changes

[ ] Voice changes after more than 30 minutes

[ ] Voice changes after less than 30 minutes, but not immediately

[ ] Constant voice changes, or they start immediately (less than 1 minute)

12. Severity of voice changes

At your worst, how severe have your voice changes been? (Nasal, hoarse, weak voice)

[ ] No voice changes

[ ] Mild changes: my voice is mostly clear

[ ] Moderate changes: it can be hard to understand me

[ ] Severe changes: it is impossible to understand me

13. Speech clarity through the day

Have you experienced difficulty pronouncing words or slurred speech? When does it occur on average?

[ ] No episodes of slurred speech

[ ] Slurred speech only in the evenings

[ ] Slurred speech starting in the afternoons

[ ] Constant slurring, or present most of the day

14. Speech clarity with prolonged conversation

How long can you talk (on average) before developing slurred speech? (Normal conversation, with pauses for other speakers)

[ ] No episodes of slurred speech

[ ] Slurred speech after 30 minutes

[ ] Slurred speech after less than 30 minutes, but not immediately

[ ] Constant slurring, or it starts immediately (less than 1 minute)

15. Severity of speech changes

At your worst, how severe have your speech changes been? (Slurring, difficulty pronouncing words)

[ ] No episodes of slurred speech

[ ] Mild slurring: It is easy to understand me

[ ] Moderate slurring: There are some difficulties understanding me

[ ] Severe slurring: It is impossible to understand me

16. Difficulty breathing

Have you experienced shortness of breath that is caused by myasthenia? (*i.e.*, not caused by asthma or other lung/heart disease) If yes, when has it occurred (at your worst)?

[ ] No shortness of breath (except for strenuous exercise)

[ ] With moderate effort (*e.g.*, walking several blocks at my own pace)

[ ] With minimal effort (*e.g.*, getting dressed, walking inside the house)

[ ] At rest or when lying on my back

[ ] Requiring assisted ventilation

GENERALIZED SYMPTOMS: Please answer regarding the past 2 weeks

17. Overall physical tiredness

Have you experienced overall physical tiredness caused by myasthenia gravis? (*i.e.*, not by sleeplessness, depression, or other medical conditions)

[ ] No physical tiredness

[ ] Overall physical tiredness only in the evenings

[ ] Overall physical tiredness starting in the afternoons

[ ] Constant physical tiredness, or present most of the day

18. Arm weakness severity

Have you experienced weakness in your arms? If yes, how severe has it been (at your worst)?

[ ] No arm weakness

[ ] Mild weakness (*e.g.*, difficulty lifting heavy objects)

[ ] Moderate weakness (*e.g.*, difficulty lifting arms above the shoulders, but I can do it)

[ ] Severe weakness (unable to lift arms above the shoulders)

19. Arm weakness with prolonged use

Have you experienced weakness in your arms after prolonged use? When does it happen (on average)?

[ ] No arm weakness

[ ] Weakness when keeping arms up for long (*e.g.*, washing or drying my hair)

[ ] Weakness with activities at the shoulder level (organizing objects on a shelf, holding a phone to the ear)

[ ] Weakness with minimal effort (*e.g.*, desk work, chopping vegetables)

20. Leg weakness severity

Have you experienced weakness in your legs? If yes, how severe has it been (at your worst)?

[ ] No leg weakness

[ ] Mild weakness (*e.g.*, difficulty standing from a squat or tying my shoes)

[ ] Moderate weakness (*e.g.*, difficulty sitting up from a chair, I need to push up with my arms)

[ ] Severe weakness (*e.g.*, unable to stand from a chair without assistance)

21. Leg weakness with prolonged use

Have you experienced weakness in your legs after prolonged use? When does it happen (on average)?

[ ] No leg weakness

[ ] Weakness when walking more than 10 blocks at my own pace

[ ] Weakness when walking less than 10 blocks at my own pace

[ ] Constant weakness or with minimal effort (standing, walking inside the house)

22. Neck weakness

Have you experienced weakness in your neck? When does it happen (on average)?

[] No neck weakness

[ ] Weakness only in the evenings

[ ] Weakness starting in the afternoons

[ ] Constant weakness or present most of the day

MYASTHENIA GRAVIS COMPOSITE SCORE (MGC SCORE) [4, 5]

Introduction

The Myasthenia Gravis Composite Score is used to quantify disease severity based on impairments of body functions and structures. Assesses various domains related to Activities and Participation in the ICF framework [4].

ICF Domain

Body functions: Muscle strength, ocular function, speech, and swallowing

Activities and participation: Mobility and self-care

Number of Items

The MGC Score comprises 13 items that assess ocular, bulbar, and limb function [5].

Instructions for Administration

Administration

Clinicians perform the MGC Score during routine clinical assessments, employing physician examinations and patient history. It is essential to conduct the evaluation in a quiet setting to ensure accurate observations.

Scoring

The scoring system involves assigning points based on the severity of symptoms for each item. The total score ranges from 0 to 50, with higher scores indicating more severe Myasthenia Gravis [5].

Interpretability

MCID (Minimal Clinically Important Difference)

The MCID for the MGC Score is considered to be a change of 2 points. This reflects a clinically meaningful alteration in a patient's Myasthenia Gravis status [5].

SEM (Standard Error of Measurement)

The SEM for the MGC Score is ±1.5 points, indicating the expected range within which an individual's true score lies with 68% confidence [5].

MDC (Minimal Detectable Change)

The MDC for the MGC Score is 4 points, suggesting that a change of 4 points or more is required to confidently infer a real change in a patient's condition [5].

Languages

Brazilian Portuguese [6].

Training Required

Healthcare professionals administering the MGC Score should possess training in neurological assessments. Familiarity with scoring criteria and interpretation guidelines is crucial for accurate evaluations [6].

Availability

The MGC Score is widely available in neurology clinics and hospitals and serves as a valuable tool for assessing Myasthenia Gravis severity [5].

Clinical Considerations

The MGC Score, which relies on both physician examinations and patient history, provides a comprehensive evaluation of Myasthenia Gravis. Clinicians should be attentive to variations in patient interpretation and the potential impact on scoring [4].

Psychometric Properties

Reliability [4, 5]

Internal consistency (Cronbach's alpha): 0.85

Test-retest reliability (intraclass correlation coefficient): 0.92

Validity

Content validity is supported by expert input, and construct validity is evidenced by significant correlations with established measures of Myasthenia Gravis severity [4].

Responsiveness

The MGC Score exhibits excellent responsiveness to changes in Myasthenia Gravis symptoms over time, making it a valuable tool for tracking disease progression or treatment efficacy [5].

Floor/Ceiling Effect

The MGC Score shows no significant floor or ceiling effects, indicating its ability to capture a broad range of disease severity levels [4 - 6].

Myasthenia Gravis Composite Score [4, 5]

Ptosis

- 45 seconds = 0
- 11-45 seconds = 1
- 1-10 seconds = 2
- Immediate = 3 (physician examination)

Double vision on lateral gaze, left or right

- 45 seconds = 0
- 11-45 seconds = 1
- 1-10 seconds = 3
- Immediate = 4 (physician examination)

Eye closure

- Normal = 0
- Mild weakness (can be forced open with effort) = 1
- Moderate weakness (can be forced open easily) = 2
- Severe weakness (unable to keep eye closed) = 3 (physician examination)

Talking

- Normal = 0 (patient history)
- Intermittent slurring or nasal speech = 2
- Constant slurring or nasal, but can be understood = 4
- Difficult to understand speech = 6

Chewing

- Normal = 0 (patient history)
- Fatigue with solid food = 2
- Fatigue with soft food = 4
- Gastric tube = 6 (patient history)

Swallowing

- Normal = 0 (patient history)
- Rare episode of choking or trouble swallowing = 2
- Frequent trouble swallowing, necessitating a change in diet = 5
- Gastric tube = 6 (patient history)

Breathing (thought to be caused by MG)

- Normal = 0
- Shortness of breath with exertion = 2
- Shortness of breath at rest = 4
- Ventilator dependence = 9

Neck flexion or extension (weakest)

- Normal = 0 (physician examination)
- Mild weakness (*i.e.*, ~50% weak, ±15%) = 3
- Moderate weakness = 4 (physician examination)
- Severe weakness = 5 (physician examination)

Shoulder abduction

- Normal = 0 (physician examination)
- Mild weakness (*i.e.*, ~50% weak, ±15%) = 2
- Moderate weakness = 4 (physician examination)
- Severe weakness = 5 (physician examination)

Hip flexion

- Normal = 0 (physician examination)
- Mild weakness (*i.e.*, ~50% weak, ±15%) = 2
- Moderate weakness = 4 (physician examination)
- Severe weakness = 5 (physician examination)

MYASTHENIA GRAVIS QUALITY OF LIFE 15-ITEMS REVISED (MG-QOL15R) [7-10]

Introduction

The Myasthenia Gravis Quality of Life 15-Items Revised (MG-QOL15r) is a validated scale designed to assess crucial aspects of a patient's experience with Myasthenia Gravis (MG). It serves as a modification of the MG-QOL15, with each of the 15 items scored on a scale of 0-2, resulting in a maximum score of 30 (compared to the MG-QOL15's maximum score of 60). The MG-QOL15r emphasizes the patient's self-report and aims to provide insights into physical, psychological, and social domains of well-being [7, 8].

ICF domain

Body Functions: Fatigue, Muscle weakness, speech, and swallowing difficulties

Activities and Participation: Mobility, self-care, social interaction

Number of Domains

- Physical Domain
- Psychosocial Domain
- Treatment Burden Domain

Procedures for Administration

Administration

Patients should be provided with the MG-QOL15r form along with instructions for self-completion. It is essential to remind patients to base their responses on the impact MG has had on their quality of life over the past 4 weeks.

Instructions

The form includes 15 questions related to how MG-related symptoms impact the patient's quality of life, as shown in Fig. (**1**). Patients are instructed to read each question, choose the answer that best describes the average impact of MG on their quality of life over the past 4 weeks, and circle the corresponding response. The patient is encouraged to consider good and bad days but to select the answer that best describes their average experience [8] (Fig. **1**).

MG-QOL15r Scale

Please indicate how true each statement has been (over the past 4 weeks).	**Not at all** **0**	**Somewhat** **1**	**Very much** **2**
1. I am frustrated by my MG			
2. I have trouble with my eyes because of my MG (e.g. double vision)			
3. I have trouble eating because of MG			
4. I have limited my social activity because of my MG			
4. My MG limits my ability to enjoy hobbies and fun activities			
6. I have trouble meeting the needs of my family because of my MG			
7. I have to make plans around my MG			
8. I am bothered by limitations in performing my work (include work at home) because of my MG			
9. I have difficulty speaking due to MG			
10. I have lost some personal independence because of my MG (*e.g.* driving, shopping, running errands)			
11. I am depressed about my MG			
12. I have trouble walking due to MG			
13. I have trouble getting around public places because of my MG			
14. I feel overwhelmed by my MG			
15. I have trouble performing my personal grooming needs due to MG			

Evaluator Signature: ______________________ Date: __________ Total MG-QOL15r score

Fig. (1). MG-QOL15r scale.

Equipment

The Myasthenia Gravis Quality of Life 15-Items Revised (MG-QOL15r) is a self-administered questionnaire designed to assess the impact of Myasthenia Gravis (MG) on an individual's quality of life.

Interpretability

MCID (Minimal Clinically Important Difference)

The MCID for the MG-QOL15r is 5 points, indicating a clinically meaningful difference in the patient's perceived quality of life [7].

SEM (Standard Error of Measurement)

The SEM for the MG-QOL15r is ±2.0 points, representing the expected range within which an individual's true score lies with 68% confidence [8].

MDC (Minimal Detectable Change)

The MDC for the MG-QOL15r is 6 points, suggesting that a change of 6 points or more is needed to confidently infer a real change in a patient's quality of life [7, 8].

Languages

Arabic [7]

French [8]

Hindi [9]

Persian [10]

Dutch [11]

Training Required

Healthcare professionals utilising the MG-QOL15r should be familiar with the administration process, patient interactions, and the interpretation of scores. Training includes understanding the patient's perspective and ensuring the patient's autonomy in completing the form [10].

Availability

The MG-QOL15r is readily available in clinical settings, and its self-report nature makes it suitable for routine patient assessments.

Clinical Considerations

The MG-QOL15r provides valuable insights into the patient's experience with MG, focusing on physical, psychological, and social aspects. Clinicians should consider the individualised nature of the responses when interpreting the scores [9].

Psychometric Properties [8 - 11]

Reliability

Internal consistency (Cronbach's alpha): 0.91

Test-Retest reliability (intraclass correlation coefficient): 0.88

Validity

Content validity is supported by the selection of items reflecting key domains. Construct validity is evidenced by significant correlations with related quality-of-life measures.

Responsiveness

The MG-QOL15r exhibits good responsiveness to changes in the patient's quality of life over time, making it a valuable tool for monitoring the impact of intervention.

Floor/Ceiling Effect

The MG-QOL15r shows minimal floor or ceiling effects, indicating its ability to capture a broad range of quality-of-life experiences among individuals with MG.

CLINICAL CONSIDERATIONS, STRENGTHS, LIMITATIONS, AND EMERGING TRENDS

Myasthenia gravis (MG) is a chronic autoimmune neuromuscular disorder characterised by fluctuating weakness, fatigability, and variable involvement of ocular, bulbar, respiratory, and limb muscles. The hallmark variability of symptoms within and across days makes assessment particularly challenging. Effective evaluation, therefore, requires tools that are sensitive to change, capture both objective impairment and patient experience, and are applicable across disease severities and treatment phases [12, 13].

Clinician-rated outcome measures such as the Myasthenia Gravis Composite (MGC) score and the Myasthenia Gravis Impairment Index (MGII) form the backbone of clinical and research assessment. The MGC integrates physician examination findings with selected patient-reported items, offering a balanced measure of disease severity that is responsive to clinical change. Its simplicity and weighting of clinically meaningful items have made it a preferred endpoint in therapeutic trials. However, the MGC may underrepresent patient-perceived fatigue and quality-of-life impact, particularly in patients with mild or predominantly ocular disease [14].

The MGII represents a more recent effort to comprehensively assess MG-related impairment by combining physical examination items with patient-reported symptom severity. Its strength lies in improved content validity and sensitivity across a broader range of disease manifestations, including bulbar and respiratory symptoms. Despite these advantages, the MGII requires more time to administer and score, which may limit its feasibility in busy clinical settings. Familiarity with the scale is also still evolving outside specialised neuromuscular centres [15].

Patient-reported outcome measures, particularly the Myasthenia Gravis Quality of Life 15-item revised scale (MG-QOL15r), capture the impact of MG on daily functioning, emotional well-being, and social participation. These instruments provide critical insight into domains that are often poorly correlated with physician-rated impairment. However, quality-of-life scores may be influenced by psychological adaptation, comorbid mood disorders, and external factors, necessitating cautious interpretation when used as standalone outcome measures [16].

A major limitation across MG assessment tools is the partial separation between impairment-based and patient-reported domains. While clinician-rated scales quantify weakness and fatigability, they may not fully reflect participation restrictions or treatment burden. Conversely, quality-of-life instruments do not directly measure neuromuscular function. Overlapping use of multiple tools without a clear framework can increase assessment burden without proportional clinical benefit. Purpose-driven selection of complementary measures is therefore essential [13, 17].

Emerging trends in MG assessment emphasise responsiveness, patient-centeredness, and integration with biomarkers. Recent clinical trials increasingly favour composite and patient-reported endpoints alongside traditional physician ratings. Digital symptom diaries and remote monitoring tools are being explored to better capture daily fluctuation and treatment response. In parallel, correlations between clinical scales, antibody status, and electrophysiological measures are being investigated to enhance prognostic accuracy and personalise therapy [18, 19].

In clinical practice, assessment strategies should be aligned with disease stage and therapeutic intent. The MGC is well-suited for routine severity grading and treatment monitoring, MGII provides a detailed assessment of impairment when a comprehensive evaluation is required, and MG-QOL15r offers essential insight into patient-perceived disease burden. An integrated but selective approach supports meaningful outcome assessment while minimising redundancy and administrative load (Table **2**).

Table 2. Comparative summary of commonly used myasthenia gravis assessment scales.

Scale	Primary Domain Assessed	Key Strengths	Major Limitations	Optimal Clinical Use
Myasthenia Gravis Composite (MGC)	Disease severity	Responsive; trial validated	Limited QoL capture	Clinical trials, routine monitoring
Myasthenia Gravis Impairment Index (MGII)	Impairment + symptoms	Comprehensive; sensitive	Time-consuming	Detailed clinical evaluation
MG-QOL15r	Quality of life	Patient-centered; brief	Subjective; no strength testing	Long-term follow-up
Antibody titers (adjunct)	Immunological activity	Biological correlation	Weak symptom correlation	Research adjunct

CONCLUSION

Accurate evaluation of the disease's severity, functional impairment, and quality of life is necessary for managing myasthenia gravis. Standardised measures such as the MGII, MGC, and MG-QOL15r provide reliable instruments for assessing psychosocial burden, patient experiences, and illness aspects. By incorporating these evaluations, patient-centred care, treatment effectiveness, and disease monitoring are all improved.

AI DISCLOSURE STATEMENT

During the preparation of this chapter, the authors used ChatGPT (OpenAI) as a support tool for language refinement, structural organisation, and clarification of ideas. All content generated with AI assistance was carefully reviewed, verified, and revised by the authors to ensure factual accuracy, originality, and consistency with the scientific literature. The authors take full responsibility for the integrity, interpretation, and final content of the published chapter.

ACKNOWLEDGEMENT

The authors sincerely acknowledge the invaluable contributions of neurologists, physiotherapists, and rehabilitation experts involved in the care and management of individuals with Myasthenia Gravis. Their dedication to improving assessment tools and refining outcome measures has greatly enhanced clinical understanding, guided more effective treatment decisions, and improved the quality of life for those living with this condition. The authors also appreciate the continued efforts of researchers and clinicians whose work inspires ongoing advancements in the field of neuromuscular rehabilitation.

REFERENCES

[1] Barnett C, Bril V, Kapral M, Kulkarni A, Davis AM. Development and validation of the Myasthenia Gravis Impairment Index. Neurology 2016; 87(9): 879-86. [http://dx.doi.org/10.1212/WNL.0000000000002971] [PMID: 27402891]

[2] Barnett C, Herbelin L, Dimachkie MM, Barohn RJ. Measuring clinical treatment response in myasthenia gravis. Neurol Clin 2018; 36(2): 339-53. [http://dx.doi.org/10.1016/j.ncl.2018.01.006] [PMID: 29655453]

[3] Pasqualin F, Barnett C, Guidoni SV, Albertini E, Ermani M, Bonifati DM. Validation of the Italian version of the Myasthenia Gravis Impairment Index (MGII). Neurol Sci 2022; 43(3): 2059-64. [http://dx.doi.org/10.1007/s10072-021-05585-5] [PMID: 34505205]

[4] Burns TM, Conaway M, Sanders DB, Sanders DB, Wolfe GI, Herrmann DN. The MG Composite. Neurology 2010; 74(18): 1434-40. [http://dx.doi.org/10.1212/WNL.0b013e3181dc1b1e] [PMID: 20439845]

[5] Barnett C, Merkies ISJ, Katzberg H, Bril V, Burns TM, Sanders DB. Psychometric Properties of the Quantitative Myasthenia Gravis Score and the Myasthenia Gravis Composite Scale. J Neuromuscul Dis 2015; 2(3): 301-11. [http://dx.doi.org/10.3233/JND-150082] [PMID: 27858737]

[6] Oliveira EF, Lima VC, Perez EA, *et al.* Brazilian-Portuguese translation, cross-cultural adaptation and validation of the Myasthenia Gravis Composite scale. A multicentric study. Arq Neuropsiquiatr 2016; 74(11): 914-20. [http://dx.doi.org/10.1590/0004-282x20160129] [PMID: 27901257]

[7] Alanazy MH, Abuzinadah AR, Muayqil T, Alharbi AA, Alghamdi FS, Alzahrani MS. Translation and validation of the arabic version of the revised 15-item myasthenia gravis quality-of-life questionnaire. Muscle Nerve 2018; 57(4): 581-5. [http://dx.doi.org/10.1002/mus.25948] [PMID: 28857210]

[8] Birnbaum S, Ghout I, Demeret S, *et al.* Translation, cross-cultural adaptation, and validation of the french version of the 15-item Myasthenia Gravis Quality Of life scale. Muscle Nerve 2017; 55(5): 639-45. [http://dx.doi.org/10.1002/mus.25381] [PMID: 27533497]

[9] Majigoudra G, Duggal AK, Chowdhury D, Koul A, Todi VK, Roshan S. Clinical profile and quality of life in myasthenia gravis using MGQOL15R (Hindi): An Indian perspective. Ann Indian Acad Neurol 2023; 26(4): 441-6. [http://dx.doi.org/10.4103/aian.aian_945_22] [PMID: 37970285]

[10] Ostovan VR, Fatehi F, Davoudi F, Nafissi S, Zamani B, Niknam R. Validation of the 15-item myasthenia gravis quality of life questionnaire (MG-QOL15) Persian version. Muscle Nerve 2016; 54(1): 65-70.
[http://dx.doi.org/10.1002/mus.25002] [PMID: 26661455]

[11] Strijbos E, Gärtner FR, Verschuuren JJ, van der Meulen MF, Westra J, Bril V. Translation and validation of the 15-item Myasthenia Gravis Quality of life scale in Dutch. Muscle Nerve 2018; 57(2): 206-11.
[http://dx.doi.org/10.1002/mus.25641] [PMID: 28271514]

[12] Gilhus NE, Tzartos S, Evoli A, Palace J, Burns TM, Verschuuren JJGM. Myasthenia gravis. Nat Rev Dis Primers 2019; 5(1): 30.
[http://dx.doi.org/10.1038/s41572-019-0079-y] [PMID: 31048702]

[13] Narayanaswami P, Sanders DB, Wolfe G, *et al.* International consensus guidance for management of myasthenia gravis: 2020 update. Neurology 2021; 96(3): 114-22.
[http://dx.doi.org/10.1212/WNL.0000000000011124] [PMID: 33144515]

[14] Burns TM, Conaway MR, Cutter GR, Sanders DB. Construction of an efficient evaluative instrument for myasthenia gravis: The mg composite. Muscle Nerve 2008; 38(6): 1553-62.
[http://dx.doi.org/10.1002/mus.21185] [PMID: 19016543]

[15] Meisel A, Saccà F, Spillane J, Vissing J. Expert consensus recommendations for improving and standardising the assessment of patients with generalised myasthenia gravis. Eur J Neurol 2024; 31(7): e16280.
[http://dx.doi.org/10.1111/ene.16280] [PMID: 38523419]

[16] Burns TM, Sadjadi R, Utsugisawa K, *et al.* International clinimetric evaluation of the MG-QOL15, resulting in slight revision and subsequent validation of the MG-QOL15r. Muscle Nerve 2016; 54(6): 1015-22.
[http://dx.doi.org/10.1002/mus.25198] [PMID: 27220659]

[17] Majigoudra G, Duggal AK, Chowdhury D, Koul A, Todi VK, Roshan S. Clinical profile and quality of life in myasthenia gravis using mgqol15 r(hindi): An indian perspective. Ann Indian Acad Neurol 2023; 26(4): 441-6.
[http://dx.doi.org/10.4103/aian.aian_945_22] [PMID: 37970285]

[18] Muppidi S, Wolfe GI, Conaway M, Burns TM, Mezei MM, Cutter GR. MG-ADL: Still a relevant outcome measure. Muscle Nerve 2011; 44(5): 727-31.
[http://dx.doi.org/10.1002/mus.22140] [PMID: 22006686]

[19] Diez Porras L, Homedes C, Alberti M A, Velez Santamaria V, Casasnovas C. Quality of life in myasthenia gravis and correlation of mg-qol15 with other functional scales. J Clin Med 2022; 11(8): 2189.
[http://dx.doi.org/10.3390/jcm11082189] [PMID: 35456281]

CHAPTER 14

Scales for Cognition

Bhumika Kashyap[1] and **Manpreet Kaur**[2,3,*]

[1] *Maharishi Markandeshwar Institute of Physiotherapy and Rehabilitation, Maharishi Markandeshwar (Deemed to be University), Mullana, Ambala, Haryana, India*

[2] *Department of Physiotherapy, University Institute of Allied Health Sciences College, Chandigarh University, Mohali, Punjab, India*

[3] *Department of Physiotherapy, Mody University of Science and Technology, Lakshmangarh (Sikar), Rajasthan, India*

Abstract: This chapter provides an overview of widely used cognitive assessment tools, with emphasis on their clinical application, target populations, psychometric strengths, and ease of use. It reviews the Mini-Mental State Examination (MMSE), Montreal Cognitive Assessment (MoCA), Saint Louis University Mental Status Examination (SLUMS), Mini-Cog, Rowland Universal Dementia Assessment Scale (RUDAS), Cognitive Assessment of Stroke Patients (CASP), and the Parkinson's Disease–Cognitive Rating Scale (PD-CRS). Each instrument is described in terms of purpose, administration, scoring, and reliability, highlighting its applicability across neurological and geriatric populations, such as dementia, stroke, Parkinson's disease, and other neurocognitive disorders. The chapter aims to guide clinicians and researchers in selecting the most appropriate cognitive screening tool for different patient groups.

Keywords: Cognition, Cognitive screening, Dementia, Neurocognitive disorders, Parkinson's disease, Psychometric properties, Stroke.

INTRODUCTION

Cognition refers to the dynamic interactions among neurons, astrocytes (the predominant type of glial cells), and other supportive cells such as microglia within the central nervous system. These neural connections are continuously shaped by an individual's engagement with their environment, influencing how information is processed and applied in daily life [1].

* **Corresponding author Manpreet Kaur:** Department of Physiotherapy, University Institute of Allied Health Sciences College, Chandigarh University, Mohali, Punjab, India; E-mail: priyuarora8427@gmail.com

Nidhi Sharma, Simranjeet Kaur & Parveen Kumar (Eds.)

Cognitive functioning spans a broad spectrum of higher-order skills, including executive abilities (planning, organizing, problem-solving, and judgment), attentional control, memory, processing speed, language, decision-making, and psychomotor coordination [1].

Memory itself is multifaceted, comprising declarative, episodic, semantic, procedural, prospective, verbal, and visual components, each supported by distinct neural circuits. When these circuits are disrupted by disease or injury, specific aspects of cognition may be impaired. Evidence from epidemiological and clinical studies shows that chronic conditions such as hypertension, cardiovascular disease, and diabetes mellitus adversely affect cerebral function, leading to measurable declines in cognition [2]. For instance, hypertension-related white matter lesions often compromise frontal lobe integrity, resulting in diminished executive function and slower reasoning capacity [3]. Such impairments can also disturb emotional regulation, leading to difficulties with impulse control, frustration tolerance, and adaptive problem-solving.

Cognitive decline can present as subtle, temporary deficits or as more severe, progressive impairments that interfere with independence and quality of life. A comprehensive neuropsychological evaluation is therefore essential, enabling clinicians to detect early signs of dementia, Alzheimer's disease, or mild cognitive impairment. Effective assessment must explore multiple domains—memory, language, abstract reasoning, attention, visuospatial ability, and processing speed—while also considering patient history and clinical examination findings [4]. Because individuals with cognitive deficits often struggle to accurately describe their difficulties, input from caregivers or family members can provide critical insight into functional abilities.

In clinical and research settings, practitioners rely on validated screening instruments to identify cognitive impairment. Widely used tools include the Mini-Mental State Examination (MMSE) and the Montreal Cognitive Assessment (MoCA), both of which offer rapid and reliable evaluation of multiple cognitive domains [5, 6]. These brief instruments remain central to routine practice, though alternative measures are available to address specific populations or contexts, ensuring that clinicians select the most appropriate tool for both the patient and the administrator [7].

SCALES AND QUESTIONNAIRES TO ASSESS COGNITION

Mini-Mental State Examination (MMSE)

Description

The Mini-Mental State Examination (MMSE) is one of the most widely adopted tools for assessing global cognition in clinical and research contexts. It evaluates multiple domains, such as orientation, registration, attention, recall, language, and visuospatial construction, with a maximum score of 30, exhibiting normal cognition [2].

The tool consists of 11 questions under 7 domains. The 7 cognitive domains covered under the MMSE are orientation to time, orientation to place, registration of 3 words, attention and calculation, recall of 3 words, language, and visual construction. The administrator asks or describes the questions to the patient and scores are given based on the answers and performance of the patient. Administration typically requires 5–10 minutes, making it practical for routine use [2].

Materials and preparation

- Plain paper and pen/pencil.
- A quiet, well-lit room free of distractions.
- A watch/pen (for naming stimuli) and a simple drawing stimulus (two intersecting pentagons or equivalent).
- Record sheet or form to score items immediately.
- Ensure patient has sensory aids (glasses, hearing aid) if needed.

Before starting, explain briefly: “I’m going to ask you some questions and have you do a few short tasks that help us understand how your thinking and memory are doing.” Confirm patient’s ability to hear/see and obtain verbal consent.

Intended Population

1. Brain Injury
2. Dementia
3. Stroke
4. Alzheimer’s Disease
5. Parkinson’s Disease
6. Older adults and the geriatric population

Administration [3]

a. Orientation — Time (5 points)

Ask the patient the current year, season, date, day of the week, and month. Scoring: 1 point for each correct answer (max 5).

b. Orientation — Place (5 points)

Ask: Which country, which state/province, which city/town, what building (or hospital/clinic name), and which floor/ward/room.

Scoring: 1 point each (max 5).

c. Registration (3 points)

Name three unrelated common objects clearly and slowly (*e.g.*, "apple — table — penny" or the stimuli you prefer). Ask the patient to repeat them immediately. Scoring: 1 point per correctly repeated word (max 3). If the patient cannot repeat after one presentation, do not repeat more than twice — note how many trials were required.

d. Attention and Calculation (5 points)

Administer one of the standard attention tests:

- **Serial sevens**: Ask the patient to subtract 7 from 100 and continue subtracting 7 for five answers (100, 93, 86, 79, 72). Score 1 point for each correct subtraction (max 5).
- **Alternative (if low education or difficulty with arithmetic):** Ask the patient to spell the word "WORLD" backwards. Score 1 point for each letter in correct reverse order (W-O-R-L-D → D-L-R-O-W). Use the alternative when serial sevens would be inappropriate [2].

e. Recall (3 points) - Ask the patient to recall the three words given in the registration task.Score 1 point per word correctly recalled (max 3).

f. Language (8 points total; several sub-tasks)

i. **Naming (2 points)** — Show two common objects (*e.g.*, watch, pen) and ask the patient to name them. 1 point each.
ii. **Repetition (1 point)** — Ask the patient to repeat a short phrase (single simple sentence). 1 point if repeated verbatim.

iii. **Three-stage command (3 points)** — Give a three-part command (*e.g.*, "Take this paper in your right hand, fold it in half, and put it on the floor") and ask the patient to carry it out. Score 1 point per correctly completed element (max 3).
iv. **Reading (1 point)** — Give a written instruction such as "Close your eyes" and ask the patient to read and follow it. 1 point if obeyed.
v. **Writing (1 point)** — Ask the patient to write a sentence of their own. Score 1 point for a meaningful sentence with a subject and verb.

g. Visuospatial / Construction (1 point) - Ask the patient to copy a simple figure (traditionally two intersecting pentagons) (Fig. **1**). Score 1 point if the copy is correct (proportions and intersections preserved).

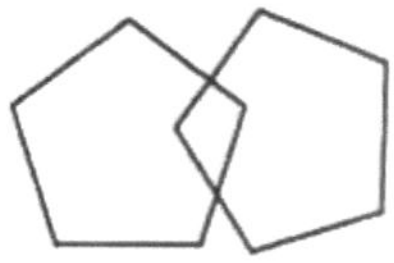

Fig. (1). Visuospatial construction.

Scoring summary [3]

- Orientation to time = 5
- Orientation to place = 5
- Registration = 3
- Attention/calculation = 5
- Recall = 3
- Language = 8
- Visuospatial = 1

Total possible = 30

Common Cut-offs and Interpretation

- A commonly used threshold: **≤23/30** suggests possible cognitive impairment and warrants further assessment [3].
- Some clinicians use more graded categories (examples used in some settings): ≥27 = normal, 21–26 = mild impairment, 11–20 = moderate impairment, ≤10 = severe impairment; however, cutoffs vary by age, education, and clinical purpose, and should be interpreted in context [3].
- **Important:** MMSE is relatively insensitive to very mild cognitive impairment (MCI) and to isolated executive dysfunction; consider MoCA or domain-specific testing when MCI is suspected [4].

Psychometric Properties [2, 4]

- Test–retest reliability and inter-rater reliability are generally high in validation studies (test–retest r ≈ 0.89–0.95; inter-rater r ≈ 0.93–0.99) [2].
- Sensitivity/specificity vary by population and chosen cutoff; systematic reviews report good accuracy for dementia screening but lower sensitivity for MCI [4].

Strengths

- Brief (5–15 minutes), widely known, easy to administer and score.
- Good utility for tracking longitudinal change when the same version and method are used.
- A large body of normative and clinical data for many populations.

Limitations and Cautions

- Affected by **education, language, and cultural background**; people with low education or non-native language speakers may score lower for reasons unrelated to true cognitive decline. Adjust interpretation accordingly [4].
- Poor sensitivity for mild impairments (executive dysfunction, early Alzheimer's pathology) — MoCA is often preferred when MCI is a concern [4].
- Tasks requiring language, writing, or motor skills can be confounded by aphasia, dysgraphia, or visual or motor disability. In such cases, use alternative or adapted instruments (CASP for aphasic stroke patients, RUDAS for multicultural populations, etc.) [4].

THE MONTREAL COGNITIVE ASSESSMENT (MOCA)

Description

The Montreal Cognitive Assessment (MoCA) was developed to improve sensitivity in detecting **mild cognitive impairment (MCI)** compared with the MMSE. While the MMSE performs well for moderate-to-severe dementia, it often fails to capture subtle deficits in executive and visuospatial functioning. The MoCA was specifically designed to address this limitation, providing a broader and more challenging range of tasks [5, 6].

MoCA includes various items under 8 domains that assess cognition. The domains under MoCA are visuospatial/executive, naming, memory, attention, language, abstraction, delayed recall, and orientation. It is a clinician-based evaluation tool, so proper expertise is required [7].

Intended Population

1. Stroke
2. Brain Injury
3. Parkinson's Disease
4. Alzheimer's Disease
5. Non-specific patient population
6. Neuromuscular Conditions
7. Older adults and geriatric patients

Administration

The MoCA is a 30-point, clinician-administered tool that requires approximately 10 minutes to complete [7]. It includes items spanning eight cognitive domains:

a. **Visuospatial/Executive (5 points):** Includes trail-making, cylinder drawing, and clock drawing (Figs. **2a-2c**).
b. **Naming (3 points):** Naming domain includes identification of three animals (Fig. **3**).
c. **Memory (5 points):** Learning and delayed recall of five words (fact, velvet, church, daisy, red) across two trials, and a recall after 5 minutes.
d. **Attention (6 points):** Digit span (forward and backward), vigilance tasks, and serial subtraction:
   - Read a list of digits/ numbers (*e.g.*: 21854) at a speed of 1 digit per second. The subject has to repeat them in the forward and backward order.
   - Read a list of numbers, the subject must tap with their hand at each specific number (*e.g.*, 1) (list of numbers: 52139411806215194511141905112). No points are given if more than 2 errors are made.
   - Subtract 7 starting from 100 (*e.g.*, 100, 93, 86, 79, 72, 65). 4 or 5 correct subtractions: 3 points, 2 or 3 correct subtractions: 2 points, 1 correct subtraction: 1 point, and no correct subtraction: 0 points.

e. **Language (3 points):** Sentence repetition and verbal fluency tasks:
f. **Abstraction (2 points):** Identifying similarities between objects (*e.g.*, banana and orange).
g. **Delayed Recall (5 points):** Recall of previously presented words, with cues if necessary. The patient has to recall the 5 words given to them earlier in the memory domain.
h. **Orientation (6 points):** Date, month, year, day, place, and city.

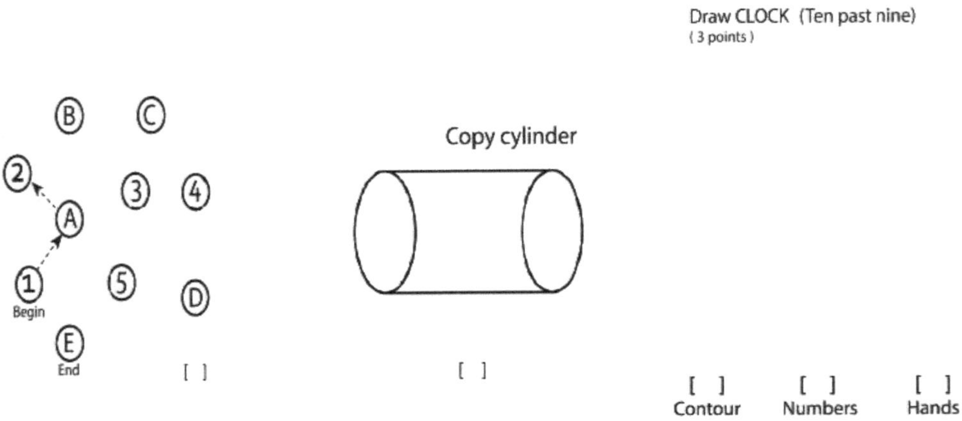

Fig. (2). (**a**) Trail-making test, (**b**) Cylinder drawing test, (**c**) Clock drawing test.

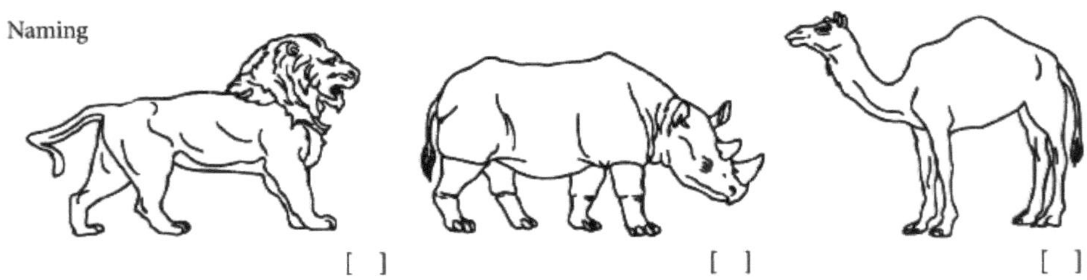

Fig. (3). Images of three different animals.

Scoring and Interpretation

MoCA scores range from 0 to 30 and are based on completing the tasks included in the scale. Score 0 indicates a poor cognitive level, and 30 indicates a high cognitive level [8].

Psychometric Properties

The MoCA demonstrates excellent internal consistency (Cronbach's α = 0.83–0.90) and high test–retest reliability (r = 0.80–0.90). Inter-rater reliability is also strong (ICC = 0.95–0.98) [6]. Compared with MMSE, MoCA shows superior sensitivity in detecting MCI and early Alzheimer's disease, with several studies reporting sensitivity >90% at the 26-point cutoff [6].

Strengths and Limitations

The MoCA is widely recognized for its ability to detect early cognitive decline across multiple conditions, including dementia, Parkinson's disease, cerebrovascular disease, and neuromuscular disorders [7]. Its comprehensive nature ensures that deficits in executive function and visuospatial skills are not overlooked. However, limitations include its reliance on literacy (*e.g.*, reading and writing tasks) and the need for trained administration. Furthermore, cultural and language adaptations are necessary to ensure validity in diverse populations, though validated translations exist in more than 40 languages [8].

SAINT LOUIS UNIVERSITY MENTAL STATUS EXAMINATION (SLUMS)

Description

The Saint Louis University Mental Status Examination (SLUMS) was introduced as an alternative screening tool to overcome limitations of the MMSE, particularly its insensitivity to mild neurocognitive deficits. SLUMS includes more challenging items that assess executive function, logical reasoning, and problem-solving, making it particularly effective for identifying **mild cognitive impairment (MCI)** [9].

Intended Population

1. Dementia
2. Alzheimer's Disease
3. Non-specific patient population
4. Older adults and the geriatric care population

Administration

SLUMS is a 30-point instrument clinician-administered outcome measure based on the interview mode. It takes about 5-10 minutes to complete. It involves 11 questions assessing attention and working memory, cognition, executive functioning, language, mental health, reasoning, and problem-solving. The domains, questions, and scoring are explained in Table **1**.

Table 1. Saint Louis University Mental Status examination (SLUMS).

Domain	Item / Question	Score Range	Patient Score
Orientation (3 pts.)	1. What day of the week is it? 2. What is the year? 3. What state are we in?	0–3	
Short-term Memory (5 pts.)	Immediate recall: Remember 5 objects (Apple, pen, tie, house, car) Delayed recall: Name the 5 objects again (1 pt. each)	0–5	

(Table 1) cont.....

Domain	Item / Question	Score Range	Patient Score
	Story recall: "Jill was a very successful stockbroker. She made a lot of money on the stock market. She then met Jack, a devastatingly handsome man. She married him and had three children. They lived in Chicago. She then stopped working and stayed at home to bring up her children. When they were teenagers, she went back to work.She and Jack lived happily ever after." Questions: Name of female? When back to work? What work? What state?	0–4	
Attention (3 pts.)	1. You have $100 – buy apples ($3) and a tricycle ($20). How much was spent? How much is left? 2. I am going to give you a series of numbers, and I would like you to give them to me backwards. For example, if I say 42, you would say 24. • Examples: 087, 1648, 08537	0–3	
Executive Function (5 pts.)	1. Problem-solving or reasoning (patterns, logic) 2. Place an X in the triangle and identify the largest shape (Fig. **4**)	0–5	
Language (6 pts.)	1. Name as many animals as possible in 1 minute. Scoring: 0–4 animals = 0; 5–9 animals = 1; 10–14 animals = 2; 15+ animals = 3 pts. 2. Sentence repetition/comprehension tasks	0–6	
Visuospatial (2 pts.)	Draw a clock (Fig. **5**). Place numbers correctly and show time at 10:50. (1 pt. for correct numbers, 1 pt. for the correct time)	0–2	
Other Cognitive Tasks (6 pts.)	Recognition, abstraction, and working memory (*e.g.*, shape identification, similarities, conceptual tasks)	0–6	
TOTAL		**0–30**	

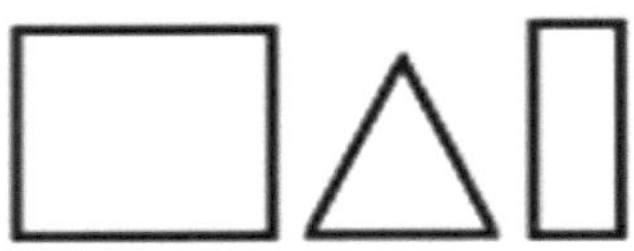

Fig. (4). Different shapes.

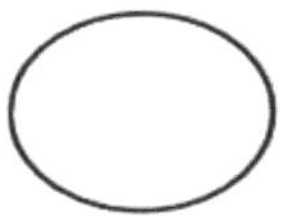

Fig. (5). Circle for drawing a clock.

Scoring and Interpretation

Unlike the MMSE and MoCA, the SLUMS scoring system accounts for **educational background**. Cutoffs vary by education level:

1. **High school education or above:** 27–30 = normal, 21–26 = mild neurocognitive disorder, 1–20 = dementia.
2. **Less than high school education:** 25–30 = normal, 20–24 = mild neurocognitive disorder, 1–19 = dementia [10].

This adjustment reduces the bias associated with formal education and provides more accurate categorization across diverse populations.

Psychometric Properties

Studies demonstrate that SLUMS has high sensitivity for detecting MCI, often outperforming the MMSE. In one validation, SLUMS correctly identified 93% of individuals with MCI compared to 71% for MMSE [10]. Reliability indices are also strong, with inter-rater reliability coefficients exceeding 0.90 [10].

Strengths and Limitations

The SLUMS offers a good balance between brevity and sensitivity. Its inclusion of story recall and logical reasoning items makes it superior in detecting early deficits that may be missed by MMSE. The education-adjusted scoring system enhances fairness across populations with different academic exposure. However, like MoCA, it requires a moderate literacy level and may still be influenced by cultural and linguistic differences. Moreover, while sensitivity for MCI is high, specificity is somewhat lower, and false positives may occur in individuals with limited education or low baseline intellectual function [10].

MINI-COG SCALE

The Mini-Cog is a brief cognitive screening tool designed to rapidly identify possible dementia in primary care and community settings. It combines a simple recall task with a clock-drawing test, making it less influenced by education and language compared to longer instruments such as the MMSE or MoCA [11].

Description

Mini-Cog consists of three-word registration, a clock drawing test, and three-word recall. It takes only three minutes to administer, making it suitable for use in a primary care setting [11, 12].

Intended Population

1. Patients with dementia
2. Older adults, especially in primary care, outpatient clinics, and community health settings, where time is limited, and a quick, reliable tool is needed..
3. Population with low literacy or limited formal education, where traditional screening tools may be less appropriate [11].

Administration

The test includes two core tasks:

1. **Three-Word Recall (3 points):** The examiner presents three unrelated words and asks the individual to repeat them to confirm registration. After a brief interval, the participant is asked to recall the words.

(Version 1: Banana, Leader, Village) (Version 2: River, Captain, Daughter) (Version 3: Sunrise, Season, Kitchen) (Version 4: Nation, Garden, Heaven)

2. **Clock Drawing Test (2 points):** The participant is instructed to draw a clock, place numbers correctly, and set the hands to a specific time (commonly "10 past 11"). Use a pre-printed circle from Fig. (**5**).

The entire test typically takes **3–4 minutes** to administer [12].

Scoring and Interpretation

- **Word Recall = 0:** Dementia suspected.
- **Word Recall = 1–2 + Abnormal Clock:** Dementia suspected.
- **Word Recall = 1–2 + Normal Clock:** Dementia less likely.
- **Word Recall = 3:** Dementia unlikely, regardless of clock result.

Total Score Range: 0–5.

- 0–2 = Possible cognitive impairment
- 3–5 = Likely normal cognition [12].

Psychometric Properties

The Mini-Cog has demonstrated high diagnostic accuracy across different populations, with sensitivity ranging from **76–99%** and specificity from **89–93%** [11]. Test–retest reliability and inter-rater reliability are both excellent (>0.90), and studies suggest it performs as well as or better than the MMSE in detecting dementia. However, while its brevity enhances practicality, it is less sensitive to mild cognitive impairment compared to MoCA or SLUMS. Additionally, subjective scoring of the clock-drawing task may introduce variability between examiners [11, 12].

Strengths and Limitations

The Mini-Cog is highly efficient (completion time 3–4 minutes), requires no formal training, and is easily understood even by individuals with limited education. It also reduces cultural and language bias by relying on simple tasks. However, it is **less sensitive** to mild cognitive impairment compared to MoCA and SLUMS. In addition, the interpretation of the clock drawing can sometimes be subjective, leading to variability between examiners [12].

ROWLAND UNIVERSAL DEMENTIA ASSESSMENT SCALE (RUDAS)

Description

The Rowland Universal Dementia Assessment Scale (RUDAS) was developed to provide a cognitive screening tool that minimizes the influence of culture, language, and educational level. It was specifically designed for use in multicultural populations where traditional instruments such as the MMSE or MoCA may not be valid due to linguistic or cultural bias [13].

Intended Population

RUDAS is particularly suited for older adults from culturally and linguistically diverse (CALD) backgrounds, including individuals with limited literacy or non-native speakers of the dominant language. It is widely used in multicultural communities and is recommended for patients where education and cultural background may confound results on standard cognitive tests [13].

Administration

RUDAS consists of six subtests and can typically be administered in about 10 minutes:

a. **Memory:** The examiner presents a short grocery list (usually three items) and asks the patient to repeat it across three trials to ensure learning. After a delay of 5–10 minutes, the patient is asked to recall the items.
b. **Body Orientation:** The patient responds to five commands involving recognition of body parts, such as pointing to the right hand, identifying the left foot, or touching the right shoulder with the left hand. One point is awarded for each correct response (maximum = 5).

c. **Praxis:** The examiner demonstrates a motor action (*e.g.*, making a fist) and asks the patient to imitate it (Table **2**). Scoring reflects accuracy and fluency: 2 points for minimal errors (Normal score), 1 point for noticeable errors (Partially adequate), and 0 if the task cannot be performed (Score as Failed).

Table 2. Scoring of praxis.

Score	Fist/ Palm Integrity	No. of Errors	Fluency	Ability to Self-Correct	Progressive Improvement	Synchrony
Normal	Good adherence to 'palm down' and 'fist' actions with few intrusions or incorrect variations	Minimal	Good	Good	Evident	Only a very slight lack of synchrony
Partially adequate	Obvious intrusions and incorrect variations in 'palm down' and 'fist' actions	Noticeable	Some attempts to maintain	Some attempt	Some indication	There may be a noticeable lack of synchrony
Failed	Barely able to identify the correct 'palm down' and 'fist' actions because of many intrusions and incorrect variations	Many	Poor or none	None	Very little or none	Little or no synchrony

a. **Visuoconstructional Drawing:** The patient is shown a cube (Fig. **6**) and asked to reproduce it. One point is awarded for each of the following: drawing based on a square, inclusion of all internal lines, and inclusion of all external lines (maximum = 3).
b. **Judgment:** The patient is presented with a scenario about crossing a busy street without pedestrian signals and asked to explain how they would look for traffic and whether they would make any additional safety proposals. Scoring awards 2 points for spontaneously mentioning key safety strategies (*e.g.*, looking for traffic), 1 point if given after prompting, and 0 if omitted.
c. **Language:** Naming and comprehension tasks are included, along with verbal fluency measures (not detailed here, but part of the complete battery).

The total possible score is **30**.

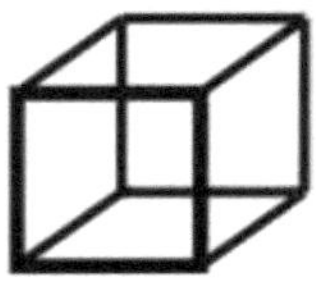

Fig. (6). A cube.

Scoring and Interpretation

A total score below 23 generally indicates possible cognitive impairment, though some studies suggest slightly higher cutoffs (*e.g.*, <25) depending on the characteristics of the population being tested [13, 14]. Due to its design, RUDAS avoids the education-related biases present in the MMSE or MoCA, thereby improving diagnostic accuracy across diverse settings.

Psychometric Properties

RUDAS has demonstrated strong psychometric reliability and validity in multiple studies. Reported sensitivity ranges from 77–89% and specificity from 82–91%, depending on the cutoff used. Both inter-rater and test–retest reliability are high (≥0.85), supporting its consistent use across different settings [13, 14].

Strengths and Limitations

RUDAS offers several strengths, including its reduced dependence on language and literacy, short administration time, and successful validation across culturally diverse populations. These features make it particularly well-suited for use in multicultural and low-resource settings [13]. However, it is not as widely recognized as MMSE or MoCA, which can limit its adoption in some health systems. Its sensitivity for mild cognitive impairment is somewhat lower than that of MoCA, which may result in missed early cases. In addition, accurate administration requires familiarity with culturally adapted versions of the test, which are not always available [14].

COGNITIVE ASSESSMENT OF STROKE PATIENTS (CASP)

Description

The Cognitive Assessment of Stroke Patients (CASP) was specifically developed to evaluate cognition in individuals with aphasia or other communication difficulties after stroke. Traditional screening tools, such as the MMSE or MoCA, rely heavily on language, making them unsuitable for patients with expressive or receptive language deficits. CASP reduces linguistic demands by incorporating tasks that rely more on visual, gestural, and nonverbal responses [15].

Intended Population

CASP is intended for stroke survivors, particularly those with aphasia or dysarthria, where standard cognitive tests may underestimate abilities due to speech limitations. It is most useful in rehabilitation and neurology settings, where accurate assessment of preserved and impaired domains is critical for therapy planning [16].

Administration — Domains (Step-by-step)

CASP is organized into specific subtests; each is administered with simple, scripted instructions and scored as indicated below. The full-scale totals **36 points** [15].

1. **Naming (3 points)**
   - Procedure: Show a set of pictures (line drawings). Ask the patient to name each image (*e.g.*, watch, spoon, butterfly). Use the exact wording: "I will show you images. Tell me what you see."
   - Scoring: Award ½ point per correct item as per the test form until the subtest total of 3 points is reached. Score immediately and record responses verbatim for qualitative interpretation.
2. **Comprehension (3 points)**
   - Procedure: Place a pen, phone, and sheet of paper in a vertical column on the table, and give a sequence of simple commands (*e.g.*, "Touch the pen," "Show me your nose," "Place the pen next to the phone," "Show me your knees," "Put the phone on the sheet of paper — don't touch the pen," "Show me your stomach").
   - Scoring: Each correctly executed action = ½ point (total possible = 3). Allow a single clear demonstration if the patient fails due to misunderstanding; document prompts used.
3. **Reproducing a Copy of a Cube (4 points)**
   - Procedure: Show the patient a three-dimensional cube drawing and ask them to draw an identical cube next to it.
   - Scoring: Up to 4 points: award 4 points if the three visible sides are reproduced and angles are preserved; otherwise, give 1 point per accurately reproduced side (0 if not recognisable).
4. **Graphic Series (2 points)**
   - Procedure: Present a short alternating pattern (*e.g.*, triangle, X, triangle, X…) and ask the patient to continue the series to the end of the row.
   - Scoring: 1 point per correctly executed suite (the test usually requires 10 correct alternations); award 0 if the suite is not completed correctly. Maximum = 2 points.
5. **Inhibition / Flexibility (4 points)**
   - Procedure: Use a paced motor inhibition/flexibility task (for example, the examiner taps once or twice, and the patient must respond with the alternate pattern — *i.e.*, when the clinician taps once, the patient taps twice, and vice

versa). This task tests inhibitory control and cognitive flexibility.
   - Scoring: Points assigned according to the number of correct sequences and error rate (structured on the test sheet); maximum = 4 points. Partial credit is given for partially correct sequences. This item detects perseveration and set-shifting impairment, common after frontal or subcortical strokes.
6. **Bisection of a Horizontal Line (2 points)**
   - Procedure: Present a single horizontal line on a sheet and ask the patient to mark the midpoint.
   - Scoring: If the bisection is reasonably centered, the patient receives full credit (2 points); marked deviations consistent with neglect or visuospatial bias reduce the score (per the manual's scoring rules). This item screens for unilateral visuospatial neglect.
7. **Image Recall (6 points)**
   - Procedure: During the naming subtest, the patient views a set of pictures; later (after intervening tasks), present a larger array of the same pictures mixed with distractors and ask the patient to identify previously seen images.
   - Scoring: Award points for correct recognition of each target image; the total for this module = 6 points. This format reduces verbal demands while assessing episodic memory/recognition.
8. **Praxis (6 points)**
   - Procedure: Examiner performs a sequence of meaningful gestures and asks the patient to imitate them (*e.g.*, show how to blow a kiss, make a fist, show a salute). Also includes pantomime for tool use.
   - Scoring: Each correctly imitated action is scored; the praxis module emphasizes motor planning and action understanding. Total = 6 points; partial credit may be given for approximations. Detailed scoring considers fluency, number of errors, and ability to self-correct.
9. **Calendar or Temporal Orientation (2 points)***(some CASP forms allocate 6 points to a related orientation/temporal task — check the local CASP version)*
   - Procedure: Ask the patient to identify the current day, date, month, and year using a calendar stimulus or direct questions.
   - Scoring: Points allocated per correct element (the standard CASP form distributes points so that the overall instrument sums to 36). Verify the local test form to assign the precise per-item points.

   Note: The exact ordering and the small scoring conventions (*e.g.*, whether naming uses ½-point increments) are taken from the official CASP form; examiners should follow their version's scoring sheet to ensure compatibility with published norms.

Scoring and Interpretation

- **Total score range:** 0–36 (higher = better cognitive function).
- **Interpretation:** Compare the patient's score with published norms or local validation samples; substantial deviation below the expected range for age and education indicates post-stroke cognitive impairment. Because CASP emphasizes nonverbal tasks, it often identifies cognitive deficits in patients whom language-based tests would falsely classify as severely impaired due to aphasia [15]. Use domain sub-scores to identify specific targets for rehabilitation (*e.g.*, praxis vs. visuospatial neglect vs. memory).

Psychometric Properties

Validation studies report good internal consistency and strong inter-rater reliability for CASP. The instrument correlates well with comprehensive neuropsychological batteries while providing the advantage of being usable in aphasic patients. Local validation studies (including Chinese-language samples) have demonstrated acceptable construct validity and sensitivity for post-stroke cognitive deficits; refer to those local norms when interpreting raw totals [15].

Strengths and Limitations

CASP's principal strength is its design for stroke populations with language impairment: by prioritizing visual, recognition, imitation, and performance-based tasks, it offers a fairer appraisal of cognitive function in people with aphasia or dysarthria. The scale provides domain-level information useful for tailoring rehabilitation and surprisingly good psychometric properties when compared with more language-dependent batteries. Limitations include a longer administration time than ultra-brief screens (often 20–30 minutes when fully administered), the need for the specific stimulus materials and scored sheets, and the requirement that examiners be trained in its scoring conventions to ensure reliable results. Finally, while CASP is well-suited to stroke clinics, its generalizability outside stroke populations is limited, and normative data vary by language and region, so local validation is recommended before clinical decision-making [15, 16].

PARKINSON'S DISEASE-COGNITIVE RATING SCALE (PD-CRS)

Description

The Parkinson's Disease–Cognitive Rating Scale (PD-CRS) was developed as a disease-specific instrument to assess both subcortical and cortical cognitive domains in patients with Parkinson's disease (PD). Unlike general screening tools such as the MMSE or MoCA, PD-CRS is tailored to capture the unique pattern of cognitive decline in PD, which often begins with deficits in executive and visuospatial abilities before progressing to cortical impairments such as memory and language [17].

Intended Population

The PD-CRS is specifically intended for use in patients with Parkinson's Disease, across all stages of the illness. It is valuable for detecting mild cognitive impairment (PD-MCI) and Parkinson's Disease Dementia (PDD), making it useful in both clinical practice and research. It is particularly helpful in monitoring cognitive changes over time in individuals undergoing pharmacological or non-pharmacological interventions [18].

Administration

The PD-CRS is a structured instrument designed to assess both subcortical and cortical cognitive functions in Parkinson's disease. It provides a balanced evaluation of executive, attentional, memory, language, and visuospatial domains. The scale is divided into two sections: the frontal-subcortical domain (seven tasks, maximum 104 points) and the posterior cortical domain (two tasks, maximum 30 points), with a total score of 134. This separation not only quantifies the overall cognitive burden but also highlights specific patterns of impairment, which are clinically useful in differentiating mild cognitive changes from dementia associated with Parkinson's disease [17, 18].

The PD-CRS comprises nine tasks, grouped into two domains. Administration usually takes 15-20 minutes.

a. Frontal-Subcortical Domain (7 tasks, max = 104)

i. Sustained Attention (max = 10)

This task evaluates the patient's ability to remain vigilant over a sequence of stimuli. The examiner presents short strings of letters or numbers and asks the patient to identify how many times a specific target occurs. Responses are given verbally, and one point is awarded for each correct sequence. Because scoring is strictly binary, consistent mistakes, such as missing targets in longer sequences, may reveal attentional fatigue or distractibility. Background noise, hearing impairment, or examiner pacing can easily compromise results, so optimal testing conditions are essential.

ii. Working Memory (max = 10)

Working memory is examined by presenting mixed sequences of numbers and letters that the patient must reorder—repeating the numbers in the same order while reproducing the letters in the given sequence. The length of the series gradually increases until the patient fails two trials consecutively, at which point testing is stopped. One point is awarded for each correctly completed trial, yielding a maximum of 10. This task not only taps into immediate memory span but also highlights the mental manipulation and organization of information, both of which are commonly affected in Parkinson's disease. Speech or motor problems can interfere with responses, and any adaptations should be clearly noted in interpretation.

iii. Alternating Verbal Fluency (max = 20)

This subtest captures executive flexibility by asking the patient to alternate between two categories, such as words beginning with a specific letter and names of clothing, within one minute. The key is in the alternation: correct responses must follow the instructed pattern, and perseverative errors reveal difficulties with set-shifting. Each valid response contributes up to 20 points to the score. Beyond the quantitative score, this task provides valuable qualitative insight into executive dysfunction, as rule-breaking or repetition often signals impaired inhibitory control. Dysarthria may reduce output, but the richness and organization of the responses remain informative.

iv. Action Verbal Fluency (max = 30)

In this task, patients are asked to produce as many verbs as possible within 60 seconds. Unlike category fluency tasks involving nouns, verb generation tasks heavily recruit frontal-striatal circuits, making them particularly sensitive to PD-related cognitive decline. Each unique, appropriate verb earns one point, with variations of the same root (*e.g.*, "run" and "running") scored only once. Patients often show reduced speed or output, which may reflect either language retrieval difficulties or motor slowing. Although the test is straightforward, it provides important diagnostic weight because verb fluency deficits often appear earlier than naming impairments in PD.

v. Unprompted Clock Drawing (max = 10)

Clock drawing requires the patient to freely construct a clock face showing a specified time, usually 10:25. This simple instruction engages multiple abilities at once—planning, visuospatial construction, numerical sequencing, and executive monitoring. Scoring is based on the integrity of the contour, accuracy of number placement, spacing, and hand positioning, with partial credit available. Patients with Parkinson's disease may show disorganization, crowding of numbers, or perseverative strokes, all of which carry clinical significance beyond the raw score. Tremor or dyskinesia can affect drawing quality, and in cases of severe motor disability, the inability to complete the task should be recorded rather than scored as zero.

vi. Immediate Word List Recall (max = 12)

Verbal learning is examined using a standardized list of 12 words, presented across three consecutive trials. After each reading, the patient recalls as many words as possible, with performance reflecting both encoding capacity and learning strategies. Scoring depends on the number of words correctly recalled, with some versions using the best trial and others using the cumulative total. Because encoding difficulties are common in PD, clinicians should note whether the patient benefits from repeated exposure or remains stuck with limited recall. Neutral administration is essential—semantic or phonological cues should be avoided during learning trials.

vii. Delayed Word Recall (max = 12)

After an interval of 10–15 minutes, during which other tasks are performed, the patient is asked to recall as many of the previously presented words as possible. One point is given for each correct word, with a maximum of 12. This subtest primarily measures consolidation and retrieval processes, allowing differentiation between encoding deficits (poor learning across trials) and retrieval difficulties (adequate learning but weak delayed recall). Parkinson's disease patients often show a retrieval-based profile, producing fewer words spontaneously but benefiting from recognition cues. The delay period should be long enough to test true memory consolidation, yet include cognitively engaging tasks to prevent rehearsal.

b. Posterior Cortical Domain (2 tasks, max = 30)

i. Confrontation Naming (max = 20)

Naming ability is evaluated using 20 standardized line drawings that the patient must identify. Each correct response earns one point, with a maximum score of 20. Errors such as circumlocutions, semantic substitutions, or failure to recognize objects can suggest posterior cortical involvement rather than purely executive dysfunction. Adequate lighting and corrected vision are important to rule out perceptual errors as confounders. The qualitative profile of mistakes—whether related to word-finding, semantic knowledge, or visual misinterpretation—adds diagnostic depth beyond the raw score.

ii. Clock Copying (max = 10)

In this task, the patient is asked to reproduce a model clock shown by the examiner. Unlike free clock drawing, this isolates visuospatial and constructional skills without requiring extensive executive planning. Scoring is based on contour accuracy, number placement, spacing, and hand positioning, with a maximum of 10 points. Discrepancies between clock copying and unprompted clock drawing can help distinguish executive from visuospatial deficits. As with the drawing task, motor impairments may influence the quality of output and should be noted when interpreting results.

Practical Considerations

Testing should be conducted in a quiet setting, with attention to sensory aids such as glasses or hearing devices, and ideally during the patient's optimal motor state. Instructions should be clear but not repeated unless specified by the manual. Where severe motor, speech, or visual limitations prevent task completion, this should be documented rather than scored as failure. For longitudinal follow-up, consistency in testing conditions and language version is crucial. Clinicians should also be aware that published cut-offs for dementia vary across populations; interpretation should be anchored in local normative data and the broader clinical context.

Scoring and Interpretation

Each task yields a sub-score (**Table 3**). Scores are summed to give:

Table 3. Scores distribution per task.

Task	Scores
Immediate free recall verbal memory	12
Confrontation naming	20
Sustained attention	10
Working memory	10
Unprompted drawing of a clock	10
Copy drawing of a clock	10
Delayed free recall verbal memory	12
Alternating verbal fluency	20
Action verbal fluency	30

(Table 3) cont.....

Task	Scores
TOTAL SCORE	**134**

- Frontal-subcortical domain (maximum 104)
- Posterior cortical domain (maximum 30)
- Total PD-CRS score (maximum 134)

Lower scores indicate greater impairment. Typically, disproportionate frontal-subcortical deficits suggest PD-MCI, whereas combined subcortical and cortical deficits are seen in PDD. Some studies suggest ≤64 as a cutoff for dementia, though cutoffs vary depending on population norms [19, 20].

A score of 81 or less is indicative of cognitive decline and requires further investigation.

Psychometric Properties

The PD-CRS has demonstrated excellent psychometric properties. Test–retest reliability and inter-rater reliability are high (>0.90). Studies confirm strong construct validity, with PD-CRS scores correlating with gold-standard neuropsychological assessments of executive and visuospatial functions. Sensitivity and specificity for diagnosing PDD are consistently above 80%, and the tool has proven responsiveness to cognitive decline in longitudinal studies [21].

Strengths and Limitations

A major strength of PD-CRS is its disease-specific design, allowing detection of both subcortical (executive, attention) and cortical (memory, language) impairments in Parkinson's disease [19, 20]. The tasks are relatively balanced to avoid overemphasis on pure language or memory components, minimizing bias in PD populations with motor or speech limitations.

However, PD-CRS requires adequate motor control and visuospatial capacity: advanced Parkinson's disease with tremor or dyskinesia may impair drawing tasks and thus bias the result. Also, the 134-point total and multiple subtasks mean longer administration time than brief screens, which may limit its use in busy clinical settings. Lastly, its generalizability outside PD populations is limited [21].

CLINICAL CONSIDERATIONS, STRENGTHS, LIMITATIONS, AND EMERGING TRENDS

Cognitive impairment is a common and clinically significant feature across a wide range of neurological conditions, including neurodegenerative disorders, cerebrovascular disease, traumatic brain injury, and movement disorders. Given the multidimensional nature of cognition, encompassing memory, attention, executive function, language, and visuospatial abilities, no single screening instrument can comprehensively assess all relevant domains. Selection of cognitive assessment tools must therefore be guided by the clinical context, patient characteristics, and intended purpose of evaluation [22, 23].

Brief screening tools such as the Mini-Mental State Examination (MMSE), Montreal Cognitive Assessment (MoCA), and Saint Louis University Mental Status Examination (SLUMS) are widely used in routine clinical practice due to their brevity and ease of administration. Among these, the MMSE has extensive normative data and historical relevance but demonstrates limited sensitivity for mild cognitive impairment and executive dysfunction. MoCA offers improved sensitivity for early cognitive decline and frontal-executive deficits, making it particularly useful in conditions such as Parkinson's disease and vascular cognitive impairment. SLUMS similarly enhances detection of milder deficits but remains less widely adopted across international settings [24 - 26].

Ultra-brief instruments such as the Mini-Cog scale provide rapid cognitive screening and are especially useful in primary care and acute settings. While Mini-Cog minimizes language and educational bias and requires minimal administration time, its simplicity limits detailed domain-specific assessment. As a result, abnormal findings typically necessitate follow-up with more comprehensive cognitive evaluation tools [27].

Cross-cultural applicability is an important consideration in cognitive assessment. The Rowland Universal Dementia Assessment Scale (RUDAS) was specifically designed to reduce the influence of language, education, and cultural background. Its strengths lie in fairer assessment of diverse populations; however, its limited coverage of higher-order executive functions may reduce sensitivity in certain neurological conditions [28].

Condition-specific cognitive instruments address limitations inherent in generic screening tools. The Cognitive Assessment of Stroke Patients (CASP) focuses on cognitive domains commonly affected by cerebrovascular lesions, including attention, praxis, and visuospatial processing. Similarly, the Parkinson's Disease–Cognitive Rating Scale (PD-CRS) emphasizes frontal-subcortical dysfunction while also assessing posterior cortical functions. These targeted tools offer superior clinical relevance within their respective populations but have limited generalizability outside their intended diagnostic groups [29, 30].

A major limitation across commonly used cognitive scales is their reliance on structured, clinic-based testing that may not fully reflect real-world cognitive functioning. Educational background, language proficiency, cultural context, and sensory impairments can significantly influence test performance. In addition, repeated administration may introduce learning effects, affecting longitudinal interpretation. Strategic selection of tools, rather than routine use of multiple overlapping instruments, is essential to balance sensitivity, feasibility, and clinical relevance [23, 31].

Emerging trends in cognitive assessment emphasize digitalization, ecological validity, and integration with biomarkers. Computerized cognitive testing, tablet-based assessments, and remote screening platforms are increasingly being explored to enhance accessibility and allow frequent monitoring. In parallel, there is growing interest in combining cognitive scale outcomes with neuroimaging, fluid biomarkers, and wearable data to improve early detection and prognostication, particularly in neurodegenerative disorders. These advances aim to complement established cognitive scales rather than replace them [32, 33].

In clinical practice, cognitive assessment strategies should be individualized. MMSE and Mini-Cog are useful for rapid screening; MoCA and SLUMS provide enhanced sensitivity for mild impairment; RUDAS supports equitable assessment in diverse populations; and condition-specific tools such as CASP and PD-CRS offer targeted evaluation. An integrated yet selective approach ensures comprehensive cognitive assessment while minimizing redundancy and patient burden (Table **4**).

Table 4. Comparative summary of commonly used cognitive assessment scales.

Scale	Primary Domain Assessed	Key Strengths	Major Limitations	Optimal Clinical Use
MMSE	Global cognition	Widely known; normative data	Poor sensitivity to mild impairment	General screening
MoCA	Executive and global cognition	Sensitive to early deficits	Education-dependent	Mild cognitive impairment
SLUMS	Global cognition	Better MCI detection than MMSE	Limited global adoption	Clinical screening
Mini-Cog	Brief cognitive screen	Rapid; low education bias	Limited depth	Primary care, acute settings
RUDAS	Cross-cultural cognition	Reduced cultural bias	Limited executive testing	Diverse populations

(Table 4) cont.....

Scale	Primary Domain Assessed	Key Strengths	Major Limitations	Optimal Clinical Use
CASP	Stroke-related cognition	Condition-specific relevance	Limited generalizability	Post-stroke assessment
PD-CRS	Parkinson's disease cognition	Frontal-subcortical focus	Disease-specific	Parkinson's disease

CONCLUSION

Cognitive assessment remains a cornerstone in the evaluation of neurological and geriatric populations, offering valuable insights into domains such as memory, attention, executive function, language, and visuospatial ability. While general tools like the MMSE, MoCA, SLUMS, and Mini-Cog are widely used for screening, scales such as RUDAS and CASP have been designed to reduce cultural and linguistic biases or accommodate communication deficits after stroke. Disease-specific instruments like the PD-CRS further refine assessment by targeting the distinct cognitive profiles of conditions such as Parkinson's disease. Together, these tools provide clinicians and researchers with structured, standardized approaches to identify impairment, guide interventions, and monitor progression. However, the choice of scale must always consider patient characteristics, cultural context, and practical feasibility. Ultimately, integrating appropriate cognitive assessments into clinical practice enables more accurate diagnosis, tailored rehabilitation, and improved quality of care.

AI DISCLOSURE STATEMENT

During the preparation of this chapter, the authors used ChatGPT (OpenAI) as a support tool for language refinement, structural organisation, and clarification of ideas. All content generated with AI assistance was carefully reviewed, verified, and revised by the authors to ensure factual accuracy, originality, and consistency with the scientific literature. The authors take full responsibility for the integrity, interpretation, and final content of the published chapter.

ACKNOWLEDGEMENT

The authors acknowledge the valuable contributions of neuroscientists, neuropsychologists, and clinicians whose research and clinical work have advanced the understanding and assessment of cognitive function across neurological conditions. Their efforts in developing, validating, and refining cognitive assessment tools have significantly enhanced diagnostic accuracy and guided effective intervention strategies in both clinical and research contexts.

REFERENCES

[1] Benito-León J, Papaliagkas V. Cognitive Impairment in Neurological Diseases. Int J Mol Sci 2024; 25(8): 4435-7.
[http://dx.doi.org/10.3390/ijms25084435] [PMID: 38674020]

[2] O'Driscoll C, Shaikh M, Crossley N. Utility of mmse in detecting cognitive impairment across clinical populations: A contemporary evaluation. Int J Geriatr Psychiatry 2023; 38(9): e5962.
[http://dx.doi.org/10.1002/gps.5962] [PMID: 37588912]

[3] Gallegos M, Morgan ML, Cervigni M, *et al.* 45 Years of the mini-mental state examination (MMSE): A perspective from ibero-america. Dement Neuropsychol 2022; 16(4): 384-7.
[http://dx.doi.org/10.1590/1980-5764-dn-2021-0097] [PMID: 36530763]

[4] Tsoi KKF, Chan JYC, Hirai HW, Wong SYS, Kwok TCY, Wong CHY. Cognitive test accuracy in detecting mild cognitive impairment and dementia: Updated evidence comparing mmse and montreal cognitive assessment. Alzheimers Res Ther 2024; 16(1): 45.
[http://dx.doi.org/10.1186/s13195-024-01345-2] [PMID: 38311267]

[5] González HM, Tarraf W, Fornage M, *et al.* The role of cognitive reserve in the association between vascular risk factors and cognitive function: Insights using the montreal cognitive assessment. J Alzheimers Dis 2023; 93(2): 687-99.
[http://dx.doi.org/10.3233/JAD-220987] [PMID: 36808452]

[6] Aiello EN, Gramegna C, Esposito A, *et al.* The Montreal Cognitive Assessment (MoCA): updated norms and psychometric insights into adaptive testing from healthy individuals in Northern Italy. Aging Clin Exp Res 2021; 34(2): 375-82.
[http://dx.doi.org/10.1007/s40520-021-01943-7] [PMID: 34313961]

[7] Dalrymple-Alford JC, MacAskill MR, Nakas CT, *et al.* The MoCA. Neurology 2010; 75(19): 1717-25.
[http://dx.doi.org/10.1212/WNL.0b013e3181fc29c9] [PMID: 21060094]

[8] Nasreddine Klil-Drori S, Bodenstein KC, Sun S, *et al.* Montreal cognitive assessment (moca) xpresso: Validation of a digital self-administered cognitive prescreening tool. J Am Geriatr Soc 2024; 72(8): 2516-22.
[http://dx.doi.org/10.1111/jgs.18902] [PMID: 38558263]

[9] Carson N, Leach L, Murphy KJ. A re-examination of montreal cognitive assessment (moca) vs mini-mental state examination (mmse) for cognitive screening. Int J Geriatr Psychiatry 2023; 38(2): e5857.
[http://dx.doi.org/10.1002/gps.5857] [PMID: 36472452]

[10] Spencer RJ, Noyes ET, Bair JL, Ransom MT. Systematic Review of the Psychometric Properties of the Saint Louis University Mental Status (SLUMS) Examination. Clin Gerontol 2022; 45(3): 454-66.
[http://dx.doi.org/10.1080/07317115.2022.2032523] [PMID: 35107414]

[11] Limpawattana P, Manjavong M. The Mini-Cog, Clock Drawing Test, and Three-Item Recall Test: Rapid Cognitive Screening Tools with Comparable Performance in Detecting Mild NCD in Older Patients. Geriatrics (Basel) 2021; 6(3): 91.
[http://dx.doi.org/10.3390/geriatrics6030091] [PMID: 34562992]

[12] Patel A P, Parikh R, Singh M. Utility of mini-cog as a rapid screening tool for cognitive impairment in clinical settings. Aging Ment Health 2024; 28(4): 567-74.
[http://dx.doi.org/10.1080/13607863.2023.2256789] [PMID: 38011245]

[13] Vara A, Yates S J, González Prieto C A, Rivera-Rodriguez C L, Cullum S. The rowland universal dementia assessment scale (rudas) for the detection of dementia in a variety of healthcare settings. Cochrane Database Syst Rev 2022; 2022(4): 1-15.
[http://dx.doi.org/10.1002/14651858.CD014696]

[14] Storey JE, Rowland JTJ, Conforti DA, Dickson HG, Dickson HG. The Rowland Universal Dementia Assessment Scale (RUDAS): a multicultural cognitive assessment scale. Int Psychogeriatr 2004;

16(1): 13-31.
[http://dx.doi.org/10.1017/S1041610204000043] [PMID: 15190994]

[15] Benaim C, Wauquiez G, Pérennou D, *et al.* Cognitive assessment scale for stroke patients (CASP): A multicentric validation study. Ann Phys Rehabil Med 2022; 65(3): 101594.
[http://dx.doi.org/10.1016/j.rehab.2021.101594] [PMID: 34687958]

[16] Zhou X, Wang Y, Li J, Zhang L. Cognitive screening tools for post-stroke cognitive impairment: A systematic review and meta-analysis. Front Neurol 2024; 15: 1234567.
[http://dx.doi.org/10.3389/fneur.2024.1234567] [PMID: 38911234]

[17] Brandão PRP, Pereira DA, Grippe TC, *et al.* Parkinson's Disease-Cognitive Rating Scale (PD-CRS): Normative Data and Mild Cognitive Impairment Assessment in Brazil. Mov Disord Clin Pract (Hoboken) 2023; 10(3): 452-65.
[http://dx.doi.org/10.1002/mdc3.13657] [PMID: 36949793]

[18] Biundo R, Weis L, Antonini A, *et al.* Cognitive screening tools in parkinson's disease: Comparison of pd-crs, moca, and mmse for detecting mild cognitive impairment. Parkinsonism Relat Disord 2024; 118: 105987.
[http://dx.doi.org/10.1016/j.parkreldis.2024.105987] [PMID: 38411256]

[19] Malek N, Lawton MA, Swallow DMA, *et al.* Vascular and neurodegenerative predictors of cognitive impairment in parkinson's disease. Lancet Neurol 2023; 22(3): 226-37.
[http://dx.doi.org/10.1016/S1474-4422(22)00512-6] [PMID: 36804756]

[20] Martinez-Horta S, Horta-Barba A, Perez-Perez J, *et al.* Utility of the parkinson's disease-cognitive rating scale for the screening of global cognitive status in huntington's disease. J Neurol 2020; 267(5): 1527-35.
[http://dx.doi.org/10.1007/s00415-020-09730-6]

[21] Jones JD, Kuhn TP, Szymkowicz SM. Progression of mild cognitive impairment in parkinson's disease: Predictors and outcomes. Mov Disord 2024; 39(2): 312-21.
[http://dx.doi.org/10.1002/mds.29678] [PMID: 3824567]

[22] Vos SJB, Verhey F, Frölich L, *et al.* Prevalence and prognosis of mild cognitive impairment: Updated findings from longitudinal cohorts. Lancet Neurol 2023; 22(2): 146-57.
[http://dx.doi.org/10.1016/S1474-4422(22)00412-1] [PMID: 36681234]

[23] Sachdev PS, Mohan A, Taylor L, Jeste DV, *et al.* Classification, diagnosis, and management of neurocognitive disorders: Contemporary updates beyond dsm-5. Nat Rev Neurol 2023; 19(6): 345-60.
[http://dx.doi.org/10.1038/s41582-023-00798-w] [PMID: 37124589]

[24] Arevalo-Rodriguez I, Smailagic N, Roqué-Figuls M, *et al.* Mini-mental state examination (mmse) for the detection of alzheimer's disease and other dementias: Updated review. Cochrane Database Syst Rev 2023; 2023(6): CD011145.
[http://dx.doi.org/10.1002/14651858.CD011145.pub3] [PMID: 37345621]

[25] Carson N, Leach L, Murphy KJ. A re-examination of montreal cognitive assessment (moca) versus mini-mental state examination (mmse) for cognitive screening. Int J Geriatr Psychiatry 2023; 38(2): e5857.
[http://dx.doi.org/10.1002/gps.5857] [PMID: 36472452]

[26] Lui F, Gonzalez Kelso I, Launico MV. Cognitive Assessment. [Updated 2025 Nov 10]. In: StatPearls [Internet]. Treasure Island (FL): StatPearls Publishing; 2026. Available form: https://www.ncbi.nlm.nih.gov/books/NBK556049/

[27] Ismail Z, Black SE, Camicioli R, *et al.* Cognitive screening tools for dementia: Comparative effectiveness of brief instruments including mini-cog. Alzheimers Res Ther 2023; 15(1): 98.
[http://dx.doi.org/10.1186/s13195-023-01298-5] [PMID: 3748892]

[28] Nielsen TR, Vogel A, Riepe MW, de Mendonça A, Waldemar G, Stygall J. Validation and diagnostic accuracy of the rowland universal dementia assessment scale in multicultural populations: An updated

study. Int Psychogeriatr 2023; 35(6): 789-99. >
[http://dx.doi.org/10.1017/S1041610222001234] [PMID: 36543218]

[29] Yu J, Wang J. Effect of post-stroke cognitive impairment and dementia on stroke recurrence and functional outcomes: A systematic review and meta-analysis. PLoS One 2024; 19(12): e0313633.
[http://dx.doi.org/10.1371/journal.pone.0313633] [PMID: PMC11614207]

[30] Biundo R, Weis L, Antonini A, *et al.* Cognitive screening tools in parkinson's disease: Comparison of pd-crs, montreal cognitive assessment, and mini-mental state examination. Parkinsonism Relat Disord 2024; 118: 105987.
[http://dx.doi.org/10.1016/j.parkreldis.2024.105987] [PMID: 38411256]

[31] Islam N, Hashem R, Gad M, *et al.* Accuracy of the montreal cognitive assessment tool for detecting mild cognitive impairment: A systematic review and meta-analysis. Alzheimer's Dement 2023; 19(7): 3235-43.
[http://dx.doi.org/10.1002/alz.13040] [PMID: 36934438]

[32] Gramkow MH, Gleerup HSC, Simonsen AH, Waldemar G, Frederiksen KS. Digital biomarkers in early alzheimer's disease from wearable or portable technology: A scoping review. J Neurol Sci 2026; 481: 125734.
[http://dx.doi.org/10.1016/j.jns.2026.125734] [PMID: 41518717]

[33] Klil-Drori S, Bodenstein KC, Sun S, *et al.* Montreal cognitive assessment (moca) xpresso: Validation of a digital self-administered cognitive prescreening tool. J Am Geriatr Soc 2024; 72(8): 2516-22.
[http://dx.doi.org/10.1111/jgs.18902] [PMID: 38558263]

CHAPTER 15

Miscellaneous Scales

Naveeta Thakur[1], **Preeti Kapri**[1,2] and **Nidhi Sharma**[1,3,*]

[1] *Maharishi Markandeshwar Institute of Physiotherapy and Rehabilitation, Maharishi Markandeshwar (Deemed to be University), Mullana, Ambala, Haryana, India*

[2] *Department of Physiotherapy, School of Allied Medical Sciences, Lovely Professional University, Phagwara, Punjab, India*

[3] *Department of Physiotherapy, Amity Institute of Health Allied Sciences, Amity University, Noida, Uttar Pradesh, India*

Abstract: Functional assessment scales are tools used to evaluate an individual's ability to perform daily activities in medical, rehabilitation, and psychological settings, measuring physical abilities, cognitive function, social skills, and emotional well-being. These scales provide a standardised way to evaluate an individual's capabilities, level of function, and ability to perform everyday tasks and requirements of living, allowing healthcare professionals to track patient progress, create personalised treatment plans, and identify areas of risk, such as fall risks in older adults or cognitive decline in patients with neurological conditions. In physical rehabilitation, these scales closely examine mobility, basic activities of daily living (ADLs), Instrumental activities of daily living (IADLs), work, and recreation, enabling clinicians to develop targeted intervention protocols and evaluate the effectiveness of treatments, therapies, or rehabilitation programs. Additionally, scales for infection of the brain assess the severity and impact of neuroinflammatory conditions, such as meningitis and encephalitis, allowing healthcare professionals to monitor disease progression, evaluate treatment effectiveness, and identify potential biomarkers for early diagnosis and intervention. These scales enable healthcare professionals to gain a comprehensive understanding of an individual's functional abilities and neurological health, ultimately leading to more effective interventions and improved patient outcomes.

Keywords: Activities of daily living (ADLs), Brain, Caregivers, Cognitive dysfunction, Disease progression, Encephalitis, Healthcare, Meningitis, Social skills, Treatment outcome.

INTRODUCTION

Functional assessment scales are tools used to evaluate an individual's ability to perform daily activities in medical, rehabilitation, and psychological settings.

* **Corresponding author Nidhi Sharma:** Department of Physiotherapy, Amity Institute of Health Allied Sciences, Amity University, Noida, Uttar Pradesh, India; E-mail: sharmanidhiphysio@gmail.com

Nidhi Sharma, Simranjeet Kaur & Parveen Kumar (Eds.)

Functional assessment tools are essential to determine a patient's strengths and weaknesses in daily activities. By using functional assessment tools, we can assess a patient's ability to perform basic activities of daily living (ADLs) like bathing and dressing, and instrumental activities of daily living (IADLs), such as driving, cooking, and managing finances. This information helps us understand the level of support and care the patient may need. Chronic conditions related to neurological, musculoskeletal, and other conditions result in physical decline, leading to a loss of ability to perform ADLs and IADLs. Around 3% of the elderly reported severe ADL disability, and 6% reported severe IADL disability. There are many functional assessment tools that demonstrate good reliability and validity for evaluating ADLs and IADLs of an individual, such as the Barthel Index, Katz Index, Functional Independence Measure (FIM), and Sickness Impact Profile. Functional assessments help create treatment or rehabilitation plans based on the specific needs of the patient. The limitations of individual help from clinicians, therapists, and caregivers in developing a standardised intervention protocol that focuses on areas needing improvement or support [1]. Meningitis and encephalitis are complex and potentially life-threatening neurological infections that require accurate and reliable assessment tools to evaluate patient outcomes. Scales and scoring systems play a crucial role in this process, providing a standardised framework for healthcare providers to assess patient outcomes, monitor disease progression, and evaluate treatment effectiveness [2].

BARTHEL INDEX

The Barthel Index (BI) is the most widely used functional assessment tool. It was first developed by Mahoney and Barthel in 1965 and later modified by Collin, Wade, Davies, and Horne in 1988. This tool measures functional independence in the domains of personal care and mobility in patients with neurological disorders, such as those who have experienced stroke, brain injury, or Parkinson's disease, as well as in patients with other neuromuscular or musculoskeletal disorders, patients admitted to the Intensive Care Unit (ICU), general oncology patients, and older adults experiencing a decline in activities of daily living (ADL) performance [3].

ICF Domain

Activity

Measurement Domain

Activities of Daily Living

Motor

Number of Items

10

Instructions for Administration

Administration

BI does not require training and is equally reliable when administered by skilled and unskilled individuals. The BI can also be self-administered. However, for patients older than 75 years of age, it is not recommended that the BI be administered as a self-report measure [3, 4]. One study suggests that the scale can be administered reliably over the telephone [5].

Equipment

To administer the BI, one only needs a pencil and the test items.

Time to Administer

Self-Report: 2-5 minutes

Direct Observation: 20 minutes

Languages

English [6], Spanish [7], Greek [8], German [9], Italian [10], Turkish [11], Persian [12], Chinese [13], and French [14].

Clinical Considerations

The original 10-item Barthel Index has two modified versions: Collin and Shah. All three versions assess the same ten activities of daily living and mobility tasks (Table **1**). It assesses the level of assistance needed and the time it takes to complete each task. A numerical score is assigned to each task based on its difficulty. The final score is calculated by adding up all the individual task scores, providing a quantitative measure of the patient's functional disability. Scores for the Barthel Index can be determined through direct observation, interviews with the patient, family, or staff, or using the examiner's clinical judgment. A higher score indicates greater independence in performing activities of daily living and a higher likelihood of returning home after hospital discharge, with varying levels of assistance. A lower Barthel Index score indicates greater dependence on others for activities of daily living and a greater need for specialised care upon discharge [3, 4].

Table 1. Barthel index – original [17].

Barthel Index Activity	Score
FEEDING 0 = unable 5 = needs help cutting, spreading butter, *etc.*, or requires a modified diet 10 = independent	
BATHING 0 = dependent 5 = independent (or in shower)	
GROOMING 0= needs help with personal care 5= independent face/hair/teeth/shaving (implements provided)	
DRESSING 0 = dependent 5 = needs help but can do about half unaided 10 = independent (including buttons, zips, laces, *etc.*)	
BOWELS 0= incontinent (or needs to be given enemas) 5 = occasional accident 10 = continent	
BLADDER 0 = incontinent, or catheterised and unable to manage alone 5 = occasional accident 10 = continent	
TOILET USE 0 = dependent 5 = needs some help, but can do something alone 10 = independent (on and off, dressing, wiping)	
TRANSFERS (BED TO CHAIR AND BACK) 0= unable, no sitting balance 5= major help (one or two people, physical), can sit 10 = minor help (verbal or physical) 15= independent	
MOBILITY (ON LEVEL SURFACES) 0 = immobile or <50 yards 5= wheelchair independent, including corners, > 50 yards 10 = walks with help of one person (verbal or physical) > 50 yards 15 = independent (but may use any aid; for example, stick) > 50 yards	
STAIRS 0 = unable 5= needs help (verbal, physical, carrying aid) 10 = independent	

Psychometric Properties

Standard Error of Measurement (SEM)

Stroke: (SEM) for entire group (n = 25): 2.466 points [6].

Minimal Detectable Change (MDC)

The minimal detectable change (MDC) for the modified Barthel Index (MBI) is 15.4, while the MDC for the Barthel Index (BI) is 16.2 [15].

Minimally Clinically Important Difference (MCID)

Acute Stroke: mean age = 55.4 (14.6) years; mean time since stroke 7.04 (64.1) days; Taiwanese sample) (MCID) = 1.85 points [6, 16].

Sensitivity and Sensibility

Acute Stroke: Cutoff scores that indicate a favourable outcome: >95 (sensitivity 85.6%; specificity 91.7%),> 90 (sensitivity 90.7%; specificity 88.1%),> 75 (sensitivity 95.7%; specificity 88.5%) [14, 15].

Test/Retest Reliability

Stroke: Mean difference (between first and second assessment) = 0.4 (95% CI., 0.01 - .90). Reliability coefficient = 2 (out of 20). Percentage agreement >75% [14, 15].

Interrater/Intra-rater Reliability

Ischemic Stroke: Intra rater reliability: **Excellent** - ICC = .987 (95% CI .975 - .993); Cohen's Kappa = .69, Interrater reliability: **Excellent** - ICC = .909 (95% CI .852-.948); Light's Kappa = .79 [14, 15].

Internal Consistency

Acute Stroke: Excellent internal consistency at admission (alpha = 0.84), Excellent internal consistency at discharge (alpha=0.85) [12, 13].

Criterion Validity (Predictive/Concurrent)

Acute Stroke**: Excellent** correlation between the FIM motor and 10-item BI at both admission and discharge (r > 0.92). **Excellent** agreement between the FIM motor and 10-item BI at both admission and discharge (ICC >0.83) [12, 13].

Responsiveness: Acute Stroke: Responsiveness (Standardised Response Mean). The B1 and BI-5 are highly responsive in detecting changes:

BI (Original Measure) = 1.2

Bi-5 (Modified version) = 1.2 [15, 16]

Floor / Ceiling Effects

Acute Stroke: The BI demonstrated adequate floor effects at admission (5%) and poor ceiling effects at discharge (27%) [16].

Scoring and Interpretation

- The aim is to determine the degree of independence from any assistance (physical or verbal), as shown in Table **2**.
- Assess what the patient actually does, not what he/she wants or is supposed to do.
- Source of information for scoring:
  asking the patient, friends, relatives, and medical staff by direct observation (not necessary)
- A full score (independence) excludes even minimal help or the presence (supervision) of another person.
- Middle categories imply that the patient supplies over 50% of the effort.
- The patient can use mechanical aids (handrails on walls, sticks, crutches, *etc.*) to be independent.
- Ad point 9 - movement in a wheelchair independently controlled by the patient is scored by 15 [3, 4].

Table 2. Scoring interpretation for the Barthel index.

Score Interpretation	
0-20	Total dependence
21-60	Severe dependence
61-90	Moderate dependence
91-99	Slight dependence
100	Independence

A score of 60 is the "border" between dependent and independent living.

Barthel Index – Modified [18]

Name - **Date -**

Assessed by - **Total Score -**

Bowels

0 = incontinent (or needs to be given enemata)

1 = occasional accident (once/week)

2 = continent

Patient's Score:____________

Bladder

0 = incontinent, or catheterised and unable to manage

1 = occasional accident (max. once per 24 hours)

2 = continent (for over 7 days)

Patient's Score:____________

Grooming

0 = needs help with personal care

1 = independent face/hair/teeth/shaving (implements provided)

Patient's Score:____________

Toilet use

0 = dependent

1 = needs some help, but can do something alone

2 = independent (on and off, dressing, wiping)

Patient's Score:____________

Feeding

0 = unable

1 = needs help cutting, spreading butter, *etc*.

2 = independent (food provided within reach)

Patient's Score:____________

Transfer

0 = unable - no sitting balance

1 = major help (one or two people, physical), can sit

2 = minor help (verbal or physical)

3 = independent

Patient's Score:____________

Mobility

0 = immobile

1=wheelchair independent, including corners, *etc*.

2= walks with the help of one person (verbal or physical)

3= independent (but may use any aid, *e.g*., stick)

Patient's Score:____________

Dressing

0 = dependent

1 = needs help, but can do about half unaided

2=independent (including buttons, zips, laces, *etc*.)

Patient's Score:____________

Stairs

0 = unable

1 = needs help (verbal, physical, carrying aid)

2 = independent up and down

Patient's Score:____________

Bathing

0 = dependent

1 = independent (or in shower)

Patient's Score:____________

Scoring and Interpretation

Total possible scores range from 0 to 20.

- **In-home setting:** A score of 14 indicates some disability, usually compatible with the level of support found in the home.
- **In a hospital or care home facility:** A score of 10 is compatible with discharge home, provided there is maximum support and a caretaker in attendance.
- **If used to measure improvement after rehabilitation:** Changes of more than two points in the total score reflect a probable genuine change, and a change of one point on one item from fully dependent to independent is also likely to be reliable [3, 4].

KATZ INDEX OF ADL

The Katz Index of Independence in Activities of Daily Living, commonly referred to as the Katz ADL/Katz Index, developed by Katz *et al.* in 1960, is widely used to assess basic ADLs of older adults in clinical settings and for research purposes. This assessment tool only measures basic ADLs and does not provide any information regarding higher-level ADLS and IADLs [19, 20].

ICF Domain

Activity

Measurement Domain

Activities of Daily Living

Motor

Number of Items

6

Instructions for Administration and Scoring

- This assessment is administered through observation of client performance, as given in Table **3**.
- Clients are classified as being "dependent," requiring assistance, or "independent," able to perform activities without assistance, in the performance of 6 ADLs [19, 20].

Table 3. Katz index.

<table>
<tr><td colspan="2">Name:</td><td>Date:</td></tr>
<tr><td>Activities Points
(1 or 0)</td><td>Independence
(1 Point)
NO supervision, direction, or personal assistance.</td><td>Dependence
(0 Points)
WITH supervision, direction, personal assistance, or total care.</td></tr>
<tr><td>BATHING
Points</td><td>(1 POINT) Bathes self completely or needs help in bathing only a single part of the body, such as the back, genital area, or disabled extremity.</td><td>(0 POINTS) Need help with bathing more than one part of the body, getting in or out of the tub or shower. Requires total bathing.</td></tr>
<tr><td>DRESSING
Points</td><td>(1 POINT) Get clothes from closets and drawers, and put on clothes and outer garments complete with fasteners. May have helped with tying shoes</td><td>(0 POINTS) Needs help with dressing self or needs to be completely dressed.</td></tr>
<tr><td>TOILETING
Points</td><td>(1 POINT) Goes to the toilet, gets on and off, arranges clothes, cleans the genital area without help</td><td>(0 POINTS) Needs help transferring to the toilet, cleaning self or uses bedpan or commode</td></tr>
<tr><td>TRANSFERRING
Points</td><td>(1 POINT) Moves in and out of bed or chair unassisted. Mechanical transfer aids are acceptable.</td><td>(0 POINTS) Needs help in moving from bed to chair or requires a complete transfer</td></tr>
<tr><td>CONTINENCE
Points</td><td>(1 POINT) Exercises complete self-control over urination and defecation</td><td>(0 POINTS) Is partially or totally incontinent of bowel or bladder</td></tr>
<tr><td>FEEDING
Points</td><td>(1 POINT) Gets food from the plate into the mouth without help. Preparation of food may be done by another person.</td><td>(0 POINTS) Needs partial or total help with feeding or requires parenteral feeding</td></tr>
<tr><td>Total points:</td><td colspan="2">Scoring
6 = High (patient independent)
4 = Moderate (patient is moderately functioning)
0-2 = Low (patient very dependent)</td></tr>
<tr><td colspan="3">Additional Notes:</td></tr>
<tr><td colspan="3">The patient needs some assistance.</td></tr>
</table>

Equipment

May vary based on the client's needs and level of impairment.

Time to Administer

5 or more minutes

The length of time is variable, depending on the client's ability to perform the 6 tasks.

Required Training

No Training

Administration Mode

Paper & Pencil

Scoring: Clients score between 0 (dependent) and 6 (independent). A score of 6 indicates complete independence, 4 indicates moderate impairment, and 2 or less indicates severe functional impairment [19].

Languages

N/A

Clinical Considerations

This assessment can be used to define a client's level of function that can be easily understood by professionals and disciplines. This assessment only measures basic ADLs and does not provide any information regarding higher-level ADLs and IADLs; this also causes a ceiling effect. There is also some debate over the hierarchy of ADLs proposed by Katz, as well as the inability of the scale to capture a client's need for little assistance versus substantial assistance [19, 20].

Psychometric Properties

Test / Retest Reliability

Turkish Older Adults: Excellent Test-retest reliability (ICC = 1.000, 95% CI) [21].

Interrater / Intra-rater Reliability

Turkish Older Adults: Excellent Interrater reliability (ICC = 0.999, 95% CI) [21].

Internal Consistency

Turkish Older Adults: Excellent internal consistency (Cronbach's alpha =0.838). Note: Internal consistency could be improved if feeding were excluded (Cronbach's alpha =0.845). Note: Internal consistency could be improved if continence were excluded (Cronbach's alpha =0.884) [21, 22].

Criterion Validity (Predictive / Concurrent)

Predictive Validity: Older Adults 2 years post-hospitalisation: (Katz, 1970), adequate predictive validity of Mobility (0.5033). Adequate predictive validity of House-Confinement (0.3882) [21 - 24].

FUNCTIONAL INDEPENDENCE MEASURE (FIM)

A technique for assessing patients' functional state during rehabilitation is the Functional Independence Measure (FIM). Measures of independence in self-care, such as sphincter control, transfers, locomotion, communication, and social cognition, are included. It is not specific to any one condition. The FIM evaluates a person's degree of disability and tracks how a patient's condition changes in response to treatment or rehabilitation. It is intended to evaluate areas of dysfunction in activities that patients with neurologic, musculoskeletal, or other illnesses—including functional mobility impairments—frequently experience. These disorders might be progressive, reversible, or persistent (Table **4**) [25].

Table 4. Functional Independence Measure (FIM).

	Admission	Discharge	Follow up
Self-Care			
A. Eating			
B. Grooming			
C. Bathing			
D. Dressing, upper body			
E. Dressing, lower body			
F. Toileting			
Sphincter Control			
G. Bladder management			
H. Bowel management			
Transfers			
I. Bed/Chair/Wheelchair			

(Table 4) cont.....

	Admission	Discharge	Follow up
Self-Care			
J. Toilet			
K. Tub/shower			
Locomotion			
L. Walk/wheelchair			
M. Stairs			
Motor subtotal score			
Communication			
N. Comprehension			
O. Expression			
Social Cognition			
P. Social Interaction			
Q. Problem Solving			
R. Memory			
Cognitive Subtotal Score			
TOTAL FIM Score			

ICF Domain: Activities of daily life

Number of items: 18 items scale, grouped into 2 subscales - motor and cognition [25].

Instructions for Administration and Scoring

Administrations

- The FIM is a clinician-administered outcome measure [25].
- The FIM assessment involves observing the individual's ability to perform daily living tasks and activities.
- The assessment is typically completed in 30-60 minutes, depending on the individual's ability and the complexity of the tasks [25].
- The FIM assessment should be conducted in a quiet and comfortable environment, free of distractions.

Equipment: Pencil and paper

Scoring

A 7-point ordinal scale, with a maximum score of 7, is used to score each item. The greater the score, the more self-sufficient the patient is in completing the task related to that item [25, 26].

1. Complete support with an assistant
2. Maximum support with an assistant
3. Moderate aid with the assistant
4. Limited help from the assistant
5. Overseeing or arranging with an assistant
6. Modified self-reliance without a caregiver
7. Total self-reliance without a helper

Leave no blanks; enter 1 if not testable due to risk [26].

Interpretability

- The FIM motor subscale has a total score range of 13 to 91, whereas the cognition subscale has a total score range of 5 to 35 [26].
- The motor and cognitive subscale scores are combined to form the overall FIM instrument score, which ranges from 18 to 126 [26].

Languages: English [26]

Training Required: No specific training required

Clinical Considerations

- The Functional Independence Measure (FIM) is a valuable tool in rehabilitation settings, used to assess the functional abilities of individuals with various conditions, including stroke, spinal cord injury, and traumatic brain injury [25].
- By providing a comprehensive understanding of an individual's functional abilities, the FIM facilitates prompt decision-making on treatment and intervention strategies. Serial FIM evaluations enable healthcare professionals to monitor progress, informing adjustments to treatment plans and optimising functional outcomes [26].
- The FIM score also serves as a prognostic indicator, approximating an individual's potential for functional recovery, with lower scores associated with a poorer prognosis and more extensive functional impairment [27].
- Furthermore, the FIM score can influence treatment decisions, including the necessity of physical, occupational, and speech therapies, as well as the level of care required [27].

Psychometric Properties

Reliability

- Excellent internal consistency (Cronbach's alpha = 0.93) [27]
- Excellent internal consistency (Cronbach's alpha = 0.95 FIM Total Score; 0.95 FIM Motor; 0.89 FIM Cognitive) [27].

Validity

- Predictive Validity- Admission motor FIM scores (β = 0.55) and admission cognitive FIM scores (β = 0.38) had the highest impact on discharge total FIM scores [28].

Responsiveness

- For the FIM motor, 15-36% of subjects showed a positive change exceeding the MDC, and 15-25% showed a negative change exceeding the MDC [29].
- In the FIM cognitive, 8-9% of subjects showed positive change exceeding the MDC, and 20-24% showed negative change exceeding the MDC [30].

Floor/Ceiling Effect

- Ceiling effect on FIM motor scale after discharge, ranging from 10% at 1 month to 15% at 12 months [30].
- Ceiling effect on the FIM cognitive scale after discharge for 70% of subjects at 1 month, reducing to 53% at 12 months [30].

SICKNESS IMPACT PROFILE

In order to assess an individual's perception of their health condition in relation to the impact of their illness, the Sickness Impact Profile (SIP), a behaviorally-based assessment of health status, was developed in 1972. It can detect variations in health conditions over time or between populations with sufficient sensitivity. It can also be used to evaluate the impact of diseases on an individual's capability to perform both physically and emotionally, as depicted in Table **5**. The evaluation of healthcare services outcomes which may be applied to planning, policy development, and program assessment, is another way SIP is helpful [31].

Table 5. Sickness impact profile-68 (SIP-68).

Category	Item Number	Item Description
Sleep and Rest	1	I am in bed most of the day.
	2	I have trouble sleeping because of my health.

(Table 5) cont.....

Category	Item Number	Item Description
	3	I need to rest more often during the day.
	4	I have trouble getting a good night's sleep.
	5	I feel tired even after resting.
	6	I have trouble relaxing.
	7	I have trouble taking naps.
Eating	8	I have trouble eating because of my health.
	9	I have lost my appetite.
	10	I have trouble preparing meals.
	11	I have trouble eating with others.
	12	I have trouble digesting food.
	13	I have trouble swallowing.
	14	I have trouble eating certain foods.
	15	I have trouble drinking enough fluids.
Work	16	I am unable to work at all.
	17	I have trouble concentrating at work.
	18	I have to take frequent breaks at work.
	19	I have trouble meeting deadlines.
	20	I have trouble doing my job.
	21	I have trouble getting to work.
	22	I have trouble staying at work all day.
	23	I have trouble doing physical tasks at work.
	24	I have trouble doing mental tasks at work.
Home Management	25	I have trouble doing household chores.
	26	I have trouble cleaning my home.
	27	I have trouble taking care of my yard.
	28	I have trouble doing laundry.
	29	I have trouble cooking meals.
	30	I have trouble managing my finances.
	31	I have trouble taking care of my pets.
	32	I have trouble doing maintenance tasks.
	33	I have trouble doing repairs.
	34	I have trouble doing yard work.
Recreation and Pastimes	35	I have trouble enjoying my hobbies.
	36	I have trouble going out with friends.

(Table 5) cont.....

Category	Item Number	Item Description
	37	I have trouble participating in sports or games.
	38	I have trouble watching TV or movies.
	39	I have trouble reading books or magazines.
	40	I have trouble listening to music.
	41	I have trouble doing crafts or arts.
	42	I have trouble traveling.
Ambulation	43	I have trouble walking.
	44	I have trouble using public transportation.
	45	I have trouble driving a car.
	46	I have trouble riding a bike.
	47	I have trouble walking up stairs.
	48	I have trouble walking down stairs.
	49	I have trouble standing for long periods.
	50	I have trouble sitting for long periods.
Mobility	51	I have trouble getting out of bed.
	52	I have trouble moving around my home.
	53	I have trouble transferring from one place to another.
	54	I have trouble standing up from a seated position.
	55	I have trouble sitting down from a standing position.
	56	I have trouble walking on uneven ground.
	57	I have trouble walking on slippery surfaces.
	58	I have trouble climbing stairs.
Body Care and Movement	59	I have trouble bathing myself.
	60	I have trouble dressing myself.
	61	I have trouble grooming myself.
	62	I have trouble moving my arms or legs.
	63	I have trouble using my hands or fingers.
	64	I have trouble using my feet or toes.
	65	I have trouble controlling my body movements.
	66	I have trouble maintaining my posture.
Social Interaction	67	I have trouble talking to others.
	68	I have trouble making friends.

ICF Domain: Body Structure, Body Function, Activity, and Participation

Number of items: SIP-68 contains 68 items [31]

Instructions for Administration and Scoring

Administration: SIP is a patient-reported outcome measure. Time required to administer is 15 to 30 minutes [31].

Equipment: Pencil and paper

Scoring: An analysis using Principal Components was used to build the SIP-68 from the items in the entire SIP. Each item on the SIP-68 is scored dichotomously (0 or 1), with higher scores indicating greater dysfunction [31].

Every item has a binomial score (yes = 1, no = 0), which is summed up at the end [32].

Interpretability: Scores range from 0 (best health) to 68 (worst health) [31, 32]

SEM: 3.79 [31]

MDC: 10.5 [31]

Languages: English [31]

Training Required: No specific training required

Clinical Considerations [31]

- For populations with brain injuries, a modified SIP has been created.
- The changes fall short of making gains that are significant enough or reliable enough to offer a useful advantage over the SIP.
- When used as long-term outcome measures, the SIP-68 is more sensitive than the Barthel Index to health-related task-specific behaviors.
- SIP-68 has been applied to patients with mild to severe traumatic brain injury.
- Cognition and awareness deficiencies may affect outcomes on this self-report questionnaire.
- The 136-item SIP served as the basis for the development of the SIP – CP (Sickness Impact Profile – Chronic Pain) assessment.
- 42 items, distributed across 7 subscales, including physical and psychosocial characteristics, make up the SIP-CP.

Psychometric Properties

Reliability

The SIP demonstrates good internal consistency:

- Cronbach's alpha values range from 0.91 to 0.95 for the overall score [31].
- For the two subscales, the alpha values range from 0.84–0.93 [31].
- Within the 12 categories, the alpha values range from 0.60 to 0.90 [31, 32]

The test-retest reliability between two administrations is also robust:

- The interviewer-administered version has a test-retest correlation of 0.97 [32]
- The self-completed version shows a correlation of 0.87 [31, 32]
- Excellent intrarater reliability (SWK = 0.87) [32]
- Excellent interrater reliability (ICC = 0.89) [32]

Validity

- Revised Strategy Application test significantly related to SIP total score $r(38) = -0.4$, $p < .05$ for mod/severe group [32].
- The R-SAT performance was related to the SIP psychosocial summary score, $r(38) = -.34$, $p < .05$ [32].

Responsiveness

- Responsiveness for the SIP-68 = 0.62 [31, 32]
- Responsiveness for the SIP-136 = 0.64 [31, 32]

Floor/ceiling effect: No floor and ceiling effect

LAWTON - BRODY INSTRUMENTAL ACTIVITIES OF DAILY LIVING SCALE (I.A.D.L.)

The Lawton-Brody Instrumental Activities of Daily Living Scale (I.A.D.L.) is a widely used assessment tool designed to measure an individual's ability to perform daily tasks that require some degree of complexity and organization [34]. The I.A.D.L. scale is a valuable tool for healthcare professionals to assess an individual's ability to perform daily tasks, which is essential for maintaining independence and quality of life.

ICF Domain: Activities of daily life

Number of items: The I.A.D.L. scale consists of 8 items, each assessing a specific instrumental activity of daily living [33]. These items include tasks such as using the telephone, shopping, and managing finances, which are essential for independent living.

Instructions for Administration and Scoring

- The I.A.D.L. scale is administered through a semi-structured interview with the individual being assessed or their caregiver [34].
- Each item is scored on a 3-point scale, with 0 indicating the individual is unable to perform the task, 1 indicating the individual requires assistance, and 2 indicating the individual can perform the task independently [34].

Equipment: No specific equipment is required to administer the I.A.D.L. scale.

Scoring: The total score ranges from 0 to 16, with higher scores indicating greater independence in instrumental activities of daily living [33].

Ability to Use Telephone

1. Operates telephone on own initiative; looks up and dials number ______1
2. Dials a few well-known numbers ______ 1
3. Answers the telephone, but does not dial ______1
4. Does not use telephone at all ______0

Shopping

1. Takes care of all shopping needs independently______1
2. Shops independently for small purchases______0
3. Needs to be accompanied on any shopping trip______0
4. Completely unable to shop______0

Food Preparation

1. Plans, prepares, and serves adequate meals independently______1
2. Prepares adequate meals if supplied with ingredients ______0
3. Heats and serves prepared meals or prepares meals but does not maintain adequate diet______0
4. Needs to have meals prepared and served______0

Housekeeping

1. Maintains house alone with occasion assistance (heavy work) ______1
2. Performs light daily tasks such as dishwashing, bed making______1
3. Performs light daily tasks, but cannot maintain acceptable level of

cleanliness______1
4. Needs help with all home maintenance tasks ______1
5. Does not participate in any housekeeping tasks______0

Laundry

1. Does personal laundry completely______1
2. Launders small items, rinses socks, stockings, *etc* ______1
3. All laundry must be done by others______0

Mode of Transportation

1. Travels independently on public transportation or drives own car______1
2. Arranges own travel via taxi, but does not otherwise use public transportation______1
3. Travels on public transportation when assisted or accompanied by another______1
4. Travel limited to taxi or automobile with assistance of another ______0
5. Does not travel at all______0

Responsibility for Own Medications

1. Is responsible for taking medication in correct dosages at correct time______1
2. Takes responsibility if medication is prepared in advance in separate dosages______0
3. Is not capable of dispensing own medication______0

Ability to Handle Finances

1. Manages financial matters independently (budgets, writes checks, pays rent and bills, goes to bank); collects and keeps track of income______1
2. Manages day-to-day purchases, but needs help with banking, major purchases, *etc* ______1
3. Incapable of handling money ______0

Interpretability

The I.A.D.L. scale scores can be interpreted as follows:

- 0-4: Severe impairment
- 5-8: Moderate impairment
- 9-12: Mild impairment
- 13-16: No impairment [34]

SEM (Standard Error of Measurement): The SEM for the I.A.D.L. scale is approximately 1.5 points [35].

MDC (Minimal Detectable Change): The MDC for the I.A.D.L. scale is approximately 3-4 points [35].

Languages: The I.A.D.L. scale has been translated into multiple languages, including English, Spanish, French, and Chinese [34].

Training Required: No specific training is required to administer the I.A.D.L. scale.

Clinical Considerations

- The I.A.D.L. scale is a useful tool for assessing an individual's ability to perform daily tasks that require some degree of complexity and organization.
- However, it may not be suitable for individuals with severe cognitive or physical impairments [34].

Psychometric Properties

Reliability

- The I.A.D.L. scale has been shown to have good internal consistency (Cronbach's alpha = 0.85) and test-retest reliability (ICC = 0.90) [34].

Validity

- The I.A.D.L. scale has been shown to have good construct validity, with significant correlations with other measures of functional ability [34].

Responsiveness

- The I.A.D.L. scale has been shown to be responsive to changes in functional ability over time [34].

Floor/Ceiling Effect

- The I.A.D.L. scale has been shown to have a moderate floor effect, with some individuals scoring at the lower end of the scale [34].

BRISTOL ACTIVITIES OF DAILY LIVING SCALE

The BADLS was developed with the help of caregivers of people with dementia to address the lack of specific measures for this population. The BADLS was designed during a period when the very early identification of dementia was not a priority. It was designed for self- completion by caregivers of people with dementia living in the community. Carers were involved both in the selection of activities for inclusion and in the design of rating levels for each activity. Items that were found to be insensitive, in that all the individuals with dementia either could or could not perform them, were removed from the scale [36, 37].

ICF Domain

Activities of daily life

Number of Items

The BADLS consist of 20 items assessing Basic ADL and IADL (food preparation, eating, drink preparation, drinking, dressing, personal hygiene, oral hygiene, bathing, toileting, transferring from bed or chair, mobility, orientation to time, orientation to place, communication, telephone use, housework/gardening, shopping, finances, games/hobbies and transport) [36].

Instructions for Administration and Scoring

The scale is usually completed by a caregiver or a close relative who is familiar with the individual's day-to-day functioning. There are 20 items covering different activities of daily living (*e.g.*, dressing, eating, using the toilet, *etc.*). For each item, the respondent selects the option that best describes the person's ability to perform the task (Table **6**).

Table 6. Bristol activities of daily living scale.

1. PREPARING FOOD	a) Selects and prepares food as required
	b) Able to prepare food if ingredients are set out
	c) Can prepare food if prompted step by step
	d) Unable to prepare food even with prompting and supervision
	e) Not applicable
2. EATING	a) Eats appropriately using correct cutlery
	b) Eats appropriately if food is made manageable and/or uses a spoon
	c) Uses fingers to eat food
	d) Needs to be fed
	e) Not applicable

(Table 6) cont.....

3. PREPARING DRINK	a) Selects and prepares drinks as required
	b) Can prepare drinks if ingredients are left available
	c) Can prepare drinks if prompted step by step
	d) Unable to make a drink even with prompting and supervision
	e) Not applicable
4. DRINKING	a) Drinks appropriately
	b) Drinks appropriately with aids, beaker/straw, *etc.*
	c) Does not drink appropriately even with aids but attempts to
	d) Has to have drinks administered (fed)
	e) Not applicable
5. DRESSING	a) Selects appropriate clothing and dresses self
	b) Puts clothes on in the wrong order and /or back to front and /or dirty clothing
	c) Unable to dress self but moves limbs to assist
	d) Unable to assist and requires total dressing
	e) Not applicable
6. HYGIENE	a) Washes regularly and independently
	b) Can wash self if given soap, flannel, towel, *etc.*
	c) Can wash self if prompted and supervised
	d) Unable to wash self and needs full assistance
	e) Not applicable
7. TEETH	a) Cleans own teeth/dentures regularly and independently
	b) Cleans teeth/dentures if given appropriate items
	c) Requires some assistance, toothpaste on brush, brush to mouth, *etc.*
	d) Full assistance given
	e) Not applicable
8. BATH/ SHOWER	a) Bathes regularly and independently
	b) Needs bath to be drawn/shower turned on but washes independently
	c) Needs supervision and prompting to wash
	d) Totally dependent, needs full assistance
	e) Not applicable

(Table 6) cont.....

9. TOILET/ COMMODE	a) Uses the toilet appropriately when required
	b) Needs to be taken to the toilet and given assistance
	c) Incontinent of urine or faeces
	d) Incontinent of urine and faeces
	e) Not applicable
10. TRANSFERS	a) Can get in/out of chair unaided
	b) Can get into a chair but needs help to get out
	c) Needs help getting in and out of a chair
	d) Totally dependent on being put into and lifted from chair
	e) Not applicable
11. MOBILITY	a) Walks independently
	b) Walks with assistance, *i.e.*, furniture, arm for support
	c) Uses aids to mobilise *i.e.* frame, sticks *etc.*
	d) Unable to walk
	e) Not applicable
12. ORIENTATION - TIME	a) Fully orientated to time/day/date, *etc.*
	b) Unaware of time/day, *etc.*, but seems unconcerned
	c) Repeatedly asks the time/day/date
	d) Mixes up night and day
	e) Not applicable
13. ORIENTATION - SPACE	a) Fully orientated to surroundings
	b) Oriented to familiar surroundings only
	c) Gets lost in the home, needs reminding where the bathroom is, *etc.*
	d) Does not recognise home as their own and attempts to leave
	e) Not applicable
14. COMMUNICATION	a) Able to hold an appropriate conversation
	b) Shows understanding and attempts to respond verbally with gestures
	c) Can make oneself understood but has difficulty understanding others
	d) Does not respond to or communicate with others
	e) Not applicable

(Table 6) cont.....

15. TELEPHONE	a) Uses the telephone appropriately, including obtaining the correct number
	b) Uses the telephone if the number given verbally/visually, or if it is predialled
	c) Answers the telephone but does not make calls
	d) Unable/unwilling to use the telephone at all
	e) Not applicable
16 HOUSEWORK / GARDENING	a) Able to do housework/gardening to the previous standard
	b) Able to do housework/gardening, but not to the previous standard
	c) Limited participation with a lot of supervision
	d) Unwilling/unable to participate in previous activities
	e) Not applicable
17. SHOPPING	a) Shops to the previous standard
	b) Only able to shop for 1 or 2 items with or without a list
	c) Unable to shop alone, but participates when accompanied
	d) Unable to participate in shopping even when accompanied
	e) Not applicable
18. FINANCES	a) Responsible for own finances at previous level
	b) Unable to write a cheque. Can sign name and recognise money values
	c) Can sign name but unable to recognise money values
	d) Unable to sign name or recognise money values
	e) Not applicable
19. GAMES /HOBBIES	a) Participates in pastimes/activities to the previous standard
	b) Participates but needs instruction/supervision
	c) Reluctant to join in, very slow, needs coaxing
	d) No longer able or willing to join in
	e) Not applicable
20. TRANSPORT	a) Able to drive, cycle, or use public transport independently
	b) Unable to drive but uses public transport, bike, *etc*.
	c) Unable to use public transport alone
	d) Unable/unwilling to use transport even when accompanied
	e) Not applicable

Each item is scored on a 4-point scale (0-3), where:

0: Independent, no help required.
1: Requires some help but can do most of the task alone.
2: Requires a lot of help or supervision.
3: Fully dependent, unable to perform the task.

Total score: Sum the scores for all 20 items. The total score will range from 0 to 60.

Interpretation: A higher score indicates greater dependency in daily activities.

0-9: Mild dependence

10-19: Moderate dependence

20-29: Severe dependence

30: Very severe dependence [36, 37]

Equipment

May vary based on the client's needs and level of impairment.

Time to Administer

The BADL takes about 10 minutes to complete and 5 minutes to score.

Required Training

No Training.

Languages

English [37], Arabic [38], Sinhalese [39].

Clinical Considerations

The BADLS is a useful tool for understanding how dementia affects a person's daily life. It can track a person's ability to manage daily tasks over time. This information helps healthcare professionals assess the severity of the dementia and plan appropriate treatment and support for both the patient and caregiver. The BADLS is often completed by caregivers who provide valuable information about the patient's daily abilities and their own stress levels. The BADLS focuses on physical abilities, not cognitive skills. To get complete information about a patient's health, it should be used with other tests that assess cognitive function, like the MMSE or MoCA [36, 37].

Psychometric Properties

Test / Retest Reliability

The BADLS correlated well with MMSE (r = -0.67, p < 0.001, 45% variance explained) and showed excellent test–retest reliability as measured both by correlation of scale totals (r = 0.95, p < 0.001, 89% variance explained) and by Cohen's kappa coefficients for each of the 20 items (seven items with fair or moderate kappa scores, 0.30–0.59; 13 with good or very good kappa scores, 0.62–0.94) [36, 37].

Criterion Validity (Predictive/Concurrent)

BADLS scores ranged from 0 to 42, with a mean of 19.2, SD of 11.2, and skewness of 0.198. BADLS correlated (r = -0.67, p< 0.001, 44.9% variance explained) with the MMSE. There were no differences in total BADLS score between men and women (t = 1.1, df 57, p = 0.30), and no relationship with years of education (r = 0.04, p = 0.75). There was a significant positive correlation between the BADLS score and age (r = 0.32, p = 0.013), explaining 10.4% of the variance. Partial correlation between MMSE and BADLS score, controlling for age, still yielded a good relationship between cognitive test performance and carer-rated ADL ability (Pearson's r = -0.72, p< 0.001, 52.3% variance explained) [36, 37].

Sensitivity and Specificity

Optimal cut-off score of the modified Bristol scale was 20 with a sensitivity of 100%, specificity of 74.2%, and the area under the curve 0.933(95% CI: 0.871-0.995) [39].

This questionnaire is designed to reveal the everyday ability of people who have memory difficulties of one form or another.

For each activity (No. 1 - 20), statements a - e refer to a different level of ability.

Thinking of the last 2 weeks, tick the box that represents your relative's/ friend's AVERAGE ability.

CLINICAL ASSESSMENT SCALE FOR AUTOIMMUNE ENCEPHALITIS (CASE)

The Clinical Assessment Scale for Autoimmune Encephalitis (CASE) is a specialized clinical scale designed to assess the severity of autoimmune encephalitis (AE) [40]. It was developed to address the limitations of existing scales, such as the modified Rankin scale (mRS), which primarily focus on motor deficits and functional independence [41].

ICF DOMAIN: The CASE assesses various aspects of AE, including cognitive, emotional, and behavioral functions, which are classified under the following ICF domains [40, 41]:

- b1: Mental functions (*e.g.*, memory, attention, executive functions)
- b2: Sensory functions (*e.g.*, perception, hallucinations)
- b3: Voice and speech functions (*e.g.*, language, communication)
- b4: Functions of the cardiovascular, hematological, immunological, and respiratory systems (*e.g.*, seizures, dyskinesia)
- b5: Functions of the digestive, metabolic, and endocrine systems (*e.g.*, appetite, sleep)
- b6: Genitourinary and reproductive functions (*e.g.*, libido, menstruation)
- b7: Neuromusculoskeletal and movement-related functions (*e.g.*, weakness, ataxia)

NUMBER OF ITEMS: The CASE consists of 9 items, each assessing a specific aspect of AE [41]:

1. Seizures
2. Memory dysfunction
3. Psychiatric symptoms (delusion, hallucination, disinhibition, aggression)
4. Consciousness
5. Language problem
6. Dyskinesia/dystonia
7. Gait instability and ataxia
8. Brainstem dysfunction
9. Weakness

SCALES

- Seizures: 0 (no seizures), 1 (controlled seizures), 2 (uncontrolled seizures) [40]
- Memory dysfunction: 0 (no memory impairment), 1 (mild memory impairment), 2 (severe memory impairment)

- Psychiatric symptoms: 0 (no psychiatric symptoms), 1 (mild psychiatric symptoms), 2 (severe psychiatric symptoms)
- Consciousness: 0 (normal consciousness), 1 (mild impairment of consciousness), 2 (severe impairment of consciousness)
- Language problem: 0 (no language problem), 1 (mild language problem), 2 (severe language problem)
- Dyskinesia/dystonia: 0 (no dyskinesia/dystonia), 1 (mild dyskinesia/dystonia), 2 (severe dyskinesia/dystonia)
- Gait instability and ataxia: 0 (no gait instability and ataxia), 1 (mild gait instability and ataxia), 2 (severe gait instability and ataxia)
- Brainstem dysfunction: 0 (no brainstem dysfunction), 1 (mild brainstem dysfunction), 2 (severe brainstem dysfunction)
- Weakness: 0 (no weakness), 1 (mild weakness), 2 (severe weakness)

INSTRUCTIONS FOR ADMINISTRATION AND SCORING

- The CASE is administered by a trained healthcare professional, typically a neurologist or psychiatrist [40].
- The scale is scored based on the patient's current symptoms and functional status, with each item rated on a 3-point scale (0-2).
- The total score ranges from 0 to 27, with higher scores indicating greater severity.

EQUIPMENT: No specific equipment is required to administer the CASE.

SCORING:

The CASE is scored by summing the ratings of each item [40].

The total score can be used to assess the severity of AE and monitor changes over time.

INTERPRETABILITY: The CASE scores can be interpreted as follows [40, 41]:

- 0-6: Mild AE
- 7-13: Moderate AE
- 14-20: Severe AE
- 21-27: Very severe AE

SEM (STANDARD ERROR OF MEASUREMENT): The SEM of the CASE has not been reported in the literature.

MDC (MINIMAL DETECTABLE CHANGE): The MDC of the CASE has not been reported in the literature.

LANGUAGES: The CASE has been translated into several languages, including English, Korean, and Chinese [40, 42].

TRAINING REQUIRED: Healthcare professionals administering the CASE should have training in neurology or psychiatry and experience in assessing patients with AE.

CLINICAL CONSIDERATIONS: The CASE should be used in conjunction with other clinical assessments and diagnostic tests to evaluate patients with suspected AE. The scale is not intended to be used as a diagnostic tool, but rather to assess the severity of AE and monitor changes over time.

PSYCHOMETRIC PROPERTIES

- **Reliability:** The CASE has demonstrated excellent inter-rater reliability (ICC = 0.96) and intra-rater reliability (ICC = 0.98) [40].
- **Validity:** The CASE has shown good construct validity, with significant correlations with the mRS (r = 0.80) [40].
- **Responsiveness:** The CASE has demonstrated responsiveness to changes in AE severity over time [40].
- **Floor/Ceiling Effect:** The CASE has not been reported to have a significant floor or ceiling effect [40].

RESPONSIVENESS METRICS

- **Effect size:** The CASE has shown a moderate to large effect size (0.5-1.0) in detecting changes in AE severity over time [40].
- **Standardized response means:** The CASE has shown a moderate to large standardized response mean (0.5-1.0) in detecting changes in AE severity over time [40].

THE LIVERPOOL OUTCOME SCORE

Japanese encephalitis (JE) is a mosquito-borne disease and the leading cause of viral encephalitis in Asia. Children bear the greatest burden of JE disease, as most adults have developed immunity to infection. In Indonesia, surveillance studies have recently confirmed JE to be an endemic human disease across the country. A simple assessment tool to measure the extent of disability after JE has recently been developed and validated. The Liverpool Outcome Score enables a rapid appraisal of the practical level of disability. A key purpose of the tool is to predict the likelihood that a child will be able to live independently. It is suitable for use by a range of health professionals, requires minimum training, and does not require any equipment for implementation; thus, it is suitable for use in developing country settings where specialized equipment is not always readily available [43].

ICF Domain

It comprises the ability to perform activities, such as walking and personal care, as well as the ability to participate in society—*e.g.*, independent transportation, the ability to work, economic self-sufficiency, and social integration [44].

Number of Items

The Liverpool Outcome Score assesses basic motor and self-care skills, as well as simple cognitive and behavioral functions, through a series of 10 questions posed to the parent or caregiver, and five observations of the child performing simple activities [43].

Languages

The Liverpool Outcome Score was translated into Bahasa (Indonesian language) and pre-tested before use [43].

Instructions for Administration and Scoring

In many questions, the interviewee is asked to compare the child's ability with that of peers of similar age in the community. The child receives a score for each question based on the grading scale for that question. For each question, a set of possible answers, scored from 2 to 5, is provided. A child whose response to a particular question is completely normal would score 5 for that question. One with minor sequelae, for example, mild behavioral problems, would score 4. A child with moderate sequelae that affect function but would not lead to dependence (*e.g.*, difficulty walking) would score 3. A child whose impairment is so great that it would lead to dependence in that setting (*e.g.*, being unable to walk in rural India) would score 2. The total score ranges from 33 to 75, while the lowest score for any single question ranges from 2 to 5.

The LOS is used to classify children into the following categories:

Liverpool Score 5: Full recovery

Liverpool Score 4: Minor sequelae

Liverpool Score <3: Moderate or severe sequelae, or death [44, 45]

Time to Administer

The amount of time needed to complete the LOS assessment varies depending on the specific questions and whether a parent or caregiver is assisting.

Required Training

Requires minimum training [43]

Clinical Considerations

The Liverpool outcome score is used across various types of encephalitis, including viral, autoimmune, and post-infectious encephalitis. Severity at presentation (coma, seizures, extensive brain involvement on imaging) is often predictive of lower LOS, guiding clinicians on the level of care and rehabilitation needed. LOS is a useful tool, but it may not capture all aspects of the patient's quality of life, such as psychological and emotional well-being.

Psychometric Properties

Inter- and Intra-observer Agreement

In the Malaysian cohort, there was very good inter-observer agreement ($K = 0.714$) on the outcome score when children were classified according to the severity of their sequelae; intra-observer agreement was also very good ($K = 0.943$). In the Indian cohort, inter-observer agreement was moderate ($K = 0.584$), and intra-observer agreement was good ($K = 0.799$) [45].

Validity

When the outcome was the child's dependence or independence, very good agreement was observed, with $K = 0.906$ and $K = 0.762$ for the Malaysian and Indian cohorts, respectively [45].

Sensitivity and Specificity

The sensitivity and specificity of the new score in identifying children likely to be dependent, as determined by clinical assessment, were 100% (95% CI: 89.1–100) and 98.4% (95% CI: 96.5–99.4), respectively, in Malaysia and 100% (95% CI: 91.2–100) and 93.8% (95% CI: 90.7–96.0), respectively, in India [45].

Liverpool Outcome Score for Assessing Children at Discharge

Name: Date of birth (dd/mm/yy): ____ _ / ___ __ /___ ___

Age: Sex: Male ☐ Female ☐ Study No.

Today's date (dd/mm/yy): ___ ___ /___ ___ /___ ___

Date of admission to hospital (dd/mm/yy): ___ /___ /____

Date of discharge from hospital ___ /___ /____

Relationship of person with child (*e.g.*, mother/aunt):

Name of person completing form – please print: ____________________

Job Title: ________________

Answer each question. Circle or underline the correct answer, and write the score in the column

Ask the parent or caregiver the following questions:

For some of these questions, you ask the parent or caregiver how the child compares with how they were immediately before the illness (irrespective of the length of time in hospital).

1. Speech or communication

Compared with before the illness, is the child's speech or communication:

- The same as before (5)
- Changed or reduced (3)
- Not speaking or communicating (2)

2. Feeding

The child's feeding is:
- The same as before the illness (5)
- Occasionally needs help (3)
- Always needs more help (2)

3. Leaving Alone

Before the illness, could this child be left alone without coming to harm?
- If **No** score 5 (5)

If **Yes**, can this child now be left alone?
- Yes (5)

• Yes, briefly in a familiar environment (3)
• No (2)

4. Behaviour

Compared with before the illness, do the caregivers think the child's behaviour is altered?
• No completely normal (5)
• Gets angry easily (4)
• Other behavioural problems (4)
• Severely abnormal (2)
If abnormal, give details:

5. Recognition

Could the child recognise their family members, other than their main carer, before the illness?
• If **No**, score 5 (5)
If **Yes**, can this child now recognise their family members, other than their main carer?
• Yes (5)
• Some (3)
• None (2)

6. School and working

Before the illness, was the child at school or working?
If **Yes**, do the carers think the child will go back to school or work?
• Yes (5)
• No (3)
If **No,** do the carers think the child will still be able to do the same tasks at home, follow the same routine, or play normally?
• Yes (5)
• Not able to (3)

7. Epilepsy/ Seizures

Did the child have any seizures during this illness?
• If **No**, score 5 (5)
If **Yes**, is the child still having seizures?
• No seizures and not on anti-epileptic drugs (5)
• No seizures and on anti-epileptic drugs (4)

• Yes, still having seizures (3)
• Yes, seizures most days (2)

8. Dressing

Can other children of this age dress themselves?
• If **No**, score 5 (5)
If **Yes**, can the child dress themselves since their illness?
• Yes, the same as before illness (5)
• Occasionally needs extra help (3)
• Needs more help than before (2)

9. Bladder and Bowel Control

Is urinary and faecal continence:
• The same as before the illness (5)
• Occasionally needs more help or occasionally is incontinent (4)
• Needs more help or is incontinent of bowel or bladder (2)

10. Hearing

Does the parent think this child's hearing is:
• Normal (5)
• Reduced in one or both ears (4)
• Cannot hear at all (3)
Observation of the child's abilities
For these questions, you observe what the child can do. If you cannot get the child to cooperate, answer these questions based on what the caregiver says.

11. Sitting

Could the child sit before the illness?
• If **No**, score 5 (5)
If **Yes**, observe, can this child sit?
• Yes independently (5)
• Needs help (3)
• Not at all (2)

12. Standing up

Could the child get from a sitting to a standing position before the illness?
• If **No**, score 5 (5)

If **Yes**, observe, can the child get from sitting to standing?
- Yes, independently (5)
- Needs help (3)
- Not at all (2)

13. Walking

Could the child walk before the illness?
- If **No**, score 5 (5)

If **Yes**, observe this child walking 5 metres across the room. The child walks:
- Normally (5)
- Abnormally, but independently +/- crutches/stick (3)
- Not able to walk (2)

14. Hands on head

Put both your hands on your head, and ask the child to copy you. Child is:
- Too young (5)
- Both hands are normal (5)
- One or both hands are abnormal (4)
- Unable to use one or both hands (3)

15. Picking Up

Ask the child to pick up a pea-sized ball of paper or a small coin. Child is:
- Too young (5)
- Normal pincer grasp of both hands (5)
- Unable with one hand (3)
- Abnormal one hand or both hands (3)
- Unable to use both hands (2)

Outcome Score =Lowest score for any single question (range 2-5):
Total Score = all the individual scores added up (range 33 –75):
(If the child died, the score = 1)
Any other Comments:
The Final Liverpool Outcome Score is the lowest number scored for any single question
Score interpretation:
5 = Full recovery
4 = Minor sequelae with no effect, or only minor effects, on physical function; or personality change; or on medication.
3 = Moderate sequelae mildly affecting function, probably compatible with independent living

2 = Severe sequelae, impairing function sufficient to make the patient dependent
1 = Death

CLINICAL CONSIDERATIONS, STRENGTHS, LIMITATIONS, AND EMERGING TRENDS

Miscellaneous functional and outcome scales are widely used across neurological and medical conditions to evaluate independence, disability, participation, and overall disease impact. These instruments are particularly valuable when disease-specific scales are unavailable or when a global assessment of functional status is required. However, the heterogeneity of constructs measured by these tools necessitates careful selection based on clinical objectives, patient characteristics, and care settings [46].

Basic activities of daily living (ADL) scales, such as the Barthel Index and the Katz Index, assess on fundamental self-care tasks, including feeding, dressing, toileting, and mobility. Their primary strengths are simplicity, rapid administration, and strong inter-rater reliability. These scales are especially useful in acute care and early rehabilitation settings. However, ceiling effects are common among higher-functioning individuals, and subtle functional changes may not be detected, limiting their usefulness for long-term outcome monitoring [47].

The Functional Independence Measure (FIM) provides a broader assessment by incorporating motor and cognitive domains, making it a cornerstone outcome measure in inpatient rehabilitation. Its standardized scoring system allows comparison across facilities and patient populations. Despite these strengths, FIM administration requires formal training, and licensing restrictions may limit accessibility. Additionally, its sensitivity to change in community-dwelling or mildly impaired individuals is limited [48].

Instrumental activities of daily living (IADL) measures, such as the Lawton–Brody IADL scale, extend functional assessment to more complex tasks, including financial management, medication use, and community mobility. These tools are particularly relevant in geriatric and cognitive disorders. However, performance may be influenced by cultural roles, gender expectations, and social context, potentially affecting interpretability across populations [49].

Global health status instruments, such as the Sickness Impact Profile (SIP), evaluate the perceived impact of illness on physical, emotional, and social functioning. While these measures provide a comprehensive overview of disease burden, their length and administrative complexity limit routine clinical use.

Shorter disease-specific or function-focused tools are often preferred for regular follow-up [50].

Condition-specific scales included in this chapter address emerging clinical needs. The Bristol Activities of Daily Living Scale was developed to assess functional decline in dementia and captures both basic and instrumental activities relevant to disease progression. The Clinical Assessment Scale for Autoimmune Encephalitis (CASE) provides a structured method for quantifying neurological and psychiatric symptom severity in autoimmune encephalitis, supporting both clinical monitoring and research applications. The Liverpool Outcome Score offers a global outcome measure across neurological conditions, emphasizing functional recovery and disability rather than diagnosis-specific impairment [51, 52].

A key limitation across miscellaneous scales is conceptual overlap, particularly among ADL measures. Using multiple tools that assess similar domains may increase assessment burden without yielding additional clinically meaningful information. Purpose-driven selection—basic ADL scales for acute care, comprehensive measures like FIM for rehabilitation, and condition-specific tools for targeted monitoring—enhances efficiency and interpretability [46, 52].

Emerging trends in functional outcome assessment emphasize streamlined tools, digital data capture, and patient-centered evaluation. Electronic health record integration, mobile-based assessments, and remote monitoring platforms are increasingly being explored to facilitate longitudinal follow-up. In parallel, newer scales such as CASE reflect a growing emphasis on structured outcome measurement in previously under-assessed neurological conditions. These developments aim to complement established instruments while reducing administrative burden and improving ecological validity [51, 52].

In clinical practice, miscellaneous scales should be selected strategically based on the stage of illness and assessment goals. Barthel Index and Katz ADL are appropriate for rapid functional screening, FIM supports comprehensive rehabilitation assessment, IADL scales inform community functioning, and condition-specific tools such as CASE and Bristol ADL enhance disease-focused monitoring. An integrated but selective approach ensures meaningful functional assessment while minimizing redundancy (Table **7**).

Table 7. Comparative summary of commonly used miscellaneous functional and outcome scales.

Scale	Primary Domain Assessed	Key Strengths	Major Limitations	Optimal Clinical Use
Barthel Index	Basic ADL	Simple; reliable	Ceiling effects	Acute care, early rehab

(Table 7) cont.....

Scale	Primary Domain Assessed	Key Strengths	Major Limitations	Optimal Clinical Use
Katz Index of ADL	Basic ADL	Quick screening	Limited sensitivity	Functional screening
FIM	Motor and cognitive function	Standardized; comprehensive	Training and licensing	Inpatient rehabilitation
Lawton–Brody IADL	Instrumental ADL	Community relevance	Cultural influence	Geriatrics, cognition
Sickness Impact Profile	Global health status	Comprehensive coverage	Lengthy; time-consuming	Research settings
Bristol ADL Scale	Dementia-related function	Disease-specific	Limited to dementia	Dementia progression
CASE	Autoimmune encephalitis severity	Structured; responsive	Limited widespread use	AE monitoring
Liverpool Outcome Score	Global neurological outcome	Broad applicability	Less diagnostic specificity	Long-term outcome

CONCLUSION

Functional and neurological assessment scales play a pivotal role in understanding the multifaceted aspects of patient health, encompassing physical, cognitive, emotional, and social domains. These tools enable healthcare professionals to quantify functional independence, monitor recovery, and evaluate the outcomes of therapeutic interventions across diverse clinical populations. In addition, scales assessing infections of the central nervous system, such as meningitis and encephalitis, provide critical insights into disease progression and treatment efficacy. Collectively, these assessment instruments facilitate a comprehensive and patient-centered approach to clinical evaluation, empowering practitioners to design individualized care strategies and optimize rehabilitation outcomes.

AI DISCLOSURE STATEMENT

During the preparation of this chapter, the authors used ChatGPT (OpenAI) as a support tool for language refinement, structural organisation, and clarification of ideas. All content generated with AI assistance was carefully reviewed, verified, and revised by the authors to ensure factual accuracy, originality, and consistency with the scientific literature. The authors take full responsibility for the integrity, interpretation, and final content of the published chapter.

ACKNOWLEDGEMENT

The authors express their sincere appreciation to the multidisciplinary teams of physicians, rehabilitation specialists, neuropsychologists, and researchers whose collective efforts have contributed to the development and validation of functional and neurological assessment scales. Their continued work in refining tools for evaluating activities of daily living, cognitive performance, and neuroinflammatory conditions has significantly improved patient care, clinical decision-making, and rehabilitation outcomes.

REFERENCES

[1] Pashmdarfard M, Azad A. Assessment tools to evaluate Activities of Daily Living (ADL) and Instrumental Activities of Daily Living (IADL) in older adults: A systematic review. Med J Islam Repub Iran 2020; 34: 33.
[http://dx.doi.org/10.47176/mjiri.34.33] [PMID: 32617272]

[2] Chauhan S, Kumar S, Bharti R, Patel R. Prevalence and determinants of activity of daily living and instrumental activity of daily living among elderly in India. BMC Geriatr 2022; 22(1): 64.
[http://dx.doi.org/10.1186/s12877-021-02659-z] [PMID: 35045809]

[3] Ocagli H, Cella N, Stivanello L, Degan M, Canova C. The Barthel Index as an indicator of hospital outcomes: a retrospective cross-sectional study. J Adv Nurs. 2021; 77(4): 1751–1761. doi:10.1111/jan.14708

[4] MacIsaac RL, Ali M, Taylor-Rowan M, Rodgers H, Lees KR, Quinn TJ. Use of a 3-Item Short-Form Version of the Barthel Index for Use in Stroke. Stroke 2017; 48(3): 618-23.
[http://dx.doi.org/10.1161/STROKEAHA.116.014789] [PMID: 28154094]

[5] Ocagli H, Cella N, Stivanello L, Degan M, Canova C. The Barthel index as an indicator of hospital outcomes: A retrospective cross-sectional study with healthcare data from older people. J Adv Nurs 2021; 77(4): 1751-61.
[http://dx.doi.org/10.1111/jan.14708] [PMID: 33277770]

[6] Della Pietra GL, Savio K, Oddone E, Reggiani M, Monaco F, Leone MA. Validity and reliability of the Barthel index administered by telephone. Stroke 2011; 42(7): 2077-9.
[http://dx.doi.org/10.1161/STROKEAHA.111.613521] [PMID: 21527755]

[7] Hsieh YW, Wang CH, Wu SC, Chen PC, Sheu CF, Hsieh CL. Establishing the minimal clinically important difference of the Barthel Index in stroke patients. Neurorehabil Neural Repair 2007; 21(3): 233-8.
[http://dx.doi.org/10.1177/1545968306294729] [PMID: 17351082]

[8] González N, Bilbao A, Forjaz MJ, *et al.* Psychometric characteristics of the Spanish version of the Barthel Index. Aging Clin Exp Res 2018; 30(5): 489-97.
[http://dx.doi.org/10.1007/s40520-017-0809-5] [PMID: 28770477]

[9] Ferfeli S, Galanos A, Dontas IA, Triantafyllou A, Triantafyllopoulos IK, Chronopoulos E. Reliability and validity of the Greek adaptation of the Modified Barthel Index in neurorehabilitation patients. Eur J Phys Rehabil Med 2024; 60(1): 44-54.
[http://dx.doi.org/10.23736/S1973-9087.23.08056-5] [PMID: 37877957]

[10] Heuschmann PU, Kolominsky-Rabas PL, Nolte CH, *et al.* [The reliability of the german version of the barthel-index and the development of a postal and telephone version for the application on stroke patients]. Fortschr Neurol Psychiatr 2005; 73(2): 74-82.
[http://dx.doi.org/10.1055/s-2004-830172] [PMID: 15685491]

[11] Galeoto G, Formica MC, Mercuri NB, *et al.* Evaluation of the psychometric properties of the Barthel

Index in an Italian ischemic stroke population in the acute phase: a cross-sectional study. Funct Neurol 2019; 34(1): 29-34.
[http://dx.doi.org/10.11138/FNeur/2019.34.1.029] [PMID: 31172937]

[12] Küçükdeveci AA, Yavuzer G, Tennant A, Süldür N, Sonel B, Arasil T. Adaptation of the modified Barthel Index for use in physical medicine and rehabilitation in Turkey. Scand J Rehabil Med 2000; 32(2): 87-92.
[http://dx.doi.org/10.1080/003655000750045604] [PMID: 10853723]

[13] Hormozi S, Alizadeh-Khoei M, Sharifi F, *et al.* Iranian Version of Barthel Index: Validity and Reliability in Outpatients' Elderly. Int J Prev Med 2019; 10(1): 130.
[http://dx.doi.org/10.4103/ijpvm.IJPVM_579_18] [PMID: 31516671]

[14] Leung SOC, Chan CCH, Shah S. Development of a Chinese version of the Modified Barthel Index — validity and reliability. Clin Rehabil 2007; 21(10): 912-22.
[http://dx.doi.org/10.1177/0269215507077286] [PMID: 17981850]

[15] Green J, Young J, Young J. A test-retest reliability study of the Barthel Index. Disabil Rehabil 2001; 23(15): 670-6.
[http://dx.doi.org/10.1080/09638280110045382] [PMID: 11720117]

[16] Yang CM, Wang YC, Lee CH, Chen MH, Hsieh CL. A comparison of test–retest reliability and random measurement error of the Barthel Index and modified Barthel Index in patients with chronic stroke. Disabil Rehabil 2022; 44(10): 2099-103.
[http://dx.doi.org/10.1080/09638288.2020.1814429] [PMID: 32903114]

[17] Mahoney FI, Barthel DW. Functional evaluation: the Barthel Index. Md State Med J 1965; 14: 61–65. PMID: 14258950 DOI: https://doi.org/10.1037/t02366-000

[18] Shah S, Vanclay F, Cooper B. Improving the sensitivity of the Barthel Index for stroke rehabilitation. J Clin Epidemiol. 1989; 42(8): 703–709. doi:10.1016/0895-4356(89)90065-6

[19] Collin C, Wade DT, Davies S, Horne V. The Barthel ADL Index: a reliability study. Int Disabil Stud 1988; 10(2): 61-3.
[http://dx.doi.org/10.3109/09638288809164103] [PMID: 3403500]

[20] Katz S, Downs TD, Cash HR, Grotz RC. Progress in development of the index of ADL. Gerontologist 1970; 10(1 Part 1): 20-30.
[http://dx.doi.org/10.1093/geront/10.1_Part_1.20] [PMID: 5420677]

[21] Katz S. Assessing self-maintenance: activities of daily living, mobility, and instrumental activities of daily living. J Am Geriatr Soc 1983; 31(12): 721-7.
[http://dx.doi.org/10.1111/j.1532-5415.1983.tb03391.x] [PMID: 6418786]

[22] Brorsson B, Asberg KH. Katz index of independence in ADL. Reliability and validity in short-term care. J Rehabil Med 1984; 16(3): 125-32.
[http://dx.doi.org/10.2340/165019778416125132] [PMID: 6494836]

[23] Arik G, Varan HD, Yavuz BB, *et al.* Validation of Katz index of independence in activities of daily living in Turkish older adults. Arch Gerontol Geriatr 2015; 61(3): 344-50.
[http://dx.doi.org/10.1016/j.archger.2015.08.019] [PMID: 26328478]

[24] Azad A, Mohammadinezhad T, Taghizadeh G, Lajevardi L. Clinical assessment of activities of daily living in acute stroke: Validation of the Persian version of Katz Index. Med J Islam Repub Iran 2017; 31(1): 178-83.
[http://dx.doi.org/10.18869/mjiri.31.30] [PMID: 29445659]

[25] Katz S, Ford AB, Moskowitz RW, Jackson BA, Jaffe MW. Studies of illness in the aged: The index of ADL. JAMA 1963; 185(12): 914-9.
[http://dx.doi.org/10.1001/jama.1963.03060120024016] [PMID: 14044222]

[26] Granger CV, Hamilton BB, Linacre JM, Heinemann AW, Wright BD. Performance profiles of the Functional Independence Measure. Am J Phys Med Rehabil. 2010; 89(3): 169–176.

doi:10.1097/PHM.0b013e3181c6f3a9

[27] Heinemann AW, Linacre JM, Wright BD, Hamilton BB, Granger C. Relationships between impairment and physical disability as measured by the functional independence measure. Arch Phys Med Rehabil 1993; 74(6): 566-73.
[http://dx.doi.org/10.1016/0003-9993(93)90153-2] [PMID: 8503745]

[28] Dodds TA, Martin DP, Stolov WC, Deyo RA. A validation of the Functional Independence Measurement and its performance among rehabilitation inpatients. Arch Phys Med Rehabil 1993; 74(5): 531-6.
[http://dx.doi.org/10.1016/0003-9993(93)90119-U] [PMID: 8489365]

[29] Hobart JC, Lamping DL, Freeman JA, *et al.* Evidence-based measurement. Neurology 2001; 57(4): 639-44.
[http://dx.doi.org/10.1212/WNL.57.4.639] [PMID: 11524472]

[30] Ng YS, Jung H, Tay SS, Bok CW, Chiong Y, Lim PAC. Results from a prospective acute inpatient rehabilitation database: clinical characteristics and functional outcomes using the Functional Independence Measure. Ann Acad Med Singap 2007; 36(1): 3-10.
[http://dx.doi.org/10.47102/annals-acadmedsg.V36N1p3] [PMID: 17285180]

[31] Coster W, Haley S, Jette A. Measuring patient-reported outcomes after discharge from inpatient rehabilitation settings. J Rehabil Med 2006; 38(4): 237-42.
[http://dx.doi.org/10.1080/16501970600609774] [PMID: 16801206]

[32] van Baalen B, Odding E, van Woensel MP, van Kessel MA, Roebroeck ME, Stam HJ. Reliability and sensitivity to change of measurement instruments used in a traumatic brain injury population. Clin Rehabil 2006; 20(8): 686-700.
[http://dx.doi.org/10.1191/0269215506cre982oa] [PMID: 16944826]

[33] Bergner M, Bobbitt RA, Carter WB, Gilson BS. The Sickness Impact Profile: development and final revision of a health status measure. Med Care 1981; 19(8): 787-805.
[http://dx.doi.org/10.1097/00005650-198108000-00001] [PMID: 7278416]

[34] Lawton MP, Brody EM. Assessment of older people: self-maintaining and instrumental activities of daily living. Gerontologist 1969; 9(3 Part 1): 179-86.
[http://dx.doi.org/10.1093/geront/9.3_Part_1.179] [PMID: 5349366]

[35] Graf C. The Lawton instrumental activities of daily living scale. Am J Nurs 2008; 108(4): 52-62.
[http://dx.doi.org/10.1097/01.NAJ.0000314810.46029.74] [PMID: 18367931]

[36] Haley SM, Fragala-Pinkham MA. Interpreting change scores of the Lawton Instrumental Activities of Daily Living Scale. J Rehabil Res Dev 2006; 43(5): 655-64.
[http://dx.doi.org/10.1682/JRRD.2005.09.0135]

[37] Alkeridy WA, Al Khalifah RA, Mohammedin AS, Khallaf R, Muayqil T, Bucks RS. The Arabic translation and cross-cultural adaptation of the Bristol Activities of Daily Living Scale. J Alzheimers Dis. 2022; 86(3): 1123–1130. doi:10.3233/JAD-215489

[38] Bucks RS, Haworth J. Bristol Activities of Daily Living Scale: a critical evaluation. Expert Rev Neurother 2002; 2(5): 669-76.
[http://dx.doi.org/10.1586/14737175.2.5.669] [PMID: 19810983]

[39] Alkeridy WA, Al Khalifah RA, Mohammedin AS, Khallaf R, Muayqil T, Bucks RS. The Arabic Translation and Cross-Cultural Adaptation of the Bristol Activity of Daily Living Scale. J Alzheimers Dis 2022; 86(3): 1123-30.
[http://dx.doi.org/10.3233/JAD-215489] [PMID: 35147542]

[40] Umayal S, Kulathunga M, Somaratne S, Srikanth S, Kathriarachchi S, De Silva R. Validation of a functional screening instrument for dementia in an elderly sri lankan population: comparison of modified bristol and blessed activities of daily living scales. BMC Res Notes 2010; 3(1): 268.
[http://dx.doi.org/10.1186/1756-0500-3-268] [PMID: 20974013]

[41] Lim JA, Lee ST, Moon J, *et al.* Development of the clinical assessment scale in autoimmune encephalitis. Ann Neurol 2019; 85(3): 352-8.
[http://dx.doi.org/10.1002/ana.25421] [PMID: 30675918]

[42] van Swieten JC, Koudstaal PJ, Visser MC, Schouten HJ, van Gijn J. Interobserver agreement for the assessment of handicap in stroke patients. Stroke 1988; 19(5): 604-7.
[http://dx.doi.org/10.1161/01.STR.19.5.604] [PMID: 3363593]

[43] Cai MT, Lai QL, Zheng Y, *et al.* Validation of the clinical assessment scale for autoimmune encephalitis: A multicenter study. Neurol Ther 2021; 10(2): 985-1000.
[http://dx.doi.org/10.1007/s40120-021-00278-9] [PMID: 34476753]

[44] Maha MS, Moniaga VA, Hills SL, *et al.* Outcome and extent of disability following Japanese encephalitis in Indonesian children. Int J Infect Dis 2009; 13(6): e389-93.
[http://dx.doi.org/10.1016/j.ijid.2009.01.009] [PMID: 19346144]

[45] Brenner J, Olijslagers SHC, Crijnen YS, de Vries JM, Mandarakas MR, Titulaer MJ. Clinical Outcome Assessments in Encephalitis. Neurol Neuroimmunol Neuroinflamm 2024; 11(1): e200168.
[http://dx.doi.org/10.1212/NXI.0000000000200168] [PMID: 38086078]

[46] Lewthwaite P, Begum A, Ooi MH, *et al.* Disability after encephalitis: development and validation of a new outcome score. Bull World Health Organ 2010; 88(8): 584-92.
[http://dx.doi.org/10.2471/BLT.09.071357] [PMID: 20680123]

[47] Yang CM, Wang YC, Lee CH, Chen MH, Hsieh CL. A comparison of test–retest reliability and random measurement error of the Barthel Index and modified Barthel Index in patients with chronic stroke. Disabil Rehabil. 2022; 44(10): 2099–2103. doi:10.1080/09638288.2020.1814429

[48] Sainsbury A, Seebass G, Bansal A, Young JB. Reliability of the Barthel Index when used with older people. Age Ageing 2005; 34(3): 228-32.
[http://dx.doi.org/10.1093/ageing/afi063] [PMID: 15863408]

[49] Jafari-Koulaee A, Mohammadi E, Fox MT, Rasekhi A, Akha O. Predictors of basic and instrumental activities of daily living among older adults with multiple chronic conditions. Bmc Geriatr 2024; 24(1): 383.
[http://dx.doi.org/10.1186/s12877-024-04947-w] [PMID: 38689212]

[50] Siavash S, Ghaffari A, Taghizadeh G, Lajevardi L, Azad A. Psychometric Properties of the Persian Version of Sickness Impact Profile-30 (SIP-30) in Community-Dwelling Older Adults. J Aging Res 2025; 2025: 9959086.
[http://dx.doi.org/10.1155/jare/9959086] [PMID: 39816625]

[51] Lim JA, Lee ST, Moon J, *et al.* Development of the clinical assessment scale in autoimmune encephalitis. Ann Neurol. 2019; 85(3): 352–358. doi:10.1002/ana.25421

[52] Brenner J, Olijslagers SHC, Crijnen YS, *et al.* Clinical outcome assessments in encephalitis. Neurol Neuroimmunol Neuroinflamm. 2024; 11(1): e200168. doi:10.1212/NXI.0000000000200168

SUBJECT INDEX

S

T

U

V

W

www.ingramcontent.com/pod-product-compliance
Lightning Source LLC
LaVergne TN
LVHW070945210926
848482LV00002B/95